Fred S. Pfahler

THE HYPNOTIC BRAIN

HYPNOTHERAPY AND
SOCIAL COMMUNICATION
PETER BROWN, M. D.

Yale University Press   *New Haven and London*

Published with assistance from the foundation established in memory of James Wesley Cooper of the Class of 1865, Yale College.

Designed by Nancy Ovedovitz and set in New Baskerville type by The Composing Room of Michigan, Inc., Grand Rapids, Michigan. Printed in the United States of America by Vail-Ballou Press, Binghamton, New York.

Library of Congress Cataloging-in-Publication Data

Brown, Peter, 1951–
    The hypnotic brain : hypnotherapy and social communication / Peter Brown.
        p.   cm.
    Includes bibliographical references and index.
    ISBN 0-300-05001-1 (alk. paper)
    1. Hypnotism—Therapeutic use. 2. Brain. I. Title.
    [DNLM: 1. Communication. 2. Hypnosis.   WM 415 B879h]
RC495.B79   1991
616.89′162—dc20
DLC
for Library of Congress   91-10346
                                                                          CIP

The paper in this book meets the guidelines for permanence and durability of the Committee on Production Guidelines for Book Longevity of the Council on Library Resources.

10   9   8   7   6   5   4   3   2   1

CONTENTS

PART THREE   USES

INTRODUCTION

In the spring of 1909, Sigmund Freud traveled to America to give a series of lectures at Clark University. During the trip he met with most of the significant figures in contemporary American psychology, including William James. Freud was not impressed. He found the Americans inadequately appreciative of the impact of his theories and far too predisposed to invoke their own models in explaining human behavior. Freud expressed considerable doubt that psychoanalysis could ever take hold in a climate as unfriendly as that of the United States (Ellenberger, 1970).

If Freud was unimpressed, James and his colleagues certainly appreciated what they had witnessed. They recognized, for all their reservations, that the future belonged to Freud and his school. As the Boston psychiatrist Morton Prince wryly observed, "Freudian psychology had flooded the field like a full rising tide and the rest of us were left submerged like clams buried in the sands at low water" (Taylor, 1983, p. 13). Prince was right. With a few notable exceptions, the first part of the twentieth century belonged to the psychoanalyst in the clinic and to the behaviorist in the laboratory. Alternate views in general, and hypnosis in particular, remained largely of peripheral interest.

The tide is now turning. The insight of dynamic theory and the methodology of behaviorism are being enriched by other approaches. Developments in cognitive psychology, anthropology, and ethology have all radically altered our view of human behavior. And the virtual explosion in the neurosciences has radically altered our understanding of how the brain functions. Although many more questions remain than have been answered, the field of human behavior is in a state of creative flux.

Hypnosis is one of the subjects that has been rehabilitated. The combination of its increasingly widespread clinical use and the scientific advances of laboratory investigators has resulted in a significant increase in its acceptability in the scientific community and among the public. Hypnosis has enjoyed periodic waves of popularity through the years, but there is now more interest in the subject than at any time since the young Freud went to Paris to study it with Charcot.

Defining Hypnosis

The term *hypnosis* is a Victorian neologism coined by James Braid in an attempt to escape from the long shadow of charlatanism cast by such terms as *mesmerism* or *animal magnetism* (Edmonston, 1986). Spiegel (1974) defines hypnosis as "a response to a signal from another or to an inner signal, which activates a capacity for a shift of awareness in the subject and permits a more intensive concentration upon a designated goal direction. This shift of attention is constantly sensitive to and responsive to cues from the hypnotist or the subject himself."

My objective is to review our changing understanding of hypnosis and its clinical use in hypnotherapy in the light of our new knowledge of human behavior and brain function. My hypothesis is that hypnotic ability is closely related to those specific brain functions that are uniquely human. The brain is, above all, designed for communication, and hypnosis is one particular manifestation of that structure. Hypnosis is a way of defining specific aspects of everyday experience. A current text describes hypnosis as "a form of attentive, receptive focal concentration with a sense of parallel awareness and a constriction in peripheral awareness. . . . The hypnotic-like experience most common in everyday life is that of becoming so absorbed in a good book, movie, or play that one loses the customary spatiotemporal orientation and enters the imagined world" (Spiegel, 1985b, p. 1389).

Despite its long history, it is difficult to be specific about hypnosis. There are several good reasons for this. First, the hypnotic state has been hard to define by any rigorous behavioral, subjective, or physiological boundaries. Second, hypnosis can mean two very different things:

It is popularly known as a distinct psychological state, with unique attributes that separate it from other states. But it is also an operation, or a label for a set of operations that constitute the hypnotic situation, or "what hypnotists do." So the word can mean either a state or an instructional set. And, in fact, the most basic theoretical difference among scientific investigators of hypnosis centers around whether hypnosis is best defined as the private, internal responses of the hypnotized subject or by external characteristics implicit in the hypnotic situation.

The definition of hypnosis has always been impure, and it is by virtue of this impurity that hypnosis is an appealing model for eliciting the effects of words on behavior, of instructions on action, and of cognitive control on performance. As an operation, it serves to magnify the subtleties of human informational control, thereby exposing them for systematic manipulation as variables. (Engstrom, 1976, p. 174)

An Outline

If our definition of hypnosis is imprecise, it is no more so than our definition of brain function. In trying to understand the human brain, we have always resorted to metaphors. In Western culture, the most popular metaphor has always been the most sophisticated piece of technology currently available. The steam engine, the telephone exchange, and the computer have all been used as models for how the brain works (Lieberman, 1984; Jeannerod, 1985). Most recently, a model has begun to emerge that stems not from our technology but from ourselves. The brain, as part of a living organism, is seen as reflecting our evolutionary past (Mayr, 1982). This metaphor (and for our purposes it is no more than that) is based not on floppy disks and microbits but on evolutionary biology. By acknowledging our nearest relatives and the patterns we share in common, we can discern a fuller and richer picture of humankind and its capacities.

The first chapter looks at our past in two ways. There is a reconstructed past in which paleontology is revealing our evolutionary origins. There is also a mirrored past, the growing evidence of the complex behavioral patterns of our primate relations. Although there are many gaps in this picture, it shows that communication in human beings arose in numerous and elaborate face-to-face interactions between members of small groups. Our ancestors' hunting, making tools, and discovering fire may be our most familiar images of human development, but more essential, if mundane, was their getting along with one another. The evidence is that social communication has been central to the development of humankind and that other, more tangible, signs of culture may have spun off from this communication.

We cannot understand any living creature without an appreciation of its environment, and a model of how the brain developed cannot be complete unless it takes into account the fact that other people were always an essential component of the human environment. Humankind evolved in an environment of constant communication, and changes in the brain and behavior reflect this. The evidence further suggests that the bulk of this communication was at first nonverbal, taking the form either of gesture or of tone. The impact of the word came only much later.

The next two chapters discuss the importance of the ability for nonverbal communication. Chapter 2 looks at the ways in which the human face communicates. The evidence suggests that emotional expression in the human face is basic and universal. Partly learned and partly neurologic, the expressions of the face are an important part of the message of the spoken word. Along with prosody, the face serves the spoken word as punctuation does the written word. In addition, I will review the evidence concerning asymmetry in the human face: the way in which the two hemispheres of the brain control the contralateral sides of the face for emotional expression. The ability of those two hemispheres to provide different expressions adds an extra dimension to facial communication. The ongoing flow of expression and tone is an important part of the rhythm of human interactions.

Chapter 3 focuses on the tonal aspects of speech and the way in which face-to-face communication is used to synchronize interactions. Intonational rhythms of speech sculpt the meaning of what we say. These rhythms reach to another person to provide a linguistic entrainment, to synchronize our communication, and then to assist in the transmission of information. Our abilities both to express and to understand intonation, chiefly mediated by the right hemisphere, comprise a vast repertoire of elaborate but, until recently, unappreciated human skills. In addition to human speech, these skills underlie much of our ability to make and appreciate music.

Chapter 4 looks to the first pinnacle of human civilization: oral cultures (societies with little or no writing). Before the advent of literacy, the ability to use the spoken word formed the matrix of such cultures. The use of face-to-face language was the mainspring in their develop-

ment. Oral skills (in both the speaker and the listener) succeeded because of their "entrancing" qualities.

That cultures can be complex and sophisticated solely on the basis of
the spoken word is difficult for us to imagine. Writing so transforms
human consciousness that it takes a considerable effort to recognize our
literate bias. Building on the long evolutionary process, the oral culture
brought personal face-to-face communication to its first great elaboration. The oral culture used what the brain was best adapted for to erect a
civilization that existed primarily in the minds of its members. This was
accomplished through the use of the powerful contextual language we
know today as poetry. The use of spoken language evolved to a high art
in which process was indistinguishable from content. The oral poetry of
nonliterate cultures forms a close parallel model to the verbal style of
Ericksonian hypnotherapy.

Chapter 5 reviews the evidence for "the common everyday trance":
the rhythmic variations in states of consciousness that occur throughout
the course of the day. It is suggested that these changes are similar to the
changes that the brain undergoes during hypnosis. They involve a total
reorganization of brain function, including subcortical structures as
well as the two cerebral hemispheres (Franklin, 1988).

Chapter 6 suggests that contextual features are mediated through
the use of metaphor. Far from being merely a poetic figure of speech,
metaphor, in its broadest sense, is a central part not only of hypnosis but
also of all normal cognition. Metaphor is the matrix for understanding.
It is the language of personal transformation.

Chapters 7 and 8 illustrate the brain's ability for trance by dealing
with two of the more popular issues in contemporary hypnosis research. Chapter 7 reviews the uses of hypnosis in altering psychophysiologic function, particularly its use in a number of medical disorders. Chapter 8 deals with the contentious issue of multiple personality
disorder. The evidence in both of these areas strongly suggests that
though there are some marked differences in individual hypnotic abilities, a significant part of this variation depends on contextual features:
the expectations of the individuals and how they are interpreted in the
face-to-face clinical situation.

The final chapter deals specifically with how language may be used
in hypnotherapy. Drawing on examples from the clinical work of Milton
Erickson, I will review the nature of hypnotic experiences and how it is
modulated by suggestion. Erickson's use of rhythmic language, elaborate syntax, and personalized metaphor and storytelling parallels the

tradition of oral poetry. The emphasis in this approach has always been that of the naturalistic and cooperative nature of trance. Each hypnotic trance is a unique personal creation, relying on prosodic and behavioral cues to create a context for hypnotherapy. The most important hypnotic suggestion of all is that the significant feature of trance is located in the interaction between therapist and patient.

I suppose that it is also salutary to note what this book does not cover. In a review of such a wide range of human behavior, most of the topics raised are not dealt with in an exhaustive fashion. The interested reader is strongly advised to consult the original sources listed in the references. They are always more detailed and generally better written. The role of this book is simply to suggest the wide range of information in the brain and behavioral sciences that is relevant in understanding the relationship between hypnosis and brain function. Given the diversity of that range, it is important that workers in various fields, whether in the clinic or in the laboratory, be aware of related work in other areas.

The brain has a story. In order to understand brain function, we must understand the context of the environment in which it originally evolved. This process is difficult, obscured both by the relative scarcity of evidence as well as by our own biases. But a story can be constructed from a number of sources, and that story reveals that hypnotic abilities emerge from the everyday processes of communication and the way those processes are organized.

The brain tells a story. Cognitive and emotional processes depend fundamentally on our ability to produce metaphor. To understand new concepts we must reutilize models from other areas. This is the essence of metaphor, to explain something in terms of another, to see the new in the guise of what is already familiar and then to make recursive, slight modifications to further our understanding. This understanding and this ability to create metaphor depends on basic physiological processes, the way we experience ourself and the world around us. In this sense, metaphor is an extension of biological processes into the domains of psychology.

The brain is hypnotic. The events that occur in hypnosis are not some isolated special case but, rather, are formed by the rhythmic changes in our everyday lives. There is no magic in hypnosis. Rather, the trance state consists of a complex interplay of cognitive, emotional, and physiologic abilities that can be overlooked or taken for granted.

We are beginning to recognize that, in its largest sense, all of psychology is social psychology. Gilligan (1987) characterizes three conceptual approaches to the hypnotic relationship:

1. The authoritarian approach, which emphasizes the "hypnotic power" of the Svengali-like individual who overwhelms the weak-willed subject
2. The standardized approach, which emphasizes that hypnotic ability is a function of the subject and, as such, is a given for each individual
3. The cooperation approach, which emphasizes that hypnotherapy is a function of the interaction between therapist and patient

The third approach looks upon hypnosis as both a brain function and a social act. Much of the difficulty in characterizing hypnosis (as well as much of the diversity in its uses) stems from this dual nature. The French anthropologist Gilbert Rouget has defined trance as "a state of consciousness composed of two components, one psychophysiological, the other cultural. The universality of trance indicates that it corresponds to a psychophysiological disposition innate in human nature, although, of course, developed to varying degrees in different individuals. The variability of its manifestations is the result of the variety of cultures by which it is conditioned" (1985, p. 3).

Many people have contributed ideas and support to this book. My thanks to Gladys Topkis and Susan Laity of Yale University Press and Cecile Watters for their careful editing of the manuscript. In particular, I would like to acknowledge the invaluable contribution of the late Thelma Law. Her patience, humor, and careful attention to detail in preparing the manuscript were inexhaustible. Without her help I doubt this work could have been completed.

PART ONE
ORIGINS

Hypnotic abilities are basic human abilities. They originate in our species' unprecedented capacity for subtle and continual face-to-face communication. Our evolutionary path and even the very structure of the brain have been profoundly influenced by the process of communication.

Face-to-face communication is a rich and powerful blend. Facial expression, gesture, and tone of voice all combine to synchronize and structure communication. Moreover, these features shape the content of communication by establishing what can be expressed and how it will be comprehended. Both speaker and listener must be fully involved both mentally and physically.

Before the advent of widespread literacy, human

cultures made use of this ability to develop elaborate and sophisticated civilizations. Poetry and music were important tools to heighten and enhance the rhythms of communication. In the absence of written records, the rhythm and imagery of poetic devices allowed important information to be retained in living memory. In this sense, culture is an evolutionary process that finds new uses for the basic biologic abilities.

LUCY'S RELATIONS: THE EVOLUTION OF INTIMATE COMMUNICATION

The combination of advanced complex brains and the interlocking lives of the group members leads to both language and culture.
Mary Maxwell, 1984

The social communication of all the higher primates—chimpanzees, gorillas, and humans—is characterized by continual and elaborate face-to-face communication among members of the group (Tanner, 1981). This flow of communication involves facial expressions, gestures, and vocalizations and serves two linked functions: ongoing expression of individual emotional states and continual adjustment of the relationship between members of the group (Grüsser, 1984; Goodall, 1986). Primates spend a lot of time not only expressing themselves but also shaping their expressions in response to the communication they receive. The content, by contrast, constitutes a relatively small proportion of the overall message even in humans (Bolinger, 1986). In a very real sense the medium is indeed the message.

It has always been so. The environment in which the human brain evolved over six million years involved intense and continual communication from the onset. The extensive growth of the association areas of the cerebral cortex enormously increased our capacity to send and respond to messages. A growing body of convincing evidence, however, suggests that speech as we know it was not anatomically possible until about one hundred thousand years ago (Lieberman, 1984). Although from a historical perspective this may seem like a long time, from an evolutionary perspective it is not. Humankind began to evolve long before the spoken word. Speech added a whole new dimension to communication and probably stimulated the beginnings of cultural development, but it did so by augmenting, not by replacing, an already well-established communication style. The human brain was neurologically committed by its evolutionary success to its talent for exquisitely sensitive, ongoing, and flexible nonverbal communication.

ORIGINS

In 1973 a team of American scientists was searching for fossils in the Hadar Formation in Ethiopia, part of a large depression that was the site of an ancient lake system. One morning while returning from a fruitless search, Donald Johanson and Tim White made a discovery that became the most famous paleontological find of the century. That discovery was recorded as AL288-1 (Johanson, 1981).

At first glance, AL288-1 seems rather unimpressive. Less than half of the skeleton is preserved and the full length could have been only 120 cm at best. Nevertheless, AL288-1, or "Lucy" as she was named by her discoverers, has a central role in contemporary paleontology. Dated at between 3 and 3.5 million years ago, she is the oldest representative of early humankind that has yet been discovered.

According to Charles Darwin, the story of evolution is the interaction between chance (random genetic mutation) and design (natural selection by the environment). The biological approach presupposes that one can understand the gradual modifications of an organism as the product of interplay between these two factors (Mayr, 1982). This interaction involves the adaptation of the organism to a particular ecologic niche (environmental opportunity). Thus, Spencer's aphorism of evolution as the "survival of the fittest" does not mean the most physically fit or the strongest organism but, rather, the organism that fits best with its particular environment. In order to understand behavior, we have to understand the environment in which it evolved (the "environment of evolutionary adaptedness"): those forces and conditions that led to that particular evolutionary response.

By the standards of the history of the world, we have only very recently diverged from our primate origins. There is evidence that a common ancestor for humans, chimpanzees, gorillas, and orangutans existed as recently as 20 million years ago (Yunis, 1982). External forces, including drastic climatic changes, produced different ecological niches, new opportunities into which these highly adaptive primates were able to fit. The best estimate is that the human branch of the primate family arose in an environment that was a mixture of forests and open grasslands (Pilbeam, 1978; Tanner, 1981). Humans may have split off from the line of great apes as they explored the fringes of the forest and moved farther into the grasslands. Under the gradual pressure of environmental change, humans appear to have made the transition from foraging (eating food as it is found) to gathering (accumulating food for later eating), an adaptation very likely prompted by the nutritional needs of females who were caring for infants for a prolonged period of time (Tanner, 1981).

The primates were characterized by significantly larger brains with greater complexity of the modular structure (Eisenberg, 1981; Steele, 1989). In less than a million years, in the mid-Pleistocene era, cranial capacity increased from an average of 1,000 cc to over 1,400 cc (Mayr, 1982). This rapid and dramatic growth further increased the mammalian development of a new style of visual processing (Jerison, 1975; Maxwell, 1984). Although basic sensory processes had not changed much, the way in which the information was processed had changed fundamentally.

Just as the eyes allow one to picture the world, through spatial coding, ears and the auditory cortex construct events in a temporal code.

. . . It is hard for us to realize the extent to which the sequencing of observed events is a novel capability, . . . because vision does not work by integrating clues temporally. But hearing does. Jerison believes that the auditory system had been evolving for about 100 million years before the mammals were able to emerge into diurnal niches. Then, they re-evolved a visual sense, based on the type of neural networks and packaging of data, which had been established in the auditory cortex. Because of this, he says, "in addition to its normal role in spatial mapping, mammalian vision would be time binding. . . . Visual images in such a system could be stored in some form for the order of seconds or longer, and could maintain 'constancy' under transformations in time and space." (Maxwell, 1984, p. 92)

In addition to these general changes in overall cortical size and cellular structure, specific changes in the human brain also occurred. The parietal-temporal areas where primary sensory input is compared and integrated underwent the greatest development and growth (LeDoux, 1982; Geschwind, 1987). The association areas produce complex polysensory models of incoming information, resulting in a far more sophisticated processing of subtle informational detail. This increased potential to receive communication forms the basis for an increasingly complex social structure (Tanner, 1981).

The integration of motor and sensory processes allows us to create an image of an object positioned dynamically in both time and space. The processing in the associational areas also influences attention and how it is to be focused (Begleiter, 1973). These abilities are a fundamental part of constructing a model of social relationships. Paul Light (1979) has demonstrated the relationship between social role–taking and abilities in spatial orientation in small children. Children who were able to "see things" from the perspective of others were the most successful at a task involving visual problem–solving. In addition, children who were the most successful at the task were more likely to come from a family environment that emphasized awareness of others' emotional states. Our cerebral development is a direct consequence of our origins as a social and gregarious species.

The cortical areas that lie between the major sensory receiving and processing centers of the brain provide the largest virgin territory for multisensory association to be established and ultimately consolidated. Most important of these is the so-called posterior association area that subtends the contiguous visual cortex (areas 17, 18, and 19 in the occipital lobe), the auditory cortex (areas 22 and 23 in the temporal lobe), and the somatosensory cortex (areas 1, 2, and 3 in the parietal lobe). Two characteristics enable the posterior association area to hold within itself the major initial associational connections among these three sensory modalities. First, there is its geographic anatomical location, central and equidistant in the processing area for these sensory modalities. Second, there is the fact that at birth the association area is almost virginally clear of any innate synaptic connections. With experience and with the exposure to widespread engram formation encroaching simultaneously from the three contiguous sensory processing areas, there is essentially no limit to the number of complex multidimensional engrams that may be formed. . . .

The anterior association area serves a function similar to that of the posterior but modified somewhat because of the nature of the processing areas it subtends. These are again the auditory and somatosensory but include also the cortical center for voluntary pyramidal motor function in the precentral frontal lobe. . . . Some recent work has suggested that cognitive material from the posterior association area is funneled through the anterior association area where cognitive information is both tied into motor activity and more importantly fed into the prefrontal lobe for major integrative involvement.

More recently, another portion of the brain, the so-called entorhinal cortex, has been identified as still a higher level of cognitive consolidation (Van Hoesen, 1982). Evidence has been cited that cognitive information from both the posterior and anterior association areas converge on the entorhinal cortex, together with motivational-emotional material from the inferior temporal lobe. Since the entorhinal cortex surrounds the hippocampus, its input into the limbic system activities, particularly attention, is highly significant. (Kissin, 1986, pp. 57–58)

There are extensive cross-modal transfer activities that occur between vision, touch, and hearing (Juurmaa, 1988). The brain's ability to construct rich models for comparison and contrast derives in large part from the way in which information can be moved back and forth from one modality to another. This ability, as we shall see in a later chapter, is the basis for the central role that metaphor plays in human cognition. It is also the basis for our remarkable skill in social communication.

BY GOMBE STREAM

Despite a diversity of environments, food sources, and other external features, the evidence for the primacy of social development appears constant. We, and all our closest relatives, have always been committed to a group structure emphasizing close but flexible relationships based partly on kinship and partly on familiarity. Daniel Dennett (1984) has described the study of primates as a form of "behavioral archaeology" that allows us to see the development of human relationships in historical perspective in much the same way that archaeology allows us to study the development of human culture. The study of the behavior of nonhuman primates is critical for our understanding of humankind.

On a functional level, the chimpanzee is closer to the human than is the orangutan or the gorilla (Tanner, 1981; Goodall, 1986). Gorillas and orangutans are both highly specialized to a particular environment and show much more anatomical specialization, including sexual dimorphism (a marked difference in body size between males and females). Humans and chimpanzees, by contrast, appear to be closer to the primate "basic anatomical plan," with a basic similarity in the body size of males and females (Maxwell, 1984). In consequence, both show considerable flexibility as to environment and diet. Behaviorally as well the chimpanzees seem remarkably similar to humans. They are active and insatiably curious as well as being relentlessly social and highly expressive. By the same token, they can be, particularly when crowded or frustrated, bad tempered, treacherous, and even murderous (Goodall, 1986).

We humans are closely related to this nearest primate branch. Similarities in basic genetic and chemical structures are one index of the degree of divergence between the branches. Biochemical studies of the similarities between organisms come primarily from two areas. In the first, structural comparisons of protein molecules, there is much evidence of convergence; for example, the protein chains in hemoglobin are identical in humans and chimpanzees (Stebbins, 1982). In the second, studies of the reconstitution of DNA, comparison of DNA structure strongly supports the notion that humans and chimpanzees have shared a common ancestor and that a split occurred only 4 to 6 million years ago (Lewin, 1984). Stebbins (1982) summarizes work showing that humans and chimpanzees have only a 2.5 percent difference in their genes, as compared to a 30 percent difference between mice and rats and a 75 percent difference between two species of the fly genus *Drosophila*. The bulk of the evidence suggests that, given our relative genetic similarity with chimpanzees, the differences in our behavioral patterns are based on relatively small initial differences that tended to reinforce themselves over time (Ghiglieri, 1987). The behavioral differences are thus dependent on quantitative, rather than qualitative, factors.

It is important to note that genetic similarity does not imply a necessary correspondence of behavioral patterns. The behavior of primates in particular is notable for its diversity (Stebbins, 1982). The primates have been successful because of their adaptability to changing environments and their requirements over time. The common thread shared by all the primates is the central role of social organization (Eisenberg, 1981). Above all, the message is that social structure is the nexus of evolution and that the ability to communicate is the matrix for social structure. Given the habits of our nearest relatives, it seems likely that our ancestors were also agile and incessant social communicators.

In 1960, Jane Goodall began her detailed study of chimpanzee behavior in the Gombe Stream National Park in Tanzania. Through years of painstaking observation, she has given us an image of chimpanzee behavior that is much richer than was previously imagined. Through her writings, individual chimpanzees with their distinctive temperaments have vividly emerged as making their unique contributions to the overall group. Goodall has followed them from birth through childhood and adolescence, monitored their relations with one another, and observed the intertwining of their lives (Goodall, 1986). What results is a strangely familiar pattern. Indeed, for a generation reared on the image of chimpanzees as portrayed in film or in the circus, the chimpanzees seem closer to us when seen in their natural habitat. There they are somehow easier to recognize as close relatives than when they have been cozened into wearing loud sports jackets, riding motorcycles, or appearing in movies with future presidents.

Observations of primate behavior also tend to highlight our previous male biases. Female chimpanzees are most often the prime movers in a wide diversity of social and behavioral settings (Tanner, 1981). Female chimpanzees are significantly more likely to prepare and use tools in food getting, largely because of their greater nutritional needs; they must be more innovative and collaborative, of necessity. Females appear to exert an important selective role in courtship behavior for sexual activity and appear to prefer for their mates males of greater social ability to those of dominant status in the group (Tanner, 1981; Ghiglieri, 1987). The absence of estrus, the florid anatomic and physiologic changes that signal sexual availability in other species, placed a further reproductive premium on the ability to interpret the meaning of ongoing communication.

Changing from time-bound to time-free sexual behavior seems to have been an event of great importance, because it led to the existence of groups of primates, young, middle-aged and old, all thrown together, in circumstances where strong erotic attraction was present more or less the whole time. As the anthropologist Ernest Becker has noted, when "mateability" ceased to be seasonal and intermittent, vertebrate behavior piled up on itself. A jumble of statuses was created, to which members of the group were forced to adjust. "This provides a welter of confusion and stimulation, a new environment that must be like Times Square to someone raised on a farm," Becker says. "At each point in the growing animal's life, he must find a new adjustment to make to those around him: young to young, male to female, male to young, young to female and so on. This need for continuing adjustment provides part of the stimulus for the emergence of a larger-brained animal. Nothing is so unpredictable as are other living organisms." (Campbell, 1986, p. 55)

The close relationships chimpanzees form with one another appear to derive from the strong and prolonged infant-mother bond. Infants are usually carried by their mothers for the first six years of life and spend most of their time with their mothers until about the age of twelve. Because of the nature of the group, this also means that they have prolonged and frequent interaction with their siblings. This forces the infant to take on a changing social role that makes it a part of the group. Infant play is rich and varied with time divided seemingly equally between exploration, imitation of adults, and general messing about. It is a schooling of sorts, a time to learn motor, sensory, and social patterns. The emotional ties that result are strong and persistent. It is also clear that mother-child interaction is one of the major ways in which behavior is transmitted in primates, especially new innovations in behavior that result from contacts with humans.

Close infant-mother interaction is not only the rule during infancy but often persists in continued ties in later life. This is also true for siblings. Young chimpanzees are breast-fed until they are around four or five years old (at which time the mother usually becomes pregnant again) and will typically remain with mother until around age ten or twelve. During this time there is constant physical, visual, and auditory communication. It is also likely that the flexible group pattern shown by chimpanzees is a product of the mother-offspring tie; it forms a natural nucleus for group formation (Tanner, 1981). Among the adult chimps at Gombe, adult pairings involving mothers with grown daughters, or brother or cousin pairs among males, were frequent.

The group organization of chimpanzees is flexible and relatively informal. Larger, stable communities (of between fifteen and eighty-five members) sharing a home area will frequently break up into smaller bands or subgroups (of up to thirty members) that vary in composition over time. The size of the smaller groups is extremely variable depending on such factors as food availability, the presence of pregnant females or small infants, and changes in social relationships. In group size and flexibility, chimpanzee groups are similar to communities of human hunter-gatherers throughout the world today (Katz, 1982). This flexibility of group organization is in contrast to that of the other large apes who have groups that tend to remain fixed over time.

The notion of a rigid hierarchy, or pecking order, does not fit for chimpanzees. Because of their loose and changing social structure, resulting in flexible population changes, factions appear to form and change according to circumstance (Goodall, 1986; Tanner, 1981). Individuals are dominant not solely for their strength or size. Other features, particularly the social skills required to form bonds with others, are important. Chimpanzees with close allies who provide support tend to do much better than those who lack these social bonds. Goodall remarks on the plight of several large and active male chimpanzees who, despite appearing to have the potential, never made it in the group because of the lack of support of others at critical times (1986).

Above all, chimpanzees are supremely social animals, highly expressive in facial expression, gesture, and vocalizations. They communicate elaborately and constantly with one another. Food gathering and foraging, which consumes most of their time, is a shared effort; it is taught by the old to the young, and all members of the group, male and female, take part. Similarly, the amount of food sharing that goes on also demonstrates a flexible and dynamic social structure. As with humans, whatever a chimpanzee is involved in quickly becomes a social event.

The ability to work together to find food and the ability to communicate with others are inextricably linked. Chimpanzees are predominantly fruit eaters, which means that food is not always uniformly available. Fruit growth is seasonal and the landscape typically alternates between large areas with little food and small bonanzas centering around a few fruit trees. The other great apes, the gorillas and orangutans, are more generalized vegetarians and are thus capable of finding consistent grazing over large areas.

Like the foragers of early humankind, chimpanzees must have an elaborate and accurate map of their environment. Consequently, they are active explorers who show good memory for spatial orientations (particularly if it relates to finding food). Moreover, they must be capable of communicating with one another about features of the environment (Menzel, 1975). Consequently, there is a built-in need to be able to express and understand relationships in space, which includes the "intellectual capacity to abstract and exchange information between different sensory modalities, specifically between vision and touch" (Tanner, 1981, p. 115; Jarvis, 1978). Previously, this capacity to transfer information from one sensory modality to another (cross-modal perception) was thought to be an exclusively human trait. This ability lies at the root of conceptualization, which is fundamental to symbolization (Tanner, 1981). The ability to name objects, a basic aspect of human language, depends on the capacity to make cross-modal transfers.

Studies of cross-modal processing in humans suggest that the various senses organize information along the dimensions of the order of events and of the overall duration (Marks, 1987a). The temporal organization of information is consistent both for individual senses and for cross-modal comparisons. Although there were wide interindividual variations in the weight of the two dimensions, individuals were consistent in these differences for all intramodal and cross-modal tasks (Marks, 1987b). There are some reliable ways in which information from different sensory systems is handled. Cross-modal interactions of sensory input from different senses show that distinctions are treated in the same way on a sensory level and on that of the metaphorical constructs arising from them. There appear to be strong similarities between the ways in which, for example, pitch and brightness, pitch and lightness, loudness and brightness, and pitch and form are processed on the levels of cross-modal perception, synesthesia, and synesthetic metaphor (Marks, 1987b).

The bulk of the human cerebral cortex is involved in the association areas that surround the primary sensory cortex. These areas can be subdivided into modality-specific (unimodal) and high-order (heteromodal) cortex (Mesulam, 1985). Whereas the modality-specific areas are reserved for processing information from one sensory modality, the heteromodal association areas integrate an admixture of information from all the modalities.

Within primary and unimodal regions, the analysis of sensory experience remains confined to single modalities. The opportunity for inter-relating the attributes of real events belonging to separate modalities occurs in the subsequent stage of sensory processing within heteromodal regions of the brain. There is a real hierarchy in the processing of sensory information. For example, the heteromodal areas in the monkey brain almost never receive their sensory information directly from primary areas. Instead, unimodal association cortex acts as an obligate intermediate relay.

Within heteromodal areas, the modality specificity of information is lost in favor of intermodal associations. Even the distinction between what is sensory and what is motor is no longer present. For example, many cells in heteromodal areas increase firing not only in response to sensory input but also in phase with motor output. It could be argued that during the process of gaining awareness of the world, sense organs are not passive portals for sensory input. Instead, they could be considered to act as tentacles or feelers for the active scanning and updating of a dynamically shifting inner representational map. At this level, the building blocks of awareness are as much motor as they are sensory phenomena, and this is clearly reflected in the physiology of heteromodal areas.

At least two essential transformations are likely to occur in heteromodal areas. First, these areas provide a neural template for intermodal associations necessary for many cognitive processes, especially language. Second, they provide the initial interaction between extensively processed sensory information and limbic-paralimbic input. Thus, another distinction that is lost in heteromodal areas is that between limbic and nonlimbic. This may initially come as a surprise, since there is a tendency to think of heteromodal cortex as a high-order association area devoted to intellectual processes and hence impervious to limbic impulses. However, the evidence obtained in the macaque brain unequivocally shows that heteromodal areas receive substantial paralimbic input. This anatomic arrangement explains how mood and drive can influence the manner in which the self and the world are experienced and also how thought and experience eventually influence mood. (Mesulam, 1985, pp. 24–25)

The development of the heteromodal association areas and their close connections with the motivational and emotional parts of the brain in the limbic system are particularly significant and point to their critical role in both face-to-face communication and in the development of altered states of consciousness. Although the amygdaloid-hippocampal system is particularly important in the identification and expression of emotional behavior in other primates, humans also receive significant input from the association areas (Kissin, 1986). As we shall see in later chapters, these capacities are intimately related to the brain's hypnotic abilities. Development of the association areas play a significant part in enriching the human ability to perform these functions.

The capacity of chimpanzees to communicate with human scientists in a subtle and complex way using sign language is well known. Chimpanzees lack a human-style supralaryngeal airway that would allow them to make the appropriate shapes necessary to produce a human-style speech; nevertheless they are capable of an extensive use of sign language by which they can express concepts that are the equivalent to those used by children of between two and three years of age. Chimpanzees demonstrate the ability to use their linguistic skills to express their emotional state, solve problems, change their minds, and even lie on occasion. (No one said that exposure to human ways was going to be morally uplifting.)

Many investigators have overstressed vocalization per se in primate communication—apparently because of their interest in the evolution of the unique human ability for speech. Primates communicate . . . by utilizing a complex constellation of many modes—postural, gestural, vocal, facial expression, movement—within a social context. But this is also true of human communication. Social context, body movements, facial expression, stylized gestures, and paralinguistic vocal qualities such as breathlessness, tone of voice, and speech speed are all exceedingly important in human communication and are essential to our evaluation of linguistic utterances. (Tanner, 1981, pp. 129–130)

In fact, what chimpanzees do most is communicate. Different forms of touch, facial expression, gesture, and vocalizations are all used in combination and virtually constantly. Even without the use of full-blown language, the amount of social communication among chimpanzees is astonishing. In addition to a remarkable amount of physical contact for reassurance, grooming, and play, facial expressions, gestures, and a wide variety of vocalizations are used both widely and persistently. Chimpanzee vocalizations are used to express emotional states, convey warnings, or adjust social relationships. There is extensive evidence that these vocalizations are not related neurologically to the areas that are the primary speech centers of the human brain (Jolly, 1983; Goodall, 1986) but are related anatomically to the prosodic elements of human speech—that is, the way in which words are delivered to convey emotional states and contextual cues and to underline importance. The content-rich and elaborately organized syntactical arrangement of human speech appears to be related to more and more complicated forms of motor behavior, which allows for conceptual manipulation in internal mental space.

Large areas of the cortex are not given over to a particular sense; rather they serve to pool information from the different senses. These association areas allow an animal to develop a polysensory image of objects. . . .

Finally, we should note the proposal that self-consciousness is a natural outcome of the information processing which is conducted by the association areas of the brain. It was mentioned above that animals can make a polysensory model of their environment. The formation of a self may have been added to this picture, as follows. In species which need to have group interaction, the "I" requires an accurate mental representation not only of other members and their interactions, but also of their likely reactions to "my" behavior. As David Oakley notes, the modeller must include a central representation of himself. Thus, he says, if consciousness and self-awareness are seen as correlates of the modelling process, there is no need to suggest a further adaptive significance for them. (Maxwell, 1984, pp. 80–81)

Much energy has gone into establishing "unique human qualities," or the differences between us and our nearest relatives. One of the more reliable distinctions appears to be the remarkable touchiness of many humans on the subject. The chimpanzees, by contrast, have expressed little opinion on the matter. The overwhelming evidence suggests that the traditional list of differences between humans and nonhuman primates has narrowed greatly with time. Ettlinger (1984), in reviewing the relevant work over the past twenty years, has concluded that "with respect to comparative differences between human and non-human primates . . . discontinuities very clearly evident in 1963 have either been resolved or have become blurred. It is argued that . . . clinical neuropsychology and experimental (animal) neuropsychology can be expected to converge increasingly during the next 20 years" (Ettlinger, 1984, p. 685).

A HUMAN VOICE

There appear to be at least two pathways taken in the evolution of man's upper respiratory system after a common pongid-like stage exhibited by the australopithecines. One line appears to have terminated with the Classic Neanderthals. The other line, encompassing those hominids with basicrania and upper respiratory structures of more modern appearance, may have given rise to modern man. (Laitman, 1979, p. 15)

Humankind as we know it makes a sudden and dramatic appearance in the fossil record about 35,000 B.C. Almost simultaneously, that record is augmented by evidence of an elaborate, relatively sophisticated culture not much different from some of the patterns currently existing on parts of the globe. What we know of this period (the Aurignacian and Magdalenian eras) reveals a picture of a diverse hunting and gathering people. Modern spears, arrowheads, and fishhooks make their first appearance. Elaborate bone carvings of human figures and animals are present as are lunar calendars and other artifacts. Most dramatic, though, are the astonishing cave paintings of Altamira and Lascaux. Rich, mysterious, and exquisitely beautiful, they, perhaps more than anything, give us a glimpse of what we can recognize as a legacy from our earliest beginnings (Stebbings, 1982; Campbell, 1984).

The appearance of this new branching corresponds with the equally dramatic disappearance of the Neanderthals, named after the Neander Valley, near Düsseldorf in West Germany, where the first identified fossils were found. The accumulation of similar fossil remains gives evidence of a form of human life that was successful and widespread from about 500,000 to 35,000 years ago. The Neanderthals were large and muscular; equally important, they had significantly larger brains than their ancestors. Archaeological finds also have revealed an extensive use of fire, a variety of stone tools, and the performance of burial practices and religious ceremonies (Kurtén, 1984).

There are some significant anatomical differences between the Neanderthals and contemporary humans. The current version of the brain is larger relative to body size (Jerison, 1975; Kurtén, 1984). More-over, the frontal cortex is significantly larger and better developed, with a much richer vascular supply (Kurtén, 1984; Lieberman, 1984). The work of Saban (1980, 1983) suggests that this is particularly true for those areas in the left hemisphere of the modern brain that are respon-sible for the production of speech. There is also a significant difference in facial structure. Whereas the face of a human today is specialized for the fine muscular movements needed for emotional expression and speech production, the Neanderthal skull, with its large jaw, was spe-cialized for efficient chewing and overall strength at the expense of individual muscle movements (Kurtén, 1984; Demes, 1987).

The final major difference is the shape of the supralaryngeal airway, the part of the vocal tract that is responsible for speech. In 1949, Victor Negus, an anatomist specializing in study of the larynx, and Sir Arthur Keith, an anthropologist, reconstructed a model of the supralaryngeal vocal tract from a Neanderthal fossil (Lieberman, 1984). They demon-strated that this near-relative of ours shows the typical primate su-pralaryngeal tract, which is relatively longer and thinner than ours, a great advantage in separating breathing from chewing. It is not likely to have been able to produce the shapes and configurations necessary for articulated speech. By contrast, our supralaryngeal airways are rela-tively shorter, rounder, and wider, with less efficient separation of the respiratory and digestive tracts. This adjustment, however, allows for the full range of distinct vowel sounds necessary for precise and articu-lated speech (Lieberman, 1984). The disadvantage of mixing the breathing and eating systems (which assured enduring fame for Dr. Heimlich and his maneuver) has been the price paid for an exponential increase in verbal communication abilities (Lieberman, 1984).

The evidence shows that relatively small adjustments in the structure of the brain, the orientation of the facial musculature, and the shape of the vocal tract resulted in massive changes in behavior. In fact, lan-guage, the "distinctive human adaptation," is a dramatic exploitation of relatively minor anatomical changes for a much greater range in face-to-face communication and the enlargement of social functions that this entails. Thus, what makes us most human is not radically different from the style of communication used by our relatives. It is just what we do best.

Human language, culture, and cognitive abilities have evolved to-gether. The actual nature of their relationship is often difficult to determine. Competing theories have usually told us more about the biases of the theorist and of the society in which the theories originate than about the relationship of these factors. Language was once held to be a supreme and uniquely human achievement that somehow allowed us to enjoy a special position in evolution. This focus on this allegedly unique difference has limited our ability to understand how language has evolved in comparison with the vocal communications of our nearest primate relatives. Language is the product of a sequence of small changes resulting in a large discontinuity, a prototype of evolutionary change and not a unique case.

The neural mechanisms that first evolved to facilitate motor control now also structure language and cognition. The rules of syntax, for example, may reflect a generalization of the automatized schema that first evolved in animals for motor control in tasks like respiration and walking. . . .

In this model, the language and cognition of human beings may be more complex than that of other animals, but it is based on similar neural mechanisms and has similar formal properties. (Lieberman, 1984, p. 35)

A HUMAN MIND

There are a number of independent, though not mutually exclusive, anatomic metaphors for the way in which the brain functions. The "hierarchic," or vertical model emphasized cortical control of more "primitive" areas in the subcortical structures, brain stem, and spinal cord. In the 1940s, MacLean described the "triune" brain, in which the human cortex coexists, with varying degrees of success, with the primate brain in the subcortex and the reptile brain in the brain stem. The emphasis is on newer or more highly evolved portions of the brain attempting to exert executive control over more primitive areas. Reversing as it does the focus on the neuromotor regulation model of a hierarchic control of behavior from the simple reflex arc up to the motor cortex, this model fits in well with traditional neurologic views of how movement is governed (Jeannerod, 1985).

In contrast, neuropsychologists have emphasized the specialized nature of specific areas in the cortex, though each still has unique connections with subcortical structures of its own. This "back-to-front" model reflects the concerns of twentieth-century psychology with perceptual and linguistic organization (Luria, 1976).

The third model of human brain function stems from the growing body of work identifying specialized ways in which the two hemispheres operate. This side-to-side dichotomy of function postulates that the two hemispheres work in complementary but different ways, the left hemisphere being involved in such matters as the specific content of speech and the precise sequencing of behavior in time. The right hemisphere is specialized to regulate the process of speech and the organization of behavior in space.

Each of these models contributes to our understanding, but none provides a complete picture of how the brain works. For most behavior patterns, the crucial control element is not a particular center in the brain but the information that arises from changes in the surrounding environment. Behavior is shaped in an ongoing interaction with the models we construct of that environment. These models are widely distributed, with different aspects being represented at different sites in the nervous system (Kissin, 1986). Information, not "higher centers," is what regulates brain function. Interpretations of this feedback, the weight we assign various elements, varies from individual to individual and also over time. Learning what stimuli to respond to and how to respond is how the subroutines of behavior are first broken down and then become automatic. Edelman (1987) has coined the term *neural Darwinism* to describe how environmental patterns in effect "select" and reinforce patterns of neural function.

The left hemisphere is specialized for precise sequencing of motor actions both in gesture and in speech. Arguing from this anatomical connection and from the similarities between problem-solving behavior in chimpanzees and conceptual thinking in humans, Reynolds has proposed a phylogenetic relationship between the two (1981). He argues that language provides a system through its structure and syntax for the manipulation of internal images of objects in the same way that the motor system allows for the manipulation of objects in the external world. As other humans form the central part of that external world and are essential for communication, language necessarily involves a social and emotional component. Thus, language is a form of social-emotional exploratory behavior. This provides a plausible strong link between our incessant curiosity about the world and our equally incessant need to communicate.

Citing Karl Pribram, Reynolds (1981) has proposed that

the evolution of the primate brain can be thought of as the progressive elaboration of cognitive mechanisms to assess both internal and external consequences of action. This functional approach crosscuts the traditional distinctions between phylogenetically older and more recent structures. Both functions are neocortically represented, both are functionally interlocked, both can call upon learned and innate behavior, and in man, at least, both are active simultaneously. These two functions can be termed here the affective modality of action and the instrumental modality of action, which regulate and evaluate internal and external consequences respectively. . . . The affective modality is highly dependent upon the rostral parts of frontal and temporal cortex and upon the limbic structures, such as hippocampus, septum, amygdala, and hypothalamus, involved with physiological homeostasis, reinforcement, inhibition, attention, and innate behavior patterns. As Pribram has stressed, these are by no means "primitive" activities, and he has delineated three dimensions of function that characterize the phylogenetically older limbic system, basal ganglia, and core brain mechanisms: (1) a *stabile* function, which regulates physiological states, . . . (2) a *protocritic* function, which mediates diffusely projecting sensory systems, like pain or temperature, . . . and (3) an *effective* function, which (a) activates the cortex in reference to significant, unexpected, or sustained stimuli . . . [and] (b) controls the basal ganglia motor systems, with their associated innate behaviors and regulation of sensory input.

In contrast, the instrumental modality of action, which assesses the external consequences of behavior, requires the cortex surrounding the major fissures— the sensory and motor cortex and related "association" areas. These structures subserve an *epicritic* function that localizes stimulation in precise points of space-time and abstracts from experience context-free patterns that are not dependent upon the internal state of the animal. . . . From this perspective, the relationship between reason and emotion, to use traditional labels, is not one of hierarchy but of specialization by function, and the human brain has as one of its major tasks the integration of such different kinds of information into a unified course of action. (Reynolds, 1981, pp. 80–81)

The conceptual change is a significant one. The traditional model shows reason trying to control more primitive emotional responses. The contemporary model emphasizes instead the integration between two equally important and equally sophisticated means of organizing behavior. Emotion is not simply a subjective internal experience; it is simultaneously a social act. As Reynolds points out, "affective systems are also specialized for the mediation of social relationships" (1981, p. 82). If play is the business of childhood, then social relationships are the play of the adult primate. Social relationships enable the individual to develop creatively the skills learned in childhood and adolescence and are equally important for continued maintenance of intellectual and emotional behavior, as critical for its maintenance as childhood play is for its development (Maxwell, 1984).

Constructing the story of human origins is a largely speculative task often influenced by the preoccupations of the present and frustrated by the sparsity of direct data. Whatever else has changed, however, we can be certain that our origins were social. For most of our history, humankind has been organized in what Robert Redfield termed the "folk society":

Such a society is small, isolated, nonliterate, and homogeneous, with a strong sense of group solidarity. The ways of living are conventionalized into that coherent system which we call "a culture." Behavior is traditional, spontaneous, uncritical, and personal; there is no legislation or habit of experiment and reflection for intellectual ends. Kinship, its relationships and institutions, are the type categories of experience and the familial group is the unit of action. The sacred prevails over the secular; the economy is one of status rather than of the market. (Redfield, 1947, p. 293)

The folk society, the beginnings of human culture, made use of the newfound capacity for speech combined with our ability for face-to-face communication. The growth of the association areas provided the cerebral basis for elaborating this combination into radically new patterns. Yet these patterns were based on the common legacy of the primate family. Our capacity for face-to-face communication (chapter 2) and for synchronizing interactions (chapter 3) was the basis of civilization until the development of literacy (chapter 4).

HYPNOTIC ORIGINS

Histories of hypnosis usually begin with the stories of such individuals as Anton Mesmer or the Abbé Faria and include some recognition of the role of the ancient Greek temple priests or perhaps the Druids (Edmonston, 1986). To begin several million years earlier, with Lucy, may seem to be overdoing it. This is not, however, a history of the social phenomenon that has been defined as hypnosis. Rather, it is a review of the evolutionary development of the underlying skills that make up hypnotic communication. The evidence shows that the brain evolved primarily for social communication, of which hypnosis is a special form. Through the interactions of our earliest relatives, the brain developed to adapt to a world of highly specialized communication (Steele, 1989). It is structured in order to be influenced by and to express face-to-face communication. All communication in general, and hypnosis in particular, derives from those basic abilities.

2

MR. DARWIN WRITES A BEST-SELLER: THE BASIS OF FACE-TO-FACE COMMUNICATION

The language of face-to-face conversation is the basic and primary use of language, all others being best described in terms of their manner of deviation from that base.

Charles J. Fillmore, 1974

The ability to recognize and respond to different facial expressions is reliable (Ekman, 1983) and appears to be universal to all cultures. It is also highly personal. Different emotional expressions elicit specific individual patterns of electrophysiologic response in people (Ekman, 1983), and these changes appear to be related to specific kinds of associated imagery (Schwartz, 1981). This is in keeping with theories that suggest that psychophysiologic patterns of response are highly specific, reliably correlate with particular emotional states (Zajonc, 1985), and are intensified by face-to-face interaction and the degree of emotional salience (Linden, 1987). Moreover, face-to-face communication is a highly complex neurologic task that provides a glimpse of the dynamic organization of the brain. That organization demonstrates the pervasive nature of automatic unconscious processes that coexist with conscious awareness.

TO FIND THE MIND'S CONSTRUCTION IN THE FACE

It is a steamy June evening in Toronto. As the orchestra begins to play, the eyes of the audience focus on the soloist, Kathleen Battle. She is singing Mozart's "Exsultate, Jubilate," a song of joy at suffering endured and transcended. The exquisite tones seem to come from deep within to rise and float above the crowd as she sings the words, "You console the griefs which make hearts sigh." While the collaboration of soloist and orchestra brings the sound of Mozart to life, her face, simultaneously displaying a number of different features, is the focus of visual attention. There is the consummate artistry producing this vibrant sound with apparent lack of effort. At the same time, she is emotionally in tune with the music, showing a quiet joy and serenity that bears the image of the music and its intentions. Third, we can read the imprint of the relationship between performer and audience, the special communication that occurs, the excitement and pleasure that come in the sharing of the creative moment. It is a form of knowledge quite different from logical description. It is powerful but fleeting, deeply personal while being shared with several hundred people.

That the human face has a special role in communication is immediately obvious. It is a uniquely individual statement of who we are and how we feel. It is also one of the most important indicators of what we share both biologically and culturally with other humans. Facial expression is a central part of everyday communication, yet much about it is poorly understood. We use the information of facial expression daily without having a clear sense of all that it reveals. Although fascination with facial expression is ageless, the beginnings of its study as a science go back only to the nineteenth century. Sources of that science may be found in a great Victorian plum-pudding of a book by Charles Darwin.

In 1872, Darwin had his only contemporary popular best-seller. *The Expression of the Emotions in Man and Animals,* though less well known today than some of his other works, was a great success with Victorian readers. Although Darwin was primarily interested in buttressing his theory of evolution with another line of evidence, the book is significant as the first detailed description of the role of the face in expressing emotional states. Building on the earlier work of the English anatomist Sir Charles Bell and the French neurologist Guillaume Duchenne, Darwin produced a wonderful pastiche derived from correspondence throughout Europe and exotic spots around the globe combined with his own meticulous observations. Correspondents contributed reports of Maori chieftains, the emotionally ill, and the primate collection of the London zoo.

Darwin had circulated in 1867 a questionnaire to scientists, missionaries, and administrators of various far-flung bits of empire. The answers he received revealed that basic emotional expression is the same throughout the world, regardless of cultural differences. Anatomical studies also show close parallels between the expressions of animals, particularly the primates, and humankind. These conclusions were important to Darwin in establishing that emotional expression has a biologic origin and, as such, can be considered an example of an evolutionary process.

The book is a panorama of nineteenth-century life: in its pages, we meet a variety of missionaries, professors, and explorers, as well as Darwin's children and the family pets. Most clearly, we see an image of Darwin in his unique ability to combine a vast theoretic overview with patient and precise sifting through innumerable observations. The core of the book is a series of unequaled descriptions of the basic facial expressions. Darwin records the muscles involved, the development of expression from infancy to adulthood, and the precise sequence in which the muscles are contracted as the expression becomes more intense.

Darwin begins by stating three principles that continue to guide investigations in the field. First is the concept of *serviceable actions,* the idea that certain behavior becomes associated with a particular state of mind and will therefore occur whenever that state of mind is present. In other words, emotional expression is not random but part of a motor program that is an attempt to reach a goal motivated by the subjective experience of the individual. This principle is related to the form of learning that Darwin called association and that is similar to both classical conditioning and state-dependent learning. It is the recognition that subjective experience is made up of particular combinations of cognitions, affects, and physiologic states with the result that "whenever the same state of mind is induced, however feebly, there is a tendency through the force of habit and association for the same movements to be performed, though they may not then be of the least use" (Darwin, [1872] 1965, p. 28).

Second is the principle of *antithesis.* Darwin suggests that emotions are organized in two pairs of opposites (for example, love-hate, joy-sorrow). He therefore suggests that the expression of these emotions would also be arranged into opposite states in a similar fashion.

The third principle is that of *actions due to the constitution of the nervous system,* the notion that the strength of an emotion will be reflected proportionately by external behavior. In other words, intense expression will usually indicate intense internal experience.

Darwin recognized the inherent difficulties in the subject. Facial expressions do not lend themselves to easy recording and analysis. We may often feel certain in recognizing an emotion, but we may have a great deal of difficulty in precisely defining the perceptions that are the basis for this certainty. Also, observations are often biased by our own subjective state. These concerns have continued to complicate the subject.

One hundred years after Darwin, in 1972, *Emotion in the Human Face,* edited by Paul Ekman, was published. Ekman and his coworkers have been responsible for the first significant steps that go beyond the observations of Darwin. Establishing the universality of facial expressions has continued to be a major thrust in the field, and eight studies have found strong common patterns of similarity in all the cultures they examined.

A number of workers have reliably identified seven major categories of emotion expressed by the face (Plutchik, 1980): happiness, surprise, fear, sadness, anger, disgust-contempt, and interest. Ekman and his coworkers (1982) concluded that although the basic emotions appear to be universal, there is significant variation in the way these emotions can be expressed not only from culture to culture but from person to person. They explain these differences on the basis of what they call *display rules.* These are the learned constraints that the individual places on emotional expression and are made up of a combination of personal, contextual, and sociocultural guidelines. They include both static and transient characteristics of the person and of the setting. For example, while observing a stressful and violent film, both Japanese and American viewers showed the same intensity of facial expressions as long as they thought they were not being observed. In the presence of another person, the facial expressions of the Americans were unaltered, but the Japanese viewers dramatically masked their facial responses (Ekman, 1972).

Individual differences in display rules are also observed. There is a wide interindividual difference in the degree of facial expressiveness as well as in the ability of individuals to recognize different facial expressions. No consistent patterns have been found except for a slight superiority of women in both aspects (Hall, 1978; Nowicki, 1988).

The work of Ekman and others in the field has finally put the study of the facial expression of emotion on a solid scientific footing. Perhaps this is their single greatest contribution to date. There are, however, a number of difficulties in the methodologies that continue to need to be worked out. Isolating facial expression from other channels of communication makes it impossible to study the contextual nature of most emotional expression. The researcher who uses still photographs or videotapes (in which the voice channel is not available) ignores the ongoing nature of social interaction. The use of facial expression to give both emphasis and punctuation to speech, the interactive nature of communication, and the expressions needed by the lower face to phonate properly remain open issues. The need to study facial expression within the social context remains the greatest ongoing challenge in the field.

When conditions are not standardized, interpretation and perception of emotional facial expressions differ dramatically. The context, the emotional state of the viewer, and the sequence in which the faces are presented will all affect the ratings of observers (Russell, 1987). Facial expression is also part of a larger communicational context. The naturalistic studies of communication of emotion support the idea that emotion is picked up through a number of different channels and that the importance given to one particular channel varies according to the context. For example, Van De Creek and Watkins (1972) showed that what was said and the prior knowledge of the subject had more impact than the visual input in terms of assessing emotional expression. Moreover, Schiffenbauer (1974) reported that the emotional state of the observer influenced the emotion he or she attributed to a facial expression. Ekman (1980) showed that the relative weight given to facial expression, speech, and body cues depended on both the judgment task and the conditions in which the behavior occurred. Interpreting an emotional expression is the composite of a number of independent judgments. Frijda (1986) has proposed a hierarchical model that emphasizes an active and ongoing judgment of facial expression rather than a static and all-or-nothing procedure.

Emotional expression in the face (either as seen by others or as felt by the individual) originates in the movement of facial landmarks caused by particular contractions of facial muscles, by accompanying changes in autonomic factors such as vascular changes resulting in skin color and tone adjustments, or by respiratory changes. Though small, the facial muscles are each capable of countless minute adjustments most of which can be both voluntary and involuntary. O'Sullivan (1982) has shown that there are literally tens of thousands of possible combinations of facial expressions. This serves to underline a basic biologic principle: simple basic units can be combined and recombined in order to produce a highly complex behavioral repertoire. Discrete muscle patterns in different parts of the face are independent and highly flexible, so that mixtures of emotion can occur either simultaneously or by rapid alternation from one expression to another. These blends of emotion are particularly important in light of the ambiguity and choice they provide for the observer. The communication of the face must be sustained and developed, providing not a message but a relationship.

The muscles of facial expression are phylogenetically related to the muscles of the gills of lower animals. Consequently, the facial muscles retain a close neurologic relationship with respiration, so that they are intimately associated with internal physiologic and emotional states (Rinn, 1984). The role of this shared autonomic nervous system in emotional experience is an important one. Changes in heart rate and breathing patterns, changes in skin color and tone, pupillary changes, and overall changes in the level of arousal—all give important communication of the emotional state and its intensity. Lanzetta (1976) has shown that increases in autonomic activity are related to increases in facial expressiveness. Malmstrom (1972) found that different patterns of heart rate coincide with different facial expressions, and Ancoli (1980) found that patterns of breathing change with different facial expressions.

On the mammalian skull, the attachments of these muscles shift from the neck to the face and become capable of much more independent movement. With the disproportionate growth in skull size in the human, the attachments of these muscles are restricted to the front of the face, leading to an even finer and more flexible variety of movements. There are two large groups of muscles in the face, those involved with eating and chewing and those that are primarily of expressive or emotional use. The former are attached to bone and ligament; the latter, to skin or connective tissue. Attachment to bone provides power; attachment to skin and other soft tissue allows for more obvious changes in appearance (Lieberman, 1984).

The upper and lower face are innervated by separate branches of the facial nerve. The lower half of the face, involved in articulation for speech, has much more voluntary control and is capable of much finer discriminations than the upper half. Because this greater discrimination means greater hemispheric specialization, the lower half of the face is also much more capable of asymmetrical action. In contrast, the upper half of the face has relatively little voluntary control and less hemispheric specialization. Proportionately it is more under the control

of the extrapyramidal system that is responsible for automatic and stereotyped motor behavior (Rinn, 1984).

The distinction between these two parts of the face is most clearly
emphasized in disorders that involve the neurologic control of the face.
Lesions that affect the voluntary motor system more often impair unilateral voluntary movement, particularly in the lower half of the face,
while spontaneous emotional responses are unimpaired. By contrast,
patients with illnesses that affect the subcortical extrapyramidal motor
system will often be able to move the facial muscles voluntarily but will
have impairment of facial expression in spontaneous emotion. Conditions that affect this area (such as pseudobulbar palsy) can result in
spontaneous and violent emotional expression in the face while the
person reports an absence of the internal experience of the feeling
(Mesulam, 1985).

Movements in the upper face are much more limited and automatic.
Movements of the forehead and brow occur throughout speech and give
significant contextual and semantic cues to the spoken word. Changes
in movement coincide with intonational changes. The eyebrows can be
to the spoken word what punctuation is to the written. They give cues to
the organization and structure of speech and indicate the points that
need to be emphasized (Rinn, 1984). Facial expression and speech
production share a common neurologic regulatory system (van Gelder,
1990).

But facial expression is not secondary to verbal communication. The
newborn are capable of a wide variety of exuberant and uninhibited
facial expressions, for the facial musculature is fully formed and functional at birth. Virtually all adult facial expressions can be seen in young
infants (Ekman, 1982). The startle reaction can be triggered in the
newborn by sudden, intense stimulation and often occurs as a spontaneous discharge in non-REM sleep (Steiner, 1973). Neonates smile
frequently, primarily during REM sleep (Emde, 1976).

Infants only a few days old are able to reliably identify and imitate
basic facial expressions to an astonishing degree (Field, 1982). Social
smiling begins around three to four weeks of age, and laughter around
four months. Simultaneously, infants will reliably give differential responses to the facial expressions of others. Imitation is an important
feature in the development of neonatal facial expression, but even infants blind from birth exhibit the same kinds of motor patterns as do
normally sighted children (Stern, 1985). Although infants can produce
virtually all the facial expressions that adults can, they are unable to

produce the constraints and asymmetries that are often seen in grown-ups (Rinn, 1984).

The recognition of emotional expression is an important part of establishing social relationships. An impaired ability to recognize facial expressions appears to be related to difficulty in establishing social contexts and disorders in social behavior. Adolescent males with a history of juvenile delinquency are significantly more likely to make errors in emotion recognition than are nondelinquent controls (McCown, 1986). Whatever the precise nature of the relationship, social skills are clearly related to the ability to identify and express emotions through the face.

FACIAL EXPRESSION AND SYNCHRONIZATION

The nature of the environment is important in determining the ratio of sensory channels used in facial communication. The size and nature of the social group, for example, will affect the nature and degree of expressiveness of an individual. Those who live a predominantly solitary or distant life do not need the ability to make subtle and continuous communication distinctions that members of an active and gregarious social group do. Redican (1982) points out:

As Gautier and Gautier (1977) expressed it, the regulation of intragroup social relations in terrestrial Old World primates of an open habitat is "ceaseless and subtle, linked with frequent looks that yield continuous information on the activity of neighbors." In Old World primates living in a woodland habitat, by contrast, "the lack of facial expressiveness and the passivity of exchanges causes reactions to be less predictable and subtle, and less susceptible to modulation." (p. 225)

Facial expressions in primates show a wide variation in intensity. They are typically a mix of two competing motives (as Darwin predicted) such as approach and avoidance. They are balanced most often by the facial expression of others, both in the polarities Darwin anticipated and in the levels of intensity. Thus the relations are fluid and responsive, constantly indicating any change in the social balance of the group.

Facial expression is used by all primates not only to convey internal states but to synchronize them as well. Movements of the upper face in particular are characteristic cues to internal states. Studies of primates (Redican, 1982) show a common frowning expression, which is part of the animal's overall alerting response when it is either concentrating on a particular stimulus or suddenly scanning the environment. The movement involves constriction of the muscles of the forehead and around the eye (orbicularis oculi and corrugator muscles), flattening the eyebrows and bringing them together. This movement improves visual acuity by stabilizing the eyes in a binocular fashion and by reducing the amount of light entering the eye (Redican, 1982; Darwin, [1872] 1965). In lower primates this movement also brings the ears forward and away from the head to improve auditory acuity as well.

In humans, slight contraction of the frontalis muscle to knit the brow occurs during periods of moderately increased arousal. Structurally similar to the alerting response seen in other primates, it is associated with increased attentiveness on a particular object and typically occurs with difficult or unpleasant experiences. With eyes closed or defocused, it reflects a stage of intense internal absorption. As Darwin noted, the frown occurs in response not only to external experiences but to internal ones as well: "A man may be absorbed in the deepest thought, and his brow will remain smooth until he encounters some obstacle in his train of reasoning, or is interrupted by some disturbance, and then a frown passes like a shadow over his brow" (Darwin, [1872] 1965, p. 221).

Gaze direction and eye contact are related means of regulating interactions. Both the direction of the gaze and the orientation of the face are important social signals. Studies suggest that the brain processes the two sorts of information separately and must synthesize and interpret their meaning. The two tasks seem to involve different groups of cells in the temporal cortex in both hemispheres (Perrett, 1985). These neural units influence evaluation of emotional response on the basis of gaze and eye contact (Perrett, 1985). Kleinke (1986) has reviewed a number of studies that suggest that gaze is critical in the expression of intimacy and rapport, the regulation of interactions, and the working out of shared tasks. The actual role of eye contact depends on the situation and the people involved in it.

Another regulatory function of gaze is the turn-taking cue. Although gaze is a relatively consistent and stable behavior, results of studies of personal factors do not always fit a meaningful pattern, largely because motivation and context have not been taken into account. Recent studies, however, suggest that gaze synchronization and the operation of gaze in turn-taking are less reliable than previously believed because they depend on the context and motives of the interactants.

The yawn, a third, related facial display described by Redican (1982), may be closely related to hypnotic behavior. The expression occurs in two stages: first, the mouth is gradually opened wider and wider as the head is drawn back and the eyes are more tightly closed, and then the head is brought forward and the eyes begin to open again as the mouth is gradually closed. Although traditionally a distinction has been made between "physiologic" and "emotional" yawns, work by Deputte (1978) relates both forms as being indicators to the relaxation phase of general arousal. Yawns are most commonly seen immediately after any form of social interaction, and most often are followed by a period of reduced activity and rest.

The yawn in primates is remarkably contagious. Usually originating with a more dominant animal, it is picked up by those in the surrounding area. Nervous yawns, usually coming from more subordinate animals, appear to be "requests" for this calming cue from the dominant members of the group. Deputte suggests that the spread of yawns is a form of social entrainment or synchronization. Thus, the yawn may be an important behavioral manifestation of the innate drive for synchronous biologic states in groups of animals. As other forms of facial expression incite other animals to increased activity, the yawn, accompanied by other physiologic manifestations of reduced activity, appears to coordinate group relaxation and reduced behavior. Sensitivity to cues for the level of arousal in the interaction is critical in maintaining synchrony (Askenasy, 1989).

In one sense, facial displays such as the stare or the yawn may be considered the rudimentary origins of hypnosis. Both indicate subjective states (the stare reflecting absorption and the yawn indicating a significant change in the level of consciousness), but they are at the same time units of social communication, altering the external behavior and internal states of other individuals. Moreover, whereas other facial displays may be related to external matters such as food or danger, these two are specifically related to the regulation of the social milieu and the relationships between members of the group. Both also have significant effects in humans. The stare is associated with intense absorption (Landau, 1989), and the yawn is a highly contagious nonverbal cue of an oncoming change in the level of consciousness, either sedating or arousing (Provine, 1987, 1989). Both are powerful "suggestions" to anyone in their vicinity.

Face-to-face communication provides context, an ongoing interaction that changes over time and develops its own history. A couple's relationship, for example, can be seen in their faces. Two people who have lived together for a long time come to resemble each other; at least they do if they are lucky. Zajonc (1987) has demonstrated this among partners in long and happy marriages. The basis for the resemblance appears to be a growing similarity in basic facial expressions, perhaps reflecting a measure of their emotional synchrony. Individuals repeatedly mimic the facial expressions of their partners.

The face also plays a role in identifying our own emotions as well as simply expressing them to others. This idea, known as self-attribution theory, has been popular since the nineteenth century. William James, the most famous exponent of this school, coined the aphorism that we feel sad because we weep and feel fear because we flee. There is a strong correlation between the intensity of facial expression and objective, emotional experience, as shown by Adelmann and Zajonc (1989). They suggest that this relationship is a two-way street. Facial expression not only reveals one's emotional state but also plays an important role in one's initiating and modulating the experience of emotion. They conclude that the kinesthetic feedback from the face is an important route in evaluating what it is that we are feeling. In this sense, each person is truly two-faced, simultaneously monitoring each facial expression while displaying it to others. Face-to-face communication quickly breaks down the arbitrary boundaries that we conceptually establish between two people, producing a field in which the roles of sender and receiver quickly merge.

By sending and receiving information on the internal state of the individual, the face provides part of the process by which the state can be both shared and altered. Communication requires that attentional processes be synchronized. That synchronization sets up an expectation of greater rapport and sensitivity to social cues. By drawing on the brain's inherent ultradian cycle of alterations in consciousness (the "everyday trance"), face-to-face communication harmonizes biologic rhythms for psychological and social ends. If hypnosis is a special state, it is one that develops out of mundane origins.

THE TWO FACES

Studies of facial expression are complicated by the fact that the two sides of the face often show separate patterns. The study of asymmetries in the human facial expression has enjoyed a recent increase in popularity that is related to the interest in hemispheric specialization in the brain. As each side of the face is predominantly under control of the opposite side of the brain, evidence of differential expression of emotion between the two halves of the face is part of a growing body of evidence of hemispheric specialization with regard to emotion.

Darwin was the first to note that some facial expressions are naturally asymmetrical, citing as examples such expressions as sneering or disdain. He proposed that the asymmetry is a natural product of giving off a mixed message. As with the rest of the body, one side of the face is controlled by the contralateral hemisphere of the brain. But the bottom half of the face, with its need for the fine sequencing of subtle movements related to speech, is under more voluntary control than the top half, which uses movements that are much more emotional and less subtle (Rinn, 1984). Thus, facial expressions can be asymmetric both from left to right and from top to bottom. These asymmetries indicate different messages being expressed simultaneously.

The Lynns (1938, 1943) studied subjects' spontaneous smiles in response to visual stimuli. They reported that the majority of the subjects had facial asymmetries in their smiles, usually with one side of the face slightly preceding the other. More recent work (Hager, 1982) using far more sophisticated techniques has generally confirmed these earlier studies. Significant facial asymmetries in the expression of some emotions have been found, but overall the studies revealed no consistent pattern in preference to right or left (Sackeim, 1978; Campbell, 1978). The left side of the face (under the control of the right hemisphere) does tend in most individuals to express emotions more intensely than the right (Sackeim, 1978; Borod, 1980; Moscovitch, 1982). Sackeim and Gur (1978) reported that negative expressions were judged as stronger on the left more often than positive emotions. Others have suggested that the increased expressiveness of the left side is true only for unpleasant emotions and that more positive emotions are expressed on the right (Sackeim, 1982; Schiff, 1989). It is clear that the relationship is not fixed but fluctuates with the emotion expressed as well as the context and the manner in which the context is interpreted (Tucker, 1985; Dane, 1985). Facial expression is a fluid mosaic highly responsive to internal states and external cues that both displays and modulates emotional states (Izard, 1990).

Thus, the asymmetries are influenced by the manner in which the brain interprets the task and by the degree of conscious involvement. G. E. Schwartz (1979) reported relatively greater muscle activity on the right zygomatic (jaw) and corrugator (forehead) muscles during positive emotions and greater activity on the left during negative emotions in the zygomatic but not in the corrugator. Muscle activity in the corrugator was greater in the left side when subjects were asked to mimic facial expressions regardless of the type. Similarly, Ekman and his coworkers (1981) reported that asymmetrical movements were more frequent in artificial smiles than in spontaneous ones. Therefore spontaneous emotional movements appear to be less asymmetrical than deliberate movements. Hager suggests that deliberate movements that are asymmetrical are more likely to be left-sided than right-sided, but that asymmetrical movements in spontaneous emotional expression do not favor one side or the other (1982).

Rinn (1984), following Luria (1973), suggests that the right hemisphere lateralization for emotion may actually be due to a left hemisphere superiority for the inhibition of emotion. In other words, the increased specialization of the left hemisphere for voluntary movements in general and language in particular may give that hemisphere an inherent skill in controlling involuntary expressions. By contrast, the right hemisphere, with its specialization for integrating and expressing varying sources of data, attempts to display the nature and intensity of the emotion as vividly as possible. These competing goals account both for asymmetries and for their fluid nature.

The asymmetry of facial expression is mirrored by hemispheric bias in the ability of the brain to "read" facial expressions (Borod, 1990a, 1990b). There is a tendency to identify the emotional state with the emotion expressed by the right side of the face, owing to the right hemisphere's specialization for processing facial information. In other words, the right side of the subject's face is picked up by the right hemisphere of the observer because it enters through the left visual field; that is, observers tend to use the side of the face in the left visual field to identify the whole face, whether it is actually the left or right half (Hager, 1982). The evidence seems to suggest a left visual field (right hemisphere) advantage in perceiving facial emotion (Etcoff, 1984). There is also evidence that the processing of emotional expression may, in fact, be more reliable when the processing occurs out of the awareness of the individual—that is, when conscious processes cannot interfere (Stambrook, 1983). There is a right hemisphere advantage in recognizing faces that is particularly pronounced when the task requires processing in terms of the overall properties of the face rather than isolated features (Campbell, 1978), or the faces to be recognized show emotional expressions rather than being emotionally neutral (Suberi, 1977).

In summary, the data suggest that the two sides of the face differ in emotional expression and that they are capable of expressing two different emotions either sequentially or simultaneously. But clearly there are no consistent findings that can be generalized for all human beings in all contexts. The degree of conscious involvement, the nature of the task, the nature of the recording devices, the simple fact of being observed and the emotional state of the observer all play significant roles. Thus asymmetries in facial expression do have a role in emotional expression, but the nature of the role seems to be much more individualized and context-bound than was originally thought.

MODULAR ORGANIZATION

Although the modules involved are found on both sides of the brain, there is a significant localization in the parietotemporal regions of the right hemisphere (Perrett, 1984, 1985; Young, 1985a, 1985b). These modules are intimately related with similar modules for the recognition of facial emotional expression and the nonverbal components of speech (Bruce, 1986). In fact, though right hemisphere damage often results in the loss of the ability to connect a name with a particular face or indeed any conscious awareness of familiarity, such patients may continue to show electrophysiologic responses to familiar individuals, which are outside of their awareness (Young, 1985b; Tranel, 1985). The evidence suggests that facial recognition and emotional processing occur in conjunction with one another to activate emotional and interpersonal patterns operating largely outside of our conscious awareness (Hansch, 1980; Strauss, 1981).

The idea that the brain breaks down tasks into distinct but interconnected modules is currently a popular one. It explains not only how complicated tasks can be done quickly, but it also explains some of the strange results seen with neurologic damage. The case of facial recognition illustrates this. Neurologic lesions affecting the right hemisphere can result in a wide variety of disorders of facial recognition. Patients may be unable to recognize faces, to recognize facial expressions, or even to lip read—that is, link what facial expressions go with what particular sounds. Moreover, the modular nature of this breakdown means that patients can often restore a particular function by adopting a different strategy (Bruce, 1986). Assal (1984) described a patient, a dairy farmer, who could not recognize people he knew, nor could he recognize the faces of his cows. He recovered the ability to recognize the faces of familiar people, but his livestock continued to look to him as if they belonged to someone else.

The modular model of any intellectual function has two great advantages: first, it explains how complicated tasks can be broken down into discrete units so that they can be performed quickly; second, it provides an explanation for how different sorts of information can be processed simultaneously with a minimum of interference. Although interference does occur in some particular forms of novel tasks, practice quickly allows for a wide degree of efficiency for any mutual combinations. Even the simplest social interaction is a bewildering combination of motor, emotional, and cognitive skills. Processing the tasks separately allows for their efficient simultaneous performance. By extension, however, it also requires an ability to synchronize that performance in a manner that is both regular and yet flexible.

A third implication of the modular model, one that is only beginning to receive sufficient attention, is the variability in cognitive strategies the modular model implies. Different connections in the sequences of the modules provide a great deal of flexibility with regard to the efficiency of a task or the time it takes to perform it. Different sequencing strategies may also explain much of interindividual variation in task efficiency and the use by an individual of different strategies in different contexts or in different states of consciousness (state-dependent learning).

This capacity is based on the brain's ability to process the same information in different ways. Processing of incoming stimuli occurs at each level in the brain, with each playing a particular role in gradually abstracting and assimilating key elements of the input. This step-by-step sequence is referred to as *serial* processing, the primary way in which information is organized by the brain. Simultaneously, the elaborate connections of the nervous system ensure that there is a gradual cascade of activation through a number of related neural centers. This system involves what is known as *parallel* processing of information.

Serial processing of information tends to be more focused and orderly, and more diffuse parallel processing is critical for integrating background knowledge and providing alternate models. The two systems normally function together. For example, in the visual system, serial processing is involved in the encoding of visual information, while parallel processing is responsible for the automatic functioning of vision and its coordination with other activities (Kissin, 1986; Marr, 1984).

Perception and learning involve simultaneous use of serial and parallel processing systems (Kissin, 1986). Although consciousness has been associated with serial processing, the evidence for unconscious learning suggests that parallel processing contributes a significant, if not decisive, element to our total understanding: "That is, language can be comprehended and responses initiated before conscious processes are activated. In other terms, conscious processes are not always necessary for highly skilled neurological and perceptual activities which include language understanding. Therefore, it is possible to understand and respond to a linguistic message without awareness of that message" (Rossi and Cheek, 1988, p. 153).

Gregory Bateson (1972) has argued that though there is obvious biologic advantage to automatic unconscious behavior, the biologic value of deliberate conscious behavior is much less obvious. Effective regulation of behavior involves automatization, not consciousness. Conscious behavior would appear to have some advantage in what is known as meta-programming—that is, in establishing priorities between competing behaviors or in altering a behavioral program when it is not working to the overall advantage of the organism. When things are running smoothly, there appears to be little advantage in conscious processing. Automatization, the transition of a learned skill from conscious to automatic behavior, is an important mechanism for ensuring the speed, efficiency, and reliability of important behavioral programs. The less conscious effort is involved in performing a particular behavior, the more likely it is to occur at the right time and in the right sequence. Descriptions of immediate subjective experience can be quite accurate, but the post hoc accounts that people provide for much of their behavior can be quite fanciful and provide little access to the basic unconscious programs (Spiegel, 1978; Lewicki, 1986; Bowers, 1986; Gazzaniga, 1985). Clearly, learning a complex neuromotor program (such as when a child learns to speak or to walk) is not primarily a conscious process. The evidence suggests that human beings learn perceptual and motor patterns as a single sequence and that the process of making a behavior automatic depends upon breaking it down into various levels of hierarchic control and effectively sequencing the subroutines (Goodman, 1980). Speech, the very mechanism we usually use to assert the preeminence of our conscious mind, is, in fact, the prototypic model of automatic behavior.

The automatic performance of a perceptual motor pattern requires that each of the individual elements be appropriately timed. This means that once one element is activated the probability is that the entire sequence will proceed. The opportunity to repeat and practice patterns is the important variable in their becoming automatic. Practice may not always make perfect, but it certainly makes probable.

THE FACE OF HYPNOSIS

The evidence suggests that facial expression is a dynamic and complex channel for communication. Facial expression changes over time to help modulate ongoing communication. Furthermore, it does not occur in isolation. It is associated with changes in tone of voice and with gesture to produce a coherent whole. In addition, the sensory cues fed back from the muscles of the face to the brain in conjunction with level of arousal, voice tone, and posture play an important role in initiating and modulating facial expression (Adelmann, 1989). Particular facial expressions are related to specific physiologic and subjective states (Levenson, 1990). Face-to-face communication is a complex amalgam that serves to express both explicit and implicit information, and it is a particularly powerful means of establishing social expectations. Face-to-face communication creates a frame for interpreting context.

From this perspective, hypnosis is a highly specialized form of face-to-face communication. The hypnotherapist monitors the hypnotic state by means of facial cues, and these cues may be important in the self-monitoring of the hypnotic subject. Face-to-face communication emphasizes the parallel activity of conscious and unconscious processes as they are interwoven in communication.

3 THE MEANING IN THE RHYTHM: SYNCHRONY IN COMMUNICATION

There has to be a meaning in the rhythm.

Ezra Pound, 1979

All the subtleties and intricacies of our ability to perceive and express nonverbal communication are in the service of one thing: our sustaining an *interactional rhythm*. These rhythms must be flexible enough to allow people to entrain with one another and strong enough to maintain that bonding (Chapple, 1982). Vocal intonation (and by extension breathing), facial expression, eye contact, and gesture are all bound together in an ongoing feedback system (Davis, 1982). Regulation of this system involves both hemispheres, as well as subcortical structures in the brain stem and hypothalamus, and arises from the basic metabolic rhythms of the brain. Chapple describes the coordination of the rhythms as a "language" (though more akin to music), having both form and meaning. "It is this body language which primarily expresses the functioning of the CNS. What we call language (verbal and nonverbal) is a cultural derivative, secondary to the cultural shaping of body language itself" (1982, p. 50). Hypnotic language is the intensification of the everyday rhythms of language to enhance rapport. It is a capacity that depends on the active involvement of both speaker and listener.

INTONATION

Molière's Bourgeois Gentilhomme describes his delight when, shortly after finding out the definition of prose, he discovers that he has been speaking it all his life. Alas, he is quite wrong (at least in English translation). Prose is a written convention of language that follows the grammatical and syntactical conventions of literacy. The spoken structure of English is far closer to blank verse, depending on the rhythms of breathing for its structure (Barton, 1984). Listeners can easily tell on the basis of the presence or absence of pauses, hesitations, and other attributes whether they are hearing spontaneous speech or a text being read aloud.

Intonation and Its Parts: Melody in Spoken English by Dwight Bolinger (1986) is a remarkable book in several respects. Bolinger takes an enormously complicated field and makes it almost deceptively accessible. Equally valuable is the wide-ranging collection of vivid illustrations he uses. Thus, the book both presents a theory and serves as a workbook in learning to be consciously sensitive to English intonation. Simply reviewing the thousands of everyday examples provides a tuning for one's ears (and brain) to the melody of the spoken word.

As we all vaguely remember from poetry appreciation classes, rhythm is produced by recurring patterns of stressed and unstressed syllables. In traditional poetry, the feet are of equal length and follow an overall pattern. This is most clearly the case in languages that derive from Latin, in which all syllables are of roughly equal length. Thus the sound patterns in such languages are much more easily structured than they are in Germanic languages.

In contrast, English has a great deal of variation in foot lengths. Its vowel system includes two grades of each vowel being either full or reduced (Bolinger, 1986, p. 37). The contrast of syllables with full and reduced vowels produces a basic rhythm in spoken English, which intonation can then vary to produce spoken melody. Hence, English has a much more varied intonational set of possibilities, whereas languages such as French or Italian have much more of a "singsong" quality to them. The intonational pattern in English is much more variable and spontaneous and much less predictable.

An important function of the rhythm of speech is to allow us to continue to breathe while speaking. We require a complex pattern of breathing movements to modify our respiration so that speech can be produced. This includes movements of the abdomen and chest as well as of the larynx and upper airway. Our breathing must coordinate with the duration and intensity of what we wish to say, and all these factors must be taken into account before we begin to speak. The pattern of breathing sustained during speech is dramatically different from the pattern of quiet breathing or breathing during physical exertion (Lieberman, 1984). Yet most of the time our breathing and speech coordinate flawlessly. When we are about to speak a long sentence, our lungs take in slightly more air—even before we are consciously aware of the need. Lieberman (1984) describes a "breath-group" that parallels the logical structure of human speech: "The breath-group theory proposes that human speakers usually segment the flow of speech into sentences, or other syntactic units, by grouping words in complete expirations. The breath-group theory further proposes that the acoustic cues that delimit the end of a sentence usually follow from articulatory gestures that represent the minimal departure from the articulatory maneuvers that would occur during quiet respiration" (Lieberman, 1984, p. 118).

Fluent speech is a neuromuscular performance of remarkable complexity. When speaking we are usually consciously aware only of a listener and of an intent to be communicated. Frequently this intent is only partial. A speaker, much like a chess player, must respond to someone else's choices as well. Despite this, not only does the correct vocabulary become instantly available, but the grammar and syntax also seem to be spontaneously present. At the same time, phonation and pronunciation (a highly complicated set of motor processes) are produced in the correct sequence. The most remarkable part of all is that we accept this complex performance in such a matter-of-fact way. Perhaps because we have been doing it all our lives and experience speech all around us, we tend to take this remarkable combination of cognitive and motor steps for granted.

The underlying story is even more complex. Simultaneous with our mustering vocabulary, grammar, syntax, and phonologic elements, we provide a continuous modulating flow in the way of gesture and intonation. Through these aspects we reveal to others (though often unknowingly) our emotions, beliefs, and judgments about what we are saying, the way it is being received, and the social context. These elements of speech are far more implicit, easily recognized and performed, but often difficult to describe. This part of speech has a great deal more to do with music than it does with prose. Intonation is the melody of speech, while gesture contributes to the rhythm with its dancelike repetitions.

PROSODY

Prosody is the name for tonal aspects of speech. This is achieved by the alternation of stressed and unstressed syllables (Bolinger, 1986). These stresses are achieved by a combination of auditory features including pitch (frequency), loudness, and tempo (Frick, 1985). Prosody provides grammatical cues about how speech is to be interpreted, frames to emphasize significant parts of the message, and ongoing expression to the speaker's emotional state. Prosodic features are capable of simultaneously underlining what is being said and providing information that complements the facial and gestural variations.

Speakers normally switch among pitch, length, and loudness (intensity or volume) to produce the overall rhythm, but pitch is the most frequently used element (Bolinger, 1986). Pitch describes the changes from sound to sound. It is produced by the vibrations of the vocal chords when air is expelled from the lungs through the larynx. Consequently, pitch can be precisely measured electrophysiologically in terms of vibrations per unit time. Pitch in adult males varies between 60 and 240 Hz, and among adult females between 180 and 400 Hz. Pitch is the most generally used cue, partly because

it is probably the most efficient cue. Length and loudness can be varied in only one dimension, more vs. less; pitch can in addition adopt a variety of shapes, including skips, glides, arrests, and combinations of these. Loudness may be distorted by wind currents, interfering objects, distance, and direction of transmission; pitch patterns are almost immune to such distortion. Length is affected by breathing, fatigue, and the phonetic influence of individual speech sounds to a greater degree than pitch. The ear is more sensitive to minute changes in pitch than to minute changes in length or loudness. And all auditory cues are more efficient than gestural ones because they do not require the receiver to be looking in a particular direction—which is why language is more speech than gesture in the first place. (Bolinger, 1986, p. 22)

Intonation is the rise and fall of pitch as it occurs along the speech chain (Bolinger, 1986). The changes in pitch, called accents or stresses, are used to mark out individual syllables (loudness or length may also be used in this). Accented or stressed syllables, and their alternation with unstressed syllables, produces the rhythm of speech. Accented syllables tend to be associated with the greater significance in communication. It is the extent of the change that gives the significance to the syllable.

Change in pitch is more important than the absolute pitch itself. Acoustically, we are able to make very precise discriminations between various pitches. These discriminations take the form of rating the pitches as higher or lower, whether a voice is going "up" or "down." The degree to which pitch changes or the rate at which it does so (whether it glides or changes abruptly) produces more brain activity than does any particular aspect of intonation. Our ability to extract content from speech depends critically on our ability to make these most minute of distinctions clearly and reliably (Cruttenden, 1986).

Cruttenden emphasizes that the relation between objective elec-trophysiologic acoustic measurement and subjective perception is not a close one. Perception is influenced by expectations evoked by previous rhythm, pitch, and content. If we must simply choose between two specific syllables, we can do so quite reliably. But if the syllables are substituted for each other in the course of ordinary conversation, the brain is likely to hear the syllable that it expected. Similarly any prosodic feature can be interpreted according to the current needs of the interaction. We may use the same change in pitch to make sense of the syntax, provide indications about the emotional import of the communication, or make judgments about the personality of the speaker. As with notes in music, the meaning assigned to one individual element also largely depends on the other sounds that accompany it.

Although it fluctuates widely around a rhythmic ideal, the rhythm of the spoken word maintains a regularity through an underlying succession of prominent stresses (Oliva, 1982). This is true whether the stress is signaled by changes in pitch, tone, volume, tempo, or contour. Although each of these elements can be recognized individually, they can be interchangeable at the level of rhythm perception. In addition, the perception can be maintained by expectation. Even a full pause does not interfere with the rhythm if the next prominent stress is close to where it should be in the succeeding line of beats.

Thus, each individual sound stands not as an independent unit but as a member of a larger aggregate. Dowling (1986) suggests that intonation is a multidimensional subjective experience in which the predictable and unpredictable elements form the structure when taken together. He likens this structure to the model of the double helix in DNA. This structure in music making appears to be universal. For our purposes, we can think of speech as a song that can be performed by one or

more voices. This song is accompanied by facial expressions and gestures based on the same rhythm. In a biologic sense, speech in an oral
culture is a multimedia display combining music, song, and dance to
enhance communication in the same way that a speaker at a scientific
conference might use her voice, slides, or videotapes in combination.

Pitch can influence speech in two ways: by driving the narrative
along with its rhythm and by providing a counterpoint to the meaning
of the words. Pitch performs the same function in music where "the
listener is conscious of pitch in two dimensions: melody and harmony.
The melody is the 'tune' and the harmony accompanies it" (Bolinger,
1986, p. 9).

Particular intonation profiles are associated with particular emotions
in the same way that facial expressions are. Higher pitch is associated
with arousal and increased tension levels; lower pitch is associated with
decreasing arousal levels and falling tension. Similar to the Darwinian
antithesis of emotional opposites, intonation follows the general human
assumption that emotions occur in polar pairs. Scherer (1979, 1981)
has reviewed the studies of vocal indicators of emotional states. There
are characteristic prosodic features for at least nine emotional states:
happiness, confidence, anger, fear, indifference, contempt, boredom,
sadness, and arousal. Each shows a characteristic pattern of pitch level,
loudness, and tempo, and there also appear to be characteristic changes
of both pitch range and variability for each.

Intonation is used simultaneously to mark the punctuation of the
spoken word and to express emotional content; there is no clear distinction between the two. It is simplest to think of the actual intonation of a
sentence as falling somewhere along a continuum between these two
usages. Most of the grammatical information provided by intonation
comes from the terminal intonation of the phrase or sentence—for
example, declarative sentences end with a gradual glide downward,
whereas a question ends with an upward glide.

Communication in the spoken world exchanges information, but it is
also a sharing of emotional state and attitudes (see chap. 4). Far from
wishing to diminish the subjective component in an attempt to make
the information more timeless and context-free (as the literate bias
encourages us), prosodic communication makes its greatest impact at
times of greatest emotional expression. The messages that are the most
subjective are the most easily responded to.

Listening is an active process in the widest sense. The absorbed listener participates in the words in an active way. Our auditory processes
select out specific components of what we hear; motor rhythms of

breathing and minor muscle movements both in the speech muscles and in the rest of the body occur in synchrony with the speaker. The quiet listener experiences a merging of the external voice with internal speech (Sheehan, 1982).

The two hemispheres process what we hear differently. The right ear (left hemisphere) has an advantage in the ability to discriminate between the distinctions of the various sound patterns of syllables that are necessary to establish the meaning of speech. In contrast, there is a left ear (right hemisphere) advantage in identifying the contour of speech, a feature that is more closely associated with the emotional meaning (Lieberman, 1984). The right ear advantage is primarily related to those features that are necessary for following the sequential order of speech (Bradshaw, 1981). This is in keeping with the function of the left hemisphere in organizing across time.

The right hemisphere has a preeminent role in the perception and expression of emotion (Chavoix, 1987). Although both hemispheres are clearly involved in the experience of emotion, the right hemisphere, with its specialized connections with the limbic system, is particularly involved in coordinating emotional states with external contextual demands (Geschwind, 1987). This role appears to be related to a particular anatomical complex that involves the parietal lobe as well as related limbic, brain stem, and thalamic connections (Mesulam, 1983). This network is responsible for a form of specific attention directed toward emotional variables in any context. It seems to involve two anatomical structures in the right hemisphere that are placed similarly to the analogous structures for perception and expression of language in the left hemisphere (Borod, 1986).

Prosody is such a pervasive element of communication that it is easily overlooked. In fact, it is easier to recognize when it is absent. Clinicians have noticed that whereas lesions in the left hemisphere result in deficits in the sensory and motor aspects of speech, injuries in the corresponding (parietotemporal) areas of the right hemisphere result in difficulties in the comprehension and expression of the emotional aspects of speech and gesture (Ross, 1985). Patients with right parietal lesions that are more anterior are likely to have difficulties in expressing prosodic features in their own speech. More posterior lesions usually result in difficulties in prosodic comprehension (Borod, 1986; Benowitz, 1983).

The right hemisphere functions to process complex linguistic structures and to interpret the context in assessing communication (Wapner, 1981). This involves the temporal processing of syllabic transitions that allow the listener to synchronize to the rhythm of the spoken word

(Molfese, 1985). As with facial expression, however, though the right hemisphere exerts a primary influence, prosodic information is processed by both hemispheres. Particular modules of neurons do perform particular elements, but the total performance of the normal brain involves the coordination of a variety of functions (Ross, 1986). The prosodic language system in the right hemisphere is closely tied both anatomically and functionally to the language systems of the dominant hemisphere (Bhatnagar, 1983).

INTERACTIONAL RHYTHMS

Rhythm is a product of biological structure (Mathiot, 1982). An accumulation of mutually entrained rhythms protects the individual components from wild fluctuations (Glass, 1988). Rhythm produces the expectation of continuity and changes in rhythm signal new experiences. These changes may be signaled by alterations in tempo or by the lengthening or shortening of the beats themselves. Obviously, varying rhythms can grow to share a common pattern only if they have the flexibility to adjust to one another. The capacity to be both repeating and flexible in the nature of that repetition is essential.

Of all the rhythms of human life, perhaps none is so central, none is more closely linked to what makes us human, as the rhythm of face-to-face interaction. The ability to create a relationship, to share a context, is the important human skill. To regulate the rhythm and tempo of the interaction is as important as the entrainment of any other cycles of activity and light, food and digestion, with the coordination of brain centers. Just as synchrony of these functions depends on the aggregation of a group of smaller elements, so too does human interaction. These rhythms provide the basis for how we know each other and share our lives.

Synchrony is the entrainment of several rhythms, so that features of the two occur within the same temporal pattern. The synchronization of various communication channels within an individual is referred to as "self-synchrony" (Condon, 1982), wherein the gestural and verbal rhythms of the individual complement each other. Changes in body movements occur with the stress rhythm of speech and serve to clarify the spoken message. Thus, gesture serves for the spoken word as punctuation does for the written.

A second form of synchrony between speaker and listener is "interactional synchrony," which takes place when the movements of the listener occur at the same rate as the gesture and verbal rhythms of the speaker. The establishment of rapport is a crucial variable in the construction of human behavior. The feeling of sharing a consensual reality serves to regulate both internal and external cohesion. The establishment of that rapport is an important feature of face-to-face communication. It is done through a process of synchrony involving motor patterns of all the interactants using gesture, posture, and speech (Chapple, 1982).

Conversation, between however many people, involves a series of sounds and movement simultaneously using a number of channels. Each member in the interaction typically shares both the content and the intonation of speech as well as bodily movements, particularly facial expressions and gestures. Simultaneously we also reveal, through the work of the autonomic nervous system, an ongoing change of pattern in breathing and heartbeat through changes in our respiratory rate, skin color, pupil size, and other features. The rhythm of conversation is made up of subcomponents of words and their structures, intonation, facial expression, gesture, and breathing. These patterns must attempt to synchronize with those of the other participants. As with other biologic patterns, these various rhythms will change tempo or intensity along the various channels until a stability can be reached.

Perhaps the single most important feature that is emphasized by all the workers in this field is the necessity for adjustment of the usual conceptual frame. Although these are descriptions of individual behavior, it is important to recognize that the unit is not the individual but the social interaction. It is not possible to appreciate the nature of the synchrony of human activity without including input from all the participants. Our usual models are too atomistic, too inclined to consider behavior as a function of each individual unit, rather than as a process involving all the elements. It is the cooperative nature of human activity that best illuminates the process of brain function:

It is striking how belatedly we have discovered the obvious. Any dancer or musician could have told us that we must share a common rhythm to sing or play or dance together. So could any athlete who plays on a team. And privately we have always known that a common rhythmicity is essential to consummate sexual union but why didn't we realize earlier that interaction rhythms were essential in every human interaction? Are scientists always the last to know what artists and others have known all along? . . .

Even in the 1950s when we did begin to conceive of communication and better appreciated that more than one person was present, we were still stuck with the habit of focusing on one person. So we watched one person and then the next one, as if we were watching a tennis match. At this point we began to conceive of communication as an interaction, as an action and reaction sequence between two "individuals" who took turns.

If we observe only one person or one person at a time, there is no way we will observe synchrony or co-action or interactional rhythm. It is interesting to note that even today we title the phenomenon of shared rhythmicity "interaction rhythms" instead of "co-action" rhythms, thereby hanging onto the notion of alternative actions in sequence. (Scheflen, 1982, pp. 14–15)

THE LEVELS OF SYNCHRONY

Beebe (1982) demonstrated the importance of both repetitive rhythmic movement and intonation patterns in shaping the mental set and maintaining attention during communication, thereby establishing a context. Context can refer to all the implicit factors influencing a situation. More narrowly, it can be used to indicate the frame of reference produced by the goals of the communication. An important part of interactional synchrony is the development of a shared goal and a resultant synchrony of contextual frames of reference. This results in the participants having the same operational syntax by which they interpret the interaction (Cicourel, 1987).

Above all, rhythms of the spoken word are actively interpreted by the brain. Mental schemata, which develop from childhood, determine the salient features, the critical cues, from the variety of fine auditory discriminations. The individual schema is a perception of the temporal organization. It is this rhythmic process that provides the link between interactional frame and cognitive schema (Kendon, 1982).

The study of human interactions became a science when we acquired the technological ability to break time up into units that are imperceptible to our conscious mind. Frame-by-frame videotape analysis of interactions reveals a complex and highly choreographed world of communication below the level of our conscious awareness. Elements of conversation that are far too brief to be noticed in real life suddenly appear when time becomes a series of images in a film. Not only do the various channels of each participant coordinate with one another, but the movements of the listener are synchronized with the structure of the speaker's language (Condon, 1982; Kendon, 1982). Furthermore the synchrony exists at several levels extending through different time frames.

This synchrony of interaction arises from basic perceptual mechanisms. For communication to be possible, our brain must be able to respond to perceptual cues that are infinitely quicker than our conscious awareness is capable of. The synchronization of the listener's body is a motoric reflection of the hearing process. As we watch and listen, attentional processes must come into play, responding to cues within milliseconds (Condon, 1982). The brain can detect sound units that are as small as six to nine microseconds, a feat that is not only far below conscious awareness but significantly faster than the time we believe it takes a message to pass from neuron to neuron—one millisecond, or one thousand microseconds. Different parts of each auditory signal are thus broken down into units that are far smaller than our perceived conscious awareness, allowing these elements to function as cues for synchronization of neural responses for the adjusting of attentional sets, muscular responses, and coordination of processing modules. Muscle responses can entrain to sounds within the ten-to-fifty-millisecond range, altering the tonic (resting) rhythm of the body (Condon, 1982). Condon hypothesizes that synchrony is a response occurring in the early phase of auditory attention in which that input is responded to by changes in motor patterns as well as by auditory processing. In effect, these features of the signal are important for discriminating what should synchronize us and what should not.

Condon (1982) also reports a further one-second rhythm cycle in behavior. These cycles appear to be related to the resting heartbeat in normal conversational interchanges. Facial expression, gesture, and speech are all coordinated in this rhythm. The result is a vehicle for the syllable with its characteristic consonant-vowel-consonant (cvc) structure, universal to spoken languages. These units of sound occur in three phases with an onset consonant, a distinguishing vowel, and a closing sound. This basic pattern makes up the building blocks of speech, each unit being discrete and each contributing to the larger rhythm of the whole (Stetson, 1951).

What is emerging is that the body is precisely locked in and integrated with this flow so that the body will hold quietly on a consonant and speed up on a vowel. You can't see it, it's so fast, but at least 80 percent of the time it looks like this happening. The body is slightly slow, speeds up on the vowel pulse, then damps down, and this rhythm occurs within other rhythms, resulting in a wider 1-second rhythm. Speech and body motion are a unity. (Condon, 1982, p. 63)

Duration, loudness, and pitch can also be identified by the brain over several time levels (Mathiot, 1982). Within a single speech contour they merge to form a beat pattern. At a macro level of several contours they produce a larger accent pattern. Thus over two time frames the same elements produce two different structures, a basic pattern that is made up of the individual beat patterns and a secondary pattern that emerges from the accents. In this way, two separate rhythms provide for a possible synchrony of patterns of thinking, feeling, or perception (Lieberman, 1984).

This is demonstrated by the characteristic pattern of autonomic nervous system activity that occurs during human speech. Stimuli that are synchronized with the phases of the cardiovascular pulse pressure produce more prominent potentials in the brain, particularly in the right hemisphere (Sandman, 1984). Alterations in the respiratory pattern can reduce measures of physiologic and psychological arousal significantly (Cappo, 1984). Moreover, these features are related to the emotional salience of the content. The actual respiratory and motor component of speech affects this autonomic (respiratory, blood volume, pulse and heart rate) pattern in a relatively minor way. But the content of speech, particularly its emotional significance, is strongly related to the autonomic variables (Linden, 1987).

SYNCHRONY IN SOUND AND GESTURE

Adam Kendon (1984) has reviewed the evidence for the idea that there are units of gesture that correspond to each tone unit (the units of speech). Each gesture phrase is made up of three stages similar to the cvc pattern of the tone unit. Cross-cultural studies have shown that this pattern is consistent across a wide variety of languages. The oscillations that produce motor behavior and those that indicate cognitive processing are both manifested in behavior. In other words, complex mental processes are reflected in patterns of body movement (Davis, 1984; Wolfgang, 1984). Not only do gestures and facial expressions demarcate the rhythm of spoken communication; they also tend to parallel pitch changes, tending in an upward direction with increases in pitch and downward with decreases in pitch (Bolinger, 1986). "Facial and manual gestures . . . will normally parallel the line of pitch: eyebrows will be arched highest as the highest pitch is approached. . . . There are limits to the dexterity of these larger muscles, of course: a gesture 'fades' more slowly than an intonation. But the collaboration is unmistakable, and the relative fixity of the gesture may be an advantage: it can precede the utterance and set the stage for it" (Bolinger, 1986, p. 212).

The "content" and function of gesture vary widely. Gestures that are frequently associated with specific facial expressions appear to be more universal than those that are used to illustrate particular aspects of speech (Kendon, 1984). With an increasing degree of literacy, gesture not only becomes a rhythmic indicator of speech sense or of punctuation for the spoken word but also provides a visual representation of the content of speech. Graham and Argyle (1975) have shown that the addition of gesture significantly improves recall of communication in Italian but not English speakers. The power of language derives from its precision in specifying what is meant. On the other hand, gesture, by its nature, is much more context-bound. What we interpret from nonverbal communication can give us a great deal more information about the current situation and cannot be generalized into other situations. In this way, the spoken word is intermediate between nonverbal communication and written communication with its precise grammar, punctuation, and spelling.

Thus, body and mind are actively involved in the synchrony of communication rhythms. The ability to entrain to these rhythms is necessary for comprehension. Mental processing requires time. Generally speaking, the more complex the data that are being processed, the longer the time (Pöppel, 1988). Registration of different types of data, whether visual, auditory, or from the other senses, has a distinctive reaction time that can be measured electrophysiologically in thousandths of a second. Although natural ability and training can influence this (superior athletes have quicker reaction times for the specific sensory input they require in their sports than do nonathletes), there is a fixed limit that is universal in healthy subjects. These fixed limits not only underscore the limits at which we are able to perceive events but also reflect the timing that is required for an event to enter into the cerebral rhythm. "Apparently, the occurrence of a sudden event and our taking cognizance of it sets in motion an oscillatory or vibratory process, each period of which has a duration of approximately . . . 0.03 or 0.04 seconds, although it can sometimes be somewhat shorter or even longer. And we must stress another point. . . . The oscillation is always present, but . . . it can be synchronized immediately with sudden events" (Pöppel, 1988, pp. 37–38).

This inherent rhythm is entirely a subjective emphasis that our brain imposes on reality. It is what transforms the identical sounds of a grandfather clock into a rhythmic tick-tock. Perception is an active process. The brain must organize input if it is to make any sense. We are capable of either building up or recognizing such rhythms up to a range of 2.5–

3 seconds (Pöppel, 1988). Significantly, this duration is about the same time required for minimal or maximal organization of a visual pattern.

The Necker cube is a form of optical illusion in which a drawing can be seen as one of two different three-dimensional cubes at any one time. If you stare at it, the image of the cube begins to reverse, alternating from one view to another in about a three-second rhythm. A number of studies have found that the ability to perceive this reversal is correlated with hypnotic ability (Wallace, 1988). The rate of reversals appears to be related to the ability to use cognitive strategies to focus attention on the object.

We conclude, therefore, that our brain furnishes an integrative mechanism that shapes sequences of events to unitary forms, and we hypothesize in relation to this integration an upper temporal limit of circa three seconds. That which is integrated is the unique content of consciousness which seems to us *present*. The integration, which itself objectively extends over time, is thus the basis of our experiencing a thing as present. The *now* has a temporal extension of maximally three seconds. . . .

The temporal machinery of our brain is not primarily in place to make time available to us, but to assure the orderly functioning of our experience and behavior. The temporal machinery provides the formal frame, the *how*, so that the *what*, the seen, the heard and the touched have the possibility of represent-ing themselves. (Pöppel, 1988, pp. 62–63)

Pöppel performed an interesting experiment to identify the nature of this periodic structuring. Subjects wore headphones and in one ear heard a sentence (for example, "Since he does not play, his old team wins"). The other ear heard a click. This click occurred at random intervals throughout the sentence and the subjects were asked to esti-mate when they heard it. Significantly, regardless of when the click actually came, the subjects identified it as occurring at the phrase boundary. The brain, following the bridge pattern, prefers a rhythmic pause.

The pause helps both speaker and listener. While the speaker organizes what comes next, the listener is allowed to anticipate on the basis of what has come before in order to be attuned to what will follow. By keeping in rhythm, this shared frame of reference can be main-tained. Otherwise, the shared understanding gradually fades out.

When a person speaks, individual consecutive units of utterance also last on the average about three seconds. Each unit of utterance is concluded with a short pause, followed in turn by the next unit. This periodic division in speaking is not, incidentally, occasioned by our need to breathe. For that reason we do not term the pauses that occur at regular intervals breathing pauses, rather more appropriately planning pauses, for in these pauses each subsequent unit of utterance is prepared. The pauses belong then properly to each subsequent unit of utterance, not to the preceding one. Of course one observes this periodic structure only in spontaneous speech. When a person reads aloud, the rhythmical pattern is often not discernible, because in reading aloud, the speaker is not obliged mentally to prepare subsequent units of utterance, since he is only repeating what has already been written. (Pöppel, 1988, p. 71).

This fundamental periodic rhythm of speech appears to be inherent. It is seen in the speech of children regardless of their age, and it appears to be the basis of poetic structure. In extensive studies of poems in English, German, French, Chinese, Japanese, Latin, and Ancient Greek (and less systematically, those in Spanish, Italian, Hungarian, Celtic, and Russian, as well as tribal languages of New Guinea and Zambia), Pöppel has found an average line duration of three seconds. Subjects who are asked to divide up pieces of music similarly do so in three-second units (Pöppel, 1988). The three-second line appears to be universal.

There is no cultural-historical reason, nor is there any syntactical reason, that could be construed as being responsible for the poet's holding his poems in the vast majority of cases to these temporal limits. The reason appears rather to be that at the outset our experience of time delineates a temporal frame within which the poetic work is able to manifest itself.
    . . . In the poetic line, the poets have devised a form that corresponds best to the formal structure of our experience of time. (Pöppel, 1988, p. 78)

As Pöppel points out, individual exceptions abound. An important component of the poetic structure is to set up an expectation of a rhythm and then subtly modify it. The exceptions all occur in one direction, however: the lines can be shorter than the three-second boundary, never longer. Rhythm and its variations require adherence to these boundaries.

Rhythmic Synchrony in Infants

The mother-infant interaction is a unit that exists within the same boundaries of variability and repetition (D. Stern, 1977). Childhood development begins with the interactional rhythm. Beatrice Beebe has shown how the rhythm developed between mother and infant serves both to regulate their interaction and to stimulate infant development (1982). This capacity exists from early infancy and is the structure by which cognitive, emotional and social learning occurs

(Beebe, 1982; D. Stern, 1982). In the developing nervous system of the infant, entrainment to external rhythms is an important feature of maturation (Brazelton, 1990). As the infant learns that certain predictable things happen in response to changes in his or her internal feelings, the building blocks of perception, motor behavior, and internal regulation develop. The newborn show an ability to pattern to the sound of particular voices and clearly prefer those voices (DeCaspar, 1984, 1986).

Using painstaking observation of films of mother-infant interaction, Beebe (1982) has shown that the synchronization is a mutual one. It is not simply a matter of the child adjusting to the mother's rhythm but of the pair learning to respond to each other. Mother-child interaction is an elaborate multichanneled process that fully involves both participants. Movements by either that cause responses when correctly timed will disrupt the pattern when they are done out of order. Rather like dancers, each correct step continues the dance, whereas a step at the wrong time breaks the rhythm. As Beebe points out, the hallmark of the rhythmic integration of mother and infant behavior is the obvious mutual pleasure derived from the process.

Stern (1982) has studied not only the regularities of mother-infant interaction but the mechanism by which transition points occur. The ability of the mother to speed up or slow down rhythms is particularly important in attracting the infant's attention. What is critical is her ability to vary the tempo of speech to emphasize emotional expression. As in musical performance, interaction is a balance between regularity and variation.

The infant's ability to synchronize to individuals in the environment is critical not only to establish communication patterns but to organize brain development. The nervous system of the infant involves a diffuse group of independent cycles that require an external patterning. It has been suggested that as anatomic organization is proceeding and nerve cells are myelinated and synapses formed, so the temporal pattern arises as these internal cycles coordinate. Because they change at rates that are independent of one another, these relationships frequently need adjustment. Consequently a consistent and powerful external rhythmic message is essential for the development of the infant brain (Fogel, 1987). Acquiring intonational and contextual abilities in speech occurs simultaneously with acquiring vocabulary and grammar in childhood (Scheflen, 1974). Fernald (1984) has shown that the dialogues between mother and child allow the child to learn not only to speak but to relate.

The rhythms of interaction and language are personal as well as universal. They become part of each person's style of expression. Tannen suggests that conversational "style is not a sophisticated skill learned late or superimposed on previously acquired linguistic forms. Rather, it is learned as an integral part of linguistic knowledge" (1984, p. 10). Children in different cultures learn language within their social context and recognize the relation between changes in language style and changes in social role at an early age (Scheflen, 1974). There is growing evidence that learning a second language also proceeds most easily when it is associated with the appropriate patterns of gesture and intonation within a specific social context (Kendon, 1984). In this way, style of conversation can be seen as the social dimension of language. "Children learn social knowledge simultaneously with language structure. . . . They simultaneously learn what to say, how to say it, and how to feel about it, which is entailed inevitably in the way to say it" (Tannen, 1984, p. 10).

Disruptions of Rhythms

Failure to achieve synchronization, for whatever reason, can be a potent source of emotional disturbance (Bowlby, 1969) and may be a particularly sensitive biological measure of stress (Chapple, 1979). These stresses, when they last long enough, can disrupt the other rhythms of the system and lead to an internal desynchronization. This implies a general loss of adaptability and coherence in the loss of temporal structure.

Observed disturbances in the balance between various rhythms reflect existing psychopathology. Individuals may show asynchrony between their various channels (Condon, 1982) or in their interactions with others (Rosenberg, 1979). Condon reports examples of asynchronies in autistic and dyslexic children as well as schizophrenic adults (1982). Autistic children, however, show evidence of a total body synchrony to minimal auditory cues (Condon, 1982), physical responses that are similar to the primitive reflexes found in normal newborn infants. Schizophrenic patients display an inability to synchronize that correlates with the severity of their illness (Steimer-Krause, 1990). Whereas the structural and syntactical organization of their speech can be disrupted, leading to bizarre, confusing communications, so too can their face-to-face interactions with others be out of synchrony, resulting in what appears to be eccentric or bizarre interpersonal behavior and emotional and social isolation (Rosenberg, 1979).

Therapeutic Rhythms

In the nonhypnotic clinical setting, physicians appear to synchronize their speech and gestures to those of their patients, according to Street and Buller (1988). In their study, the patient's sex, education, or previous contact with the doctor had relatively little effect on the degree of physician accommodation. They also found a strong positive correlation between patients' overall ratings of satisfaction with their health care and the individual physician's ability to respond nonverbally (1987).

Studies of psychotherapy showed increased rapport when the therapist made interventions that did not interfere with the tempo or content of the patient's narrative (Chapple, 1982). Davis (1982, 1984) showed that not only did different gestural patterns indicate specific themes in therapy, but these themes emerged at the same time during the course of the therapeutic hour. Moreover, the gestures became more elaborate and more detailed as the rapport developed over time. This particular "dance" between the therapist and patient was characterized by an elaborate confrontation in which the therapist could be seen to "stay with" the patient following her postural shifts and actions until the interpretation was confirmed (Davis, 1984).

The notion that adoption of identical or similar postures (posture mirroring) is a nonverbal indicator of increased rapport between individuals has been proposed by Scheflen (1973). Imitation is generally understood as a means for achieving empathy into another's internal world or for sharing a similar experience. It would appear that posture mirroring and adopting the breathing rate or voice tone of another in conversation are additional features used in obtaining a synchrony complementing the motor and verbal interplay of turn taking. Psychotherapists, such as Fromm-Reichman (1950), have suggested that such changes are important in achieving clinical rapport. As with adoption of similar facial expressions, sharing postures may contribute to shared emotional experiences.

Dabbs (1969) reported that subjects identified more with the experimenter when the interaction involved their behavior being mimicked than when it did not. Charney (1966) reported a significant association between the degree of mirroring in upper body postures and positive speech content during psychotherapy.

LaFrance (1982) suggested that posture mirroring not only may be reflective of increased rapport but may actually be instrumental in achieving it. In a series of studies, she showed that posture mirroring is significantly related to increased rapport in small groups. Furthermore, in analyzing the sequencing of events, LaFrance reported that the mirroring appears to precede the increase in rapport. This investigator suggested that the mirroring of body positions may be a special form of the interactional synchrony that occurs when people move with the same rhythm. She also suggested that the value of posture mirroring seems to be strongest in the early phases of the group's functioning. The correlation between posture mirroring and rapport decreased from week to week. It is likely that in a new social context, greater emphasis on synchronization is necessary to initiate interaction, but with time the cues can be used in a much more flexible and individual way.

Waxer has reviewed the evidence for the complex nature of total communication:

Mehrabrian and Ferris (1967) presented the argument that in the communication of attitude, total information conveyed was a function of verbal, paralinguistic and nonverbal components in the ratio of 7% verbal, 38% vocal and 55% facial. Waxer (1981) was curious to see if the same proportions held in the instance of emotional communication. In addition, the issue of channel combination was examined to see whether such combinations (e.g., audio-visual) acted synergistically to yield greater communication accuracy. In this study, raters evaluated the anxiety levels of 20 psychiatric patients under 6 different channel conditions, full audio-visual, visual, full audio, patient audio-visual (with therapist's input deleted), patient audio and patient transcript. When single channels of communication were examined, results in this study indicated that nonverbal cues were both more potent and accurate than content or paralinguistic cues in a manner almost identical to the proportions reported by Mehrabrian and Ferris. When channel combinations were examined, it was found that in no instance did these combinations act synergistically to yield greater accuracy. In one instance (i.e., combined nonverbal and paralinguistic cues) channel combination actually generated poorer results than those obtained for nonverbal cues alone. This study paralleled findings supported by Strahan, Zytowski (1976) reporting the notion that "the whole . . . may sometimes be less than one of its parts." (Waxer, 1984, p. 232)

It is clear that no single channel is more important than the others. Synchrony is typically maintained by a combination of gesture, facial expression, posture, the rate of speech, and prosody, and although individuals do not usually pay conscious attention to these features, their ratings of a sense of involvement in the conversation are strongly correlated with them (Coker, 1987). The ability to utilize these features either consciously or unconsciously is critical for the development of rapport.

Rhythmic interaction, then, appears to be a critical if complex element of psychotherapy. Of course, psychotherapy is but one culturally defined form of personal and social healing. There are other rhythmic processes that are more widely used by humans to achieve synchrony and repair.

MUSIC, SOCIAL RHYTHM, AND TRANCE

There is no characteristic single rhythm for interactions. We can adjust our rhythms according to circumstance and pattern the responses of others. Speech and behavior are rhythmic, but variations in rate or intensity are equally important in expressing the message and maintaining the synchrony. Communication shares the rhythmic variety of music. "So the rhythms become musical, not in the strict and literal sense always, but in spacing individuals in places relative to one another and in combining their movements in space with the responses or nonresponses as they act as the oscillators require. The language of music utilizes the infinite variations which the rhythm timing provides, shifting the volume to accentuate the melodic contrasts mediated by pitch changes" (Chapple, 1982, p. 48).

Music is a cultural elaboration of a primary and personal cerebral structure that is as fundamental to human awareness as is language (Clynes, 1986). As with language, music involves the coordination of both hemispheres with fundamental and largely unconscious processes being mediated by the right hemisphere and culturally elaborated musical "literacy" being mediated by the left (Geschwind, 1987). As Suhor (1986) suggests, music improvisation and language performance are parallel competencies. Throughout human cultural history, music has been an integral part of work, child rearing, and social activity (Stern, 1982).

The microstructure that underlies our emotional expression and forms the basis for our synchronization of interactional rhythms is the same process that allows us both to produce and to appreciate music (Clynes, 1986). This microstructure is responsive to extremely subtle differences in rhythm and tone, and our ability to manipulate these small differences is the reason we can produce highly sophisticated musical productions (Longuet-Higgins, 1979). Manfred Clynes has shown that this microstructure can function as a type of fingerprint (1984). Each composer has a different characteristic microstructural pulse, and musicians approach sound similarly. Thus, like a conversation, a performance of a piece of music is indeed an active collaboration and synchronization of composer and performer.

The measurable acoustic qualities of sound relate to the psychological experience of these qualities in a complex way (Deutsch, 1982; Howell, 1985; Dowling, 1986). Each of these elements can interact in an ongoing way to color the experience. At the same time, the subjective state of the listener provides a structure of expectation and understanding. Thus, the nervous system can make many fine discriminations among each of the separate aspects of prosody, and it is also capable of synthesizing them into a personal and subjective experience.

There also appears to be a time interval of the order of a few seconds over which perceptual events (such as the contents of a musical phrase) tend to be integrated into what William James called the "psychological present." Composers manipulate steadiness of tempo and the constancy of other rhythmic factors to keep a piece within the real-time framework of the world outside or by creating temporal ambiguity, dissociate time within the piece from time in the world. (Dowling, 1986, p. 201)

The temporal organization of music relates to a physiologic internal sense of time. In order to be satisfying, the sound must be both predictable, meeting the framework of expectations, and novel, providing slight differences from those expectations. The slight violation of expectancies produces a state of arousal and a cognitive push to resolve the incompleteness.

The violation of (largely unconscious) expectancy brings about nonspecific arousal, which in turn triggers a search for an interpretation of the arousing event. That search provides the content of the emotional experience—the musical meaning. In our discussion of emotion and meaning, we reviewed evidence that listeners agree on the emotional meanings of pieces of music in styles with which they are familiar. Indeed, they were able to agree on very subtle shades of meaning when provided with sufficient context. (Dowling, 1986, p. 224)

In his studies of music from over four hundred cultures, Lomax (1982) found structural musical features characteristic to each culture that relate to specific behavioral patterns. The length of phrases used correlate with the regularity of the meter. Short phrases are associated with a more regular meter, whereas the longer phrases are found in cultures with a more irregular meter. It also appears that these rhythms relate to the structure of the society: agricultural societies have highly rhythmic music and dance, whereas cultures that use other forms of food gathering tend toward more individual variation.

Lomax postulates that meter arises from the different patterns of coordinating the rhythms between the right and left side of the body. The rhythm of breathing changes as the ratio of movements from side to side changes. In addition, more complicated rhythms are produced when there is alternation not only between left and right but between upper limb and lower limb. Thus, derivatives of movement, music, and dance have long been intrinsic parts of social cohesion. Every form of communal enterprise has a particular rhythm and song. Each society associates particular tasks with sounds that help to coordinate action and provide a sense of community. The work song and the lullaby are as universal a part of human rhythmic experience as the rising and setting of the sun.

These features emphasize the social role of rhythmic and metrical style in music. Rhythm is a way in which groups both define themselves and synchronize their behavior. The rhythmic aspect of music not only expresses a worldview but allows all individuals to experience it both within themselves and in connection with other people. Cultures with simple rhythmic patterns in music are the societies that are the most cohesive and closely bound.

Smaller "folk" groups tend to have more predictable patterns with simple rhythms and a great deal of repetition. As cultures grow in size, they also grow in complexity. Repetition remains, but it becomes far more elaborate. As the number of voices increases, the pattern interweaves in polyphonic form. Again and again, the basic building blocks are reiterated to produce a world of sound that exists as a scaffolding for the building of a richer world of human creation. Rhythm, repetition, and tempo all begin to be used as independent variables, the elements of an architecture of sound.

Our musical ability emerges from our evolutionary development of face-to-face communication. Rhythmic speed and precision form the basis for the brain's astonishing skill at appreciating and producing music (Clynes, 1984). Music is, in a real way, as much a manifestation of this prowess as is our ability to mutually synchronize states of consciousness (Gilligan, 1987). The neurobiology of hypnosis overlaps with the neurobiology of music. This is underlined by anthropological evidence that suggests an intimate linking of music and trance in a wide variety of cultures (Rouget, 1985).

Throughout the world, the trance state is associated with dance and music, but the relationship is not a simple one. The types of dance and music vary markedly from culture to culture, as does their role (Rouget, 1985). Music is used variously to induce, deepen, or end trance. As Rouget has shown convincingly, it is not simply a question of some music being "hypnotic"; rather, variations in rhythm and sound have been assigned a particular meaning by the people who use them.

Music will ultimately appear as the principal means of manipulating the trance state, but by "socializing" much more than by triggering it. This process of socialization inevitably varies from one society to another, and it takes place in very different ways according to the systems of representations—or, if one prefers, the ideological systems—within which trance occurs. In each case a different logic determines the relationship between trance and music. Rouget, 1985, p. xviii)

Music serves to synchronize and socialize. It derives from the rhythm of everyday life, and in that sense, it is to our interactional rhythms what poetry is to our everyday conversation: a more heightened and stylized form of the daily pattern. Our ability to produce that rhythm occurs at the interface between the psychological and the physiologic. It bespeaks not a separation between mind and body but their fundamental connection in the brain.

The music also "means" something at a physiologic level. Rouget (1985) has found in his worldwide study of the relationship between trance and music that the music invariably demonstrates two characteristics. The first is a heavily patterned and rhythmic structure that unites the various phases. The second is the presence of abrupt breaks or changes of rhythm that balance against the overall structure. These features tie the use of music in trance to the hypnotic use of words by the great oral poet.

Above all, music, song, and dance are physical. By participating in the music, each individual is physically connected with the trance and with the experience of the rest of the community. "It is both the subject's own singing and dancing that lead him to trance" (Rouget, 1985, p. 317). Thus, trance is both deeply personal and quintessentially social at the same time. "This means that the role of the music is much less to produce the trance than to create conditions favorable to its onset, to regularize its form, and to ensure that instead of being a merely individual, unpredictable, and uncontrollable behavioral phenomenon, it becomes, on the contrary, predictable, controlled, and at the service of the group" (Rouget, 1985, p. 320).

Highly hypnotizable subjects report more absorption in music than do subjects with less hypnotic ability, says Snodgrass (1989). All subjects in this study reported more imagery with music that stimulated imaginative processes, but the highly hypnotizable subjects were particularly reactive. Thus the effect was influenced both by individual ability and by the nature of the music itself.

The brain is highly sensitive to music. In another study, the responses to music of trained and untrained subjects showed considerable differences, as did those of men and women; and the nature of the music itself produced further differences. A significant component was the degree of attention required by a musical task (Petsche, 1988). As we shall see in a later chapter, the characteristic changes in brain activity in the alpha, beta, and theta range are similar to those found in hypnotic subjects while in trance.

HYPNOTIC RHYTHM

Our auditory processes are complex, active, and varied. Sound waves are translated into neural impulses, but in the process, they are also translated into personal experiences. Rather than simply reproducing a sound, the brain actively constructs a pattern that is largely guided by expectations of what the sound ought to be like and what it means. Hearing is not simply the reception of a message; it is a process that T. S. Eliot described as "auditory imagination." Meaning, like rhythm, must be shared by speaker and listener. That sharing is a form of poetic communication that relates to the original source of the word *prosody:* "The Greek *prosoidia* had two meanings: 'a song sung to or accompanied by music; the tone or accent of a syllable' . . . what, in the broadest sense, we understand as the music of poetry; and, in a narrower sense, as the specific organization of the syllables, that is, the meter" (Gross, 1979, p. 8).

Most poetry in English is blank verse (unrhymed iambic pentameter)—five feet of alternating stressed and unstressed syllables. It is the style of poetry that is closest to conversational English and represents a balance between the formalism of verse and the spontaneity of the spoken word. In order to coordinate breathing with speaking and listening, the segments of speech must be sculpted to fit the available breath patterns. Consequently, the production of speech has an inherent rhythm linked to other physiologic patterns. These patterns form part of the expectation of the listener (which, as we shall see, is an important hypnotic induction technique). As with music, the rhythm of poetry can be used to link everyone within range of the spoken word in a synchronized physiologic pattern. It is the dramatic accentuation of rhythm that primarily distinguishes poetry from other forms of verbal expression. Poetry and song form the transition between music and conversation, but the differences are quantitative rather than qualitative.

Meter is what results when the natural rhythmical movements of colloquial speech are heightened, organized, and regulated so that pattern—which means repetition—emerges from the relative phonetic haphazard of ordinary utterance. Because it inhabits the physical form of the words themselves, meter is the most fundamental technique of order available to the poet. . . .

The pleasure which universally results from foot tapping and musical time-beating does suggest that the pleasures of meter are essentially physical and as intimately connected with the rhythmic quality of our total experience as the similarly alternating and recurrent phenomena of breathing, walking, or love-making. (Fussell, 1979, pp. 4–5)

Rhythm is a means by which the listener can be drawn into the words of the speaker, participating in the immediate contact and thus joining the subjective experience and point of view of the speaker. A "moving" argument may be exactly that. By linking the synchrony of body and ideas, parallel physiologic changes begin to occur. The original rhythm of all music is the heartbeat (before the invention of the metronome, musicians used the resting heartbeat as a baseline). Conversational synchrony, absorbing narrative, and a gradual unfolding of emotional experiences are reflected in physiologic, emotional, and cognitive changes. William Butler Yeats describes the function of meter as being to "lull the mind into a waking trance." I. A. Richards says, "Many of the most characteristic symptoms of incipient hypnosis are present in a slight degree. Among these, susceptibility and vivacity of emotion, suggestibility, limitations of the field of attention, marked differences in the incidence of belief—feelings closely analogous to those which alcohol and nitrous oxide can induce—and some degree of hyperaesthesia (increased power of discriminating sensations) may be noted" (1979, p. 75).

The purpose of a heightened rhythm in the spoken word is to produce what W. H. Auden described as "memorable speech." As we remember the rhythm, we remember the words. Content can be embedded in human memory more powerfully when it is aided by a repeated rhythm. In a world without writing, the memorable speech of poetic rhythm provided the only available way of recording and maintaining information over time by ensuring ease of transmission from one individual to another. "'Expectancy must be thought of as a very complex tide of neural settings . . . [a] texture of expectations, satisfactions, disappointments, surprisals.' Meter, on the other hand, focuses our response; through it we become 'patterned ourselves'" (Richards, 1979, p. 68).

But none of this is absolute. Spoken language, like other features of human behavior, follows no fixed and predictable pattern. Possessing the flexibility to compromise between competing needs is the great hallmark of human social behavior in general and speech in particular. The finished product is usually a blend of all the features. Too little rhythm, and speech is unintelligible; a too regular rhythm becomes monotonous and becalms the listener.

In fact, in spoken language rules are made to be broken. Once a certain rhythm sets up an expectation in the listener, powerful effects can be produced by slight variations. In the same way that variations on a theme of music can build the emotional intensity of the experience, a gradual accumulation of minor differences catches the listener up in a combination of expectation and surprise, anticipation and novelty. The most powerful effects of poetry are achieved not by a relentlessly perfect rhythm but, rather, by subtle and unexpected reversals that provide a much more powerful sense of psychological completion than simple, rigid symmetry. Shakespeare does this continually, setting up a rhythm and then fitting in an unexpected variation (Barton, 1984). The variation sets up an internal rhythm reminding us of what has been said before, a kind of meta dialogue (or in the terms of Ericksonian hypnotherapy, "an interspersed suggestion"). It is the rhythm of language, the poetry of everyday words, that synchronizes human imagination (Friedrich, 1979).

Tannen (1984) emphasizes the frequency of what we think of as poetic devices in normal conversation. While the conversation is flowing, the speakers in turn tend to echo the rhythm and rhyme of the previous speaker. Intonational patterns are usually shared between two people in a conversation. One person sets up an intonational pattern, and the reply completes the rhythm. A simple question-and-answer pair is a good example. This serves to remind us that poetry and music both originate in the rhythms of the spoken word; they are not isolated entities. Both are simply a heightening and emphasis of the features that are normally used in conversation to facilitate the flow.

In the same way, storytelling (also known as narrative strategy) shows the same basic elements of conversation shared between two or more people. Coming from these common roots, storytelling, poetry, and music were the first media used to enhance cultural transmission and cultural growth.

Conversation, like epic poetic performance, derives its impact from processes of identification between audience and speaker, to similar ends. In other words, face to face conversation . . . seeks primarily to move an audience by means of involvement, as opposed to (typically) expository prose (in Havelock's terms, literacy), which seeks to convince an audience while maintaining distance between speaker/writer and audience. (Tannen, 1984, p. 153)

The ability to communicate is based on the capacity to orient to social cues and to remain in rhythm with them. This orientation involves a process of selective attention to the important features of the context (Ziller, 1988). It is focused by the frame provided by nonverbal communication as well as by preexisting cognitive schemata. In order to be sustained, it must be synchronized to both the ongoing rhythm of the brain and the concurrent rhythm of the interaction.

Communication is active, and an interaction such as hypnosis involves the skill of everyone involved. Otherwise the creation of a frame by the nonverbal communication cannot occur. The ability to establish and maintain a rhythm (as demonstrated by musical absorption or visually by the Necker cube reversals) is associated with hypnotic ability. Our ability to attend to and produce nonverbal communication becomes rhythm, and that rhythm sustains context, orientation, attention, and meaning. The rhythm that maintains the interaction is the rhythm that maintains the trance state. The various forms of hypnosis, including self-hypnosis, are based on the rhythm that maintains interpersonal interaction. As the brain is a social organ, we are social, even when we are alone.

4 THE SPOKEN WORLD

It is the more poetic levels and processes of language, however defined, that massively model, constrain, trigger, and otherwise affect the individual imagination.

Paul Friedrich, 1979

Cultural development exploited humankind's unprecedented capacity for face-to-face communication. Oral cultures, based solely on the spoken word, flourished long before the development of literacy. These cultures depended on the highly sophisticated verbal skills of oral poets to store and transmit knowledge. Oral poets in turn relied on vivid imagery, complex verbal patterns, and the repetition of well-loved stories that dealt directly with basic everyday concerns to produce their entrancing effects. This capacity to absorb attention and share a personal construction based on the spoken word is related to the contemporary uses of hypnotherapy.

A FIELD TRIP TO UZBEKISTAN

In 1931, Alexander Luria, a neuropsychologist, left Moscow for an extensive period of fieldwork in Uzbekistan. The Soviet Union was undergoing a phase of "radical restructuring" (Luria, 1976, p. v), and Luria decided to take the opportunity to study the effects of the "modernization program" among the Uzbekis, far away from politically tumultuous Moscow. The trip gave him the opportunity to observe the impact of learning to read and write on a well-established society.

Luria defined some of the basic differences in cognitive style between literate and oral cultures. Apart from its significance to cognitive psychology, his work is a wonderful example of the collisions of cultures. Samples of the interactions between Luria's team of urban psychologists and the villagers are full of a rich offbeat humor with a Zen-like quality of pervasive misunderstanding. But as the psychologists attempted to understand the thought processes of the natives, their subjects worked equally hard to unravel the hidden meanings behind the apparently idiotic questions. They automatically assumed there was some sort of pattern or game that these queries were supposed to initiate. Once they felt they had caught on they played it with great gusto.

The following syllogism is presented: "There are no camels in Germany. The city of B. is in Germany. Are there camels there or not?"
    Subject repeats syllogism exactly.
    "So, are there camels in Germany?"
    "I don't know, I've never seen German villages."
    The syllogism is repeated.
    "Probably there are camels there."
    "Repeat what I said."
    "There are no camels in Germany, are there camels in B. or not? So probably there are. If it's a large city, there should be camels there."
    "But what do my words suggest?"
    "Probably there are. Since there are large cities, there should be camels."
    "But if there aren't any in all of Germany?"
    "If it's a large city, there will be Kazakhs or Kirghiz there."
    "But I'm saying that there are no camels in Germany, and this city is in Germany."
    "If this village is in a large city, there is probably no room for camels." (Luria, 1976, p. 112)

Members of a flourishing and prosperous community, the villagers were intelligent, lively, and successful. But attempts to demonstrate these qualities using standard intelligence tests quickly ran up against a brick wall. Luria's subjects saw things that belonged to their world, not abstract geometrical figures. A circle would be identified as a wheel if placed next to a picture of a horse, but became the sun if placed next to a crescent. They focused on context and answered questions on the basis of their own personal experience or not at all. When presented with the syllogism "In the Far North, where there is snow, all bears are white.

Novaya Zemlya is in the Far North. What color are bears there?" the most common answer was "I don't know, I've never been there" (p. 107).

Not only were abstraction and generalization not used; they were seen as breaking up the unity of context demands. The villagers saw connections between sets of objects not as members of independent classes but as things that could be connected for a particular task. They had no place for definitions that did not relate to an immediate real-life situation. Objects, facts, and conceptual or logical processes that did not serve this orientation were of no interest—they were literally non-sense. For example, the request to identify which of four objects—hammer, saw, log, and hatchet—did not belong in the group produced the following exchange:

"They're all alike. I think all of them have to be there. See, if you're going to saw, you need a saw, and if you have to split something you need a hatchet. So they're all needed here."

We tried to explain the task by another, simpler example.

"Look, here you have three adults and one child. Now clearly the child doesn't belong in this group."

"Oh, but the boy must stay with the others! All three of them are working, you see, and if they have to keep running out to fetch things, they'll never get the job done, but the boy can do the running for them. . . . The boy will learn; that'll be better, then they'll all be able to work well together." (p. 55)

Our use of language is central to who we are as a species, but the relationship is a dynamic one. Newer innovations—writing, the printing press, the electronic media—all serve to extend and elaborate this process. As McLuhan (1969) has pointed out, the various technologies of communication exert a significant influence over the content of communication and, by extension, over our modes of thinking. The very way in which experience is represented is altered; there is a change in what McLuhan called "the ratio of the senses." In the case of literacy, this meant a significant shift toward a visual representation of language and away from the auditory world.

Sight presents surfaces (it is keyed to reflected light; light coming directly from its source, such as fire, an electric lamp, the sun, rather dazzles and blinds us). . . .

Sound, on the other hand, reveals the interior without the necessity of physical invasion. Thus we tap a wall to discover where it is hollow inside, or we ring a silver-colored coin to discover whether it is perhaps lead inside. To discover such things by sight, we should have to open what we examine, making the inside the outside, destroying its interiority as such. Sound reveals interiors because its nature is determined by interior relationships. The sound of a violin is determined by the interior structure of its strings, of its bridge, and of the wood in its soundboard, by the shape of the interior cavity in the body of the violin, and other interior conditions. (Ong, 1977, p. 140)

The transition to literacy also involves a shift of knowledge from personal awareness to objective record. In a literate culture, information can be stored permanently, independent of human minds. Facts can be recorded and written down "in black and white." But though this cultural transition occurred over the past fifteen hundred years (which is nearly instantaneous in evolutionary terms), our brains continue to retain their capacity to create a world that depends on oral face-to-face communication.

To suppose that after a million years, vision employed on a physical artifact—a piece of writing—could suddenly replace the biologically programmed habit of responding to acoustic messages, that is, that reading could replace hearing, automatically, and easily, without profound and artificial adjustments of the human organism, is to fly in the face of the evolutionary lesson.
. . . An act of vision was offered in place of an act of hearing as the means of communication, and as the means of storing communication. The adjustment that it caused was in part social, but the major effect was felt in the mind and the way the mind thinks as it speaks. (Havelock, 1986, pp. 99–100)

Embedded as we are in a culture that depends on the written word, it is difficult for us to recognize the influence of literacy on our consciousness. We describe individuals who do not use the alphabet as being "illiterate," the very word suggesting that there is something intrinsically defective about depending solely on the spoken word (Ong, 1982). But comparative studies reveal to us complex and highly successful cultures that flourished before the advent of the written word (Havelock, 1982; Ong, 1982; Logan, 1986). Because nothing could be written down, these cultures depended on what could be retained in living human memory. For this, they relied on poets who as artisans of words were as valued for their technical skills as the blacksmith or potter. The original Greek term for the oral poet is *rhapsodizer* (from which we get our word *rhapsody*), from a root that means "to stitch together." Oral poets stitched together words and sounds to create meaning. They were the living heritage of the culture, combining in one individual entertainer, physician, public library, and court of justice. The oral poet was expected to provide tales that would guide both the individual and the group in any endeavor. To do this, their performance had to be "entrancing"—deeply relevant and totally memorable.

By way of illustration, Homer's *Iliad* existed as an oral epic long before it was written down. As well as being an engrossing tale, the poem gives step-by-step instructions for many important functions: how a ship should be launched, how a dispute should be settled, how men and women can be expected to behave (Havelock, 1982).

Havelock described the impact of literacy on thinking in ancient Greece. In *Preface to Plato* (1963), he describes the transition from the predominantly oral world of Homer to the literate world of Plato. Specifically, Plato's rejection of poetry in *The Republic* was a signal of a shift to a new type of society that was based on objective, analytic, and individual standards. This marked a great departure from the subjective, synthetic, and communal world of the oral poets.

Although we are accustomed to think of poetry as being a combination of rhythm and meaning, we are generally unaccustomed to the idea of its having any real importance. In Western twentieth-century culture, poetry is typically seen as a minor art form with some sort of vague aesthetic contribution to make. In this light, Plato's recommendation in *The Republic* that the first order of business in establishing a utopian state is to eliminate the poets does not sound to us like the most urgent of priorities. In fact, Plato was describing the impact of the greatest cultural change in humankind's story: the invention of literacy (Havelock, 1963).

LITERACY

The earliest writing systems were visually based, more or less idealized drawings of the objects they stood for. Cuneiform and hieroglyphics and other types of pictograms all represent images of the thing itself. The Semitic alphabet, by contrast, was the culmination of a gradual transition toward a representation of the sound of words. Moving from a visual portrayal of objects to a phonetic (sound-based) writing that represented language provided another level of abstraction, a much more efficient and flexible means of communication. But the system also remained complex and ambiguous (Logan, 1986).

The true revolution occurred with the Greek modification that added vowels to the system: a simple method for recording any of the sounds of the spoken word. The earliest example of Greek writing dates from around 700 B.C. The earliest coherent text (written on a wall) dates from about 450 B.C. (Havelock, 1982). The Greek system provided a tool that could reliably reproduce all of the sounds of spoken language in a way that was unambiguous. Simultaneously it provided a means of storage that was infinitely more efficient, flexible, and lasting than anything available to a purely oral culture.

The transition from orality to literacy cannot be immediate but requires a gradual development of reading skills throughout the population (Ong, 1982). It is not sufficient to have writers; the literate society also requires a minimum number of readers. Until the invention of the printing press, books were intended to be read aloud, usually by a professional reader to an illiterate audience. Even an individual reading to himself recited aloud what he read. Reading without moving one's lips was so unusual that it was invariably commented upon by historians (Clanchy, 1979).

For most of the history of Western civilization, the two traditions have coexisted. The oral style continues to be a part of the way we live our lives day by day. Literacy has only recently become a widespread phenomenon. At the same time, until recently, only literacy provided a record. When literacy becomes widespread, oral traditions simply disappear. It is only with the advent of modern recording technology that the concept of "oral history" as an ongoing record has been possible.

Literacy does change cognitive processes. The development of literacy increases the acoustic ability of readers to distinguish between phonemes and to comprehend language under difficult listening conditions, as compared to nonreaders (Morais, 1987). Both children and adults, as they acquire the ability to read, develop a parallel ability to distinguish between what is said and what is meant (Olson, 1987). In other words, they are able to see meaning as something that exists independently of communication and that must be interpreted.

The transition from orality to literacy was a crisis in the true sense of the word: a turning point after which the perceptions, thinking, and behavior of humanity were changed forever. Literacy transformed memory and, with memory, awareness. Facts and events could be recorded and retained independently of ongoing thought. This separation of thoughts and thinkers, of memory and remembering, provided the scope for a new form of objectivity. A distinctive "correct" version of a story was available; an argument could be analyzed in detail and contrasted immediately with earlier or later versions.

Literacy creates a system of language in which words are independent of people. By virtue of being written down, words become things. "Information" becomes material that can be enumerated, weighed, and broken down into composite parts. Literacy results in a more static, canonical use of language in which spelling, grammar, and syntax are formalized in an objective way. In this sense, literacy is truly a tool, an extension of ourselves that gives us greater flexibility.

The tools for objectivity and analysis resulted in the creation of new disciplines: literature, philosophy, science, and mathematics. These changes pervaded every level of society even while a majority of humankind remained illiterate. Not only thought, but nature and even time could be taken apart and examined. History arose beside myth, justice and ethics beside traditional tribal codes, and science beside technical skills. By changing the ways in which language was used, changes in thinking occurred—the most dramatic example of how our technical abilities can change the environment in which we live.

Literacy also changes the social role of memory. Literacy is a form of artificial memory, allowing us to retain a great deal more while freeing up psychological resources for other tasks. Freed from the burden of memorization and provided with texts that can be studied at leisure, we can develop new cognitive skills. Abstraction and analysis lead to a style of thinking that is objective—no longer based in a particular individual and freed from the constraints of immediate context. The transition to print is typified by the slow development of what McLuhan (1969) described as "linear thinking." The flow of sound can be stopped and transformed into an object that can be examined critically.

ORAL CULTURE

Orality is not simply an absence of literacy but a style in its own right. This style reflects the nature of composition in an oral culture as well as the state of mind and of society that is the backdrop for that style (Ong, 1982). The spoken word is immediate, transitory, and inherently interpersonal. Its goal is not the transmission of information but the creation of a shared experience. The syntax of the spoken culture is fluid and heuristic. It is closely tied to the physical rhythms of the body and is judged not for "correctness" but for the impact it has on the listener.

As Ong has pointed out, oral cultures are in essence profoundly conservative, intent upon preserving the tradition that is handed down from person to person (1982). Retaining all knowledge in living memory severely limits personal originality and encourages consensus. The basis of oral communication is to repeat what is already known. It relies heavily on the shared heritage, and it advances only by elaborating on the consensual information. By its drawing on a standard group of known and universally understood experiences in day-to-day life, the flow of ideas is maintained. By moving from one familiar experience to another, the individuals are tied more strongly together.

ORAL POETRY

In the oral world, poetry was the principal vehicle of learning. It was the only effective system by which information could be retained, organized, and transmitted to others. This emphasis on memorization had an effect on the style of communication. The more memorable knowledge could be made, the greater the likelihood of it being retained (Ong, 1982). Well-known stories, colorfully and rhythmically told, and with layers of rich and repetitive language, produced the closest equivalent to a permanent record available in the absence of convenient writing. The oral poet was a performer serving a living community tradition.

The oral Greek epic poet was very much part of the workaday world, simultaneously entertainer, chronicler and historian, recorder of genealogies and deeds, cheer leader, ethician, philosopher, and schoolmaster. . . . Not only was the epic poet involved in real-life concerns, but real-life concerns were akin to epic. Ordinary talk and practical thought processes consisted largely of the same proverbs, exempla, epithets, and formulas of all sorts which the epic poet or narrator stitched into his more elaborate and exquisite art forms in a somewhat variant language. (Ong, 1977, p. 278)

The work of the oral poets was a balance between remembrance and improvisation. Tales were handed down from living memory to living memory, with each individual modifying and elaborating according to current needs. The style of the oral poets was designed to arrest the attention, allow for easy sharing and remembering, and encourage active and personal participation.

In the 1920s, Milman Parry was the first to recognize the complexity of composition without writing. He pointed out the distinctive features in the *Iliad* that suggest it was composed by oral methods and only much later written down (Parry, 1971). Albert Lord came to similar conclusions in his studies of living Yugoslavian oral poets (1960). Oral poetry involved not a poet in our sense of the word but a performer who could weave words together in the style of a modern jazz improvisation.

In a primary oral culture, to solve effectively the problem of retaining and retrieving carefully articulated thought, you have to do your thinking in mnemonic patterns, shaped for ready oral recurrence. Your thought must come into being in heavily rhythmic, balanced patterns, in repetitions or antitheses, in alliterations and assonances, in epithetic and other formulary expressions, in standard thematic settings, . . . in proverbs which are constantly heard by everyone so that they come to mind readily and which themselves are patterned for retention and ready recall, or in other mnemonic form. Serious thought is intertwined with memory systems. Mnemonic needs determine even syntax. (Ong, 1982, p. 34)

Memorization in an oral culture is quite unlike what we, as literates, are used to. There can be no verbatim memorization as there was no original text to memorize to begin with. Each repetition of a story in an oral culture reproduces only one-half to two-thirds of the previous telling (Lord, 1960; Ong, 1982). (Our standards are quite different. Imagine a performance of *Hamlet* that is only 50 percent verbatim.) What the oral poet memorizes is not a text but a certain number of themes and a style, a certain number of implicit linguistic patterns. Each work is the combination of a once-only performance and an accumulation of the work of generations. The difference in performance is analogous to the difference between a string quartet playing from a musical score and a jazz group improvising on a theme. Both involve "making music," but the intellectual demands of the tasks involved are quite different.

The memory feats of these oral bards are remarkable, but they are unlike those associated with memorization of texts. Literates are usually surprised to learn that the bard planning to retell the story he has heard only once wants often to wait a day or so after he has heard the story before he himself repeats it. In memorizing a written text, postponing its recitation generally weakens recall. An oral poet is not working with texts or in a textual framework. He needs time to let the story sink into his own store of themes and formulas, time to "get with" the story. In recalling and retelling the story, he has not in any literate sense "memorized" its metrical rendition from the version of the other singer—a version long gone forever when the new singer is mulling over the story for his own rendition. The fixed materials in the bard's memory are a float of themes and formulas out of which all stories are variously built.

   Basically the same formulas and themes recurred, but they were stitched together or "rhapsodized" differently in each rendition even by the same poet, depending on audience reaction, the mood of the poet or of the occasion, and other social and psychological factors. (Ong, 1982, pp. 59–60)

The actual oral performance is the product of a great deal of personal and communal know-how coupled with the spontaneity of the live performance. As a result, the performer relies on familiar themes and standardized formulae of composition and language rather than a text repeated verbatim. Behind the use of formulae are clusters of images and ideas that provide a general program for the choice of words and the directions the story will take (Ong, 1982).

The oral culture encourages, rather than a consciously plotted narrative with a developed sense of personal continuity, intense personal involvement in the current situation, focusing on content and external custom, not on an individual viewpoint. The need is for vivid flashbacks, a recollection that draws on well-learned patterns but also adds present concerns. The result is the stuff of memory and is irresistible: it is both what everyone has always known (the well-loved story) and what everyone can see, hear, and feel (the current context).

For the oral culture, meaning is embedded in events. Significance is produced by the interaction between the current situation and active memory, which creates a matrix of similar situations (metaphor); this significance can stem only from a synchronized agreement between speaker and listener. There can be no knowledge that exists independent of the context. "The memories are personal, belonging to every man, woman, and child in the community, yet their content, the language preserved, is communal, something shared by the community as expressing its tradition and its historical identity" (Havelock, 1986, p. 70).

The style of communication and, consequently, the style of thinking in the oral culture depend upon the creation of natural clusters of ideas. Ideas that need to be conveyed and preserved are more easily available if they are part of a sequence of a story. The action of the narrative provides a framework from which information is not only preserved but sequenced so that it can be easily transformed into action. The story is built not with the straightforward narration of one event following another that is the paradigm of the story in a literate culture but with a number of rather loosely connected elements hung together by other, common elements and the verbal skill of the poet. "The epic is built like a Chinese puzzle, boxes within boxes" (Ong, 1982, p. 27).

Thematic echo on a far larger scale is employed everywhere in the Homeric poems: to give one of the more obvious examples, all the conferences between Achilles and his mother recurring throughout the extent of twenty-four books have a family resemblance. Yet within the resemblances, something new also occurs. The echo connection between them assists the memory to pass on easily from the first example to the second and to the third. The sequence registers itself as a sequence. (Havelock, 1986, p. 73)

This redundancy has the paired advantage of both repeating what is already known and providing a connecting pathway so that the flow can be maintained. The continuity that is critical in the spoken word depends on repetition both of rhythm and of meaning. This cumulative process, by a gradual overlapping of ideas, builds a bridge from what is already shared toward new constructions and new understandings. It is "a difference contained within the same." The apparent redundancy is in fact a recursive process, an organic cumulative change.

By its vividness and personal attractiveness as much as by its repetition and elaboration, the style of the language is designed to assist memorization and retention. What connects one oral performance with another is not precision in reproduction of the words but a similarity in pattern. The elements of a story may differ, but the stock phrases and the rhythms used for each element do not vary. The work of the oral poets is replete with antithesis, contrasting separate elements. Holding the two opposites together makes the whole more memorable and maintains a dramatic tension to hold the listener's attention (a device Shakespeare uses effectively—for example, "To be or not to be").

To store and retrieve its knowledge, an oral culture must think in heavily patterned forms facilitating recall—antitheses, epithets, assertive rhythms, proverbs, and other formulas of many sorts. Without these, in a purely oral culture thinking is impossible, for, without writing, unless one's articulated thoughts occur in heavy mnemonic patterns they cannot be retained or retrieved. Oral cultures do not add antitheses, proverbs, and other formulas and mnemonic patterning to their thought: their thought consists in such elements from the start. In a completely oral noetic economy, thought which does not consist in memorable patterns is in effect nonthought: you can normally never get it back again. Not merely poetry, but serious discourse of all sorts in such a culture is thus of necessity formulaic—mythology, jurisprudence (consisting in maxims, proverbs, and other sayings and formulas), administrative directives, and the rest.

. . . Oral epic, as Havelock has shown, is of a piece with the rest of oral noetic activity: the epic poet uses superlatively, in his own fashion and for his own artistic purposes, the kinds of thought processes and concurrent expressions that other formal verbalizers in his culture use for their purposes—administrators, mothers teaching their children, messengers, judges, and witch doctors. (Ong, 1977, pp. 191–192)

The works of the oral poets are highly patterned. Rate and tempo of voice are rhythmic, the choice of words depending on fitting the rhythm of breathing, the rhythm of the poetic line. Stock expressions are used (such as Homer's "wine-dark sea") to maintain both the verbal flow and the expectations of the listener. The stories are of heroes and their deeds, well-known figures in familiar situations, typically told at a time when they resonate with the ongoing situation in the community. The oral poet combines what is uniquely contemporary with something old and familiar—all represented as the living wisdom of the community.

Acoustic rhythm is a component of the reflexes of the central nervous system, a biological force of prime importance to orality. Very early, it induced a secondary effect, by encouraging a supplementary habit of semantic rhythm, or balancing of ideas (or better, balancing of "notions," since "idea" is a literate term). One perceives it in the construction of certain maxims through balance of oppositions (as also in familiar Greek idiom "on the one hand . . . on the other") and again in the responsive balancing of narrative episodes that have a family likeness, forming the thematic "patterns" observed by scholars of Homeric epic. Such compositional "systems" (another literate term) extend the echo device to the ideological level. (Havelock, 1986, p. 72)

In order for this to be so, rhythm must be both physical and pleasurable. The patterns of the spoken word must remain nested in the rhythms of speech, breathing, and gesture. In ancient Greece, *musical* and *unmusical* were used as equivalent terms for *educated* and *uneducated* (Strate, 1986). Music functions as a kind of proto-literacy in assisting memorization among oral peoples. The enhanced rhythm encourages the use of stock phrases just as writing locks the sequence of words in syntax.

A musical accompaniment is only one of the more obvious manifestations of the manner in which, in the oral world, words never exist separate from behavior. The spoken word is accompanied by physical rhythms including facial expression and gesture as well as the movements of the respiratory system and the vocal organs. Words do not exist by themselves in a dictionary waiting to be used but are always related to a particular circumstance. "The oral word, as we have noted, never exists in a simply verbal context, as a written word does. Spoken words are always modifications of a total, existential situation, which always engages the body" (Ong, 1982, p. 67).

The style of an oral culture emphasizes gaining the attention of the listener, holding it, and making what is transmitted easy to assimilate. Bound together by much repetition, a flowing rhythm, and a constant reference to shared experience, the result is a matrix of words, memories, and feelings, each element supporting the others.

Oral poetry is thus an elaboration of everyday language. It is based on the rhythms of conversation but heightened to maximize the impact of rhythmic features, vivid imagery, and the absorbing nature of metaphor. The language is "heightened"—that is, based on but not equivalent to everyday language. Language that is heightened and stereotyped increases both the ease of use for the oral poet and the ease with which it can be understood. Ideas cluster together in an easy and predictable way. Suggestion of one component leads via these connections to elaborating the entire chain. Ideas, experiences, and motivations follow one another in a hypnotic inevitability.

"Once upon a time," we begin. The phrase lifts you out of the real world. Homer's language is "once upon a time" language. It establishes a fictional world. But the fictionalizing in oral epic is directly limited by live interaction, as real conversation is. A real audience controls the narrator's behavior immediately. Students of mine from Ghana and from western Ireland have reported to me what I have read and heard from many other sources: a given story may take a skilled or "professional" storyteller anywhere from ten minutes to an hour and a half, depending on how he finds the audience relates to him on a given occasion. "You always knew ahead of time what he was going to say, but you never knew how long it would take him to say it," my Irish informant reported. The teller reacts directly to audience response. Oral storytelling is a two-way street. (Ong, 1977, p. 69)

HYPNOSIS AND LITERATE CONSCIOUSNESS

The story of literacy is the story of the growth of self-awareness transforming the nature of relationships between people: a record of both a gradually more pervasive literate consciousness and a gradually deepening "interiorization," a clear sense of the self and its separateness from others (Ong, 1986). By promoting this cleavage, literacy restructured the modes of expression and consciousness, providing the tools for a new sense of the individual (although, as Ong points out, this alienation provided the opportunity for a potentially richer reintegration of shared awareness, for a deeper sense of the connections between people and of the ways of relating). Says Havelock, "As language became separated visually from the person who uttered it, so also the person, the source of the language, came into sharper focus and the concept of selfhood was born. The 'self' was a Socratic discovery or, perhaps we should say, an invention of the Socratic vocabulary" (1986, pp. 113–114).

The change in McLuhan's "ratio of the senses" is a change in the modes of consciousness. Each sensory system has a characteristic way of representing and processing the contents of awareness. Visual, auditory, and kinesthetic processing moves along a continuum toward greater personal subjective involvement. The shift from a predominantly oral culture, which occurred with the greater emphasis on visual understanding, emphasized the visual characteristics of objectivity, distance, and the primacy of empirical evidence. Objective sciences rose to the fore replacing personal understanding. The rise of empiricism and the scientific method sprang from the analogy of thinking as vision (Ong, 1977, p. 124).

The development of objective modes of thought with the new visual predominance is also the story of conscious, rational development. Above all, it is the development of the personal voice, the voice of the narrator. The individual creator producing unique and original works becomes possible. Perhaps the most critical of these works is the individual's sense of self, for the personal sense is above all a narration, a continuity that depends on a much more highly developed awareness of individuality than is possible in an oral culture.

At the same time, a greater identification with the conscious mind leads to a deemphasis of unconscious processes. The conscious mind identifies itself with what is explicitly known and what can be put into words. Other types of awareness, other ways of knowing, are not only devalued but actively mistrusted—they are not under conscious control.

This is the other side of the coin. For it is the unconscious, grounded so largely in communally processed experience, that logic undertakes to move away from, if always with only limited success. The emergence of logic sets up a new variance between consciousness and the unconscious. Logic establishes new interior distances within the mind. Attempts to describe in depth what happened to the Western European psyche . . . inevitably find themselves dealing with dissociations—T. S. Eliot's "dissociation of sensibility," for example—which logic registers and defends. (Ong, 1977, pp. 211–212)

But though the various senses are different, as are the styles of cognition they define, they do not function in isolation. Although our sensory apparatus is not much different (except in some cases somewhat inferior) to those of other animals, there is a massive change in the size of the association areas. The brain organizes around the antithetical tasks of breaking down and building up information. Polysensory integration of information produces cognitive models that are rich and flexible. Our cognition reflects the external world where sound, sight, and tactile and kinesthetic information are simultaneously available. We can describe music as "bright" or a color as "quiet," using one modality to extend another. The metaphoric brain extends itself and its understanding by blending experiences.

THE ORAL TRADITION AND HYPNOSIS

Oral cultures are guided by what works in a given context, what is relevant to the current situation (Ong, 1982). Analysis, tightly reasoned logical argument, and arbitrary rules that are independent of present concerns are the legacy of literacy. The contrasts between oral and literate states of mind are similar to those used to distinguish between right and left hemisphere function, or between hypnotic and normal states of consciousness. The features that oral poetry highlights are inherently "hypnotic," aimed at synchronizing and patterning cognition and behavior to ensure close, personal collaboration.

Although the oral world is obscured by literacy, our brains retain their capacity to create and respond to acoustic rhythms. Indeed, oral structures become even more powerful by virtue of their hidden impact. Absorption is based on our ability to experience directly, without an intermediary. Trance and related altered states of consciousness, which are universally recognized and institutionalized in all known cultures, become rare and exotic. Normal human abilities take on an almost magical quality and can even be feared as the manifestations of some unknown power.

In discouraging analysis, the oral style depends upon thought processes similar to trance logic found in hypnotic subjects (Spanos, 1986a). Hypnotic subjects can entertain two mutually exclusive ideas at the same time without perceiving any inconsistency. For example, a subject may see a hallucination of a person beside the real person and accept this as not unusual.

Oral learning requires a total participation involving both conscious and unconscious levels of attention. As we shall see later (with the hypnotherapeutic work of Milton Erickson), the ability to absorb attention is rooted in the use of metaphor, the ability to explain one idea in terms of another. This allows for the drawing of distinctive parallels between the story and the listener. Unexpected complexities and connections could be revealed in a dramatic fashion, with the connections made not by overt, logical analysis but by a shared emotional state and present experience.

What we see revealed in poetry is, I suggest, the best way of guessing what in fact our language mind is really like, is really capable of. As will be described later, there appear to be fairly distinct mechanisms in the brain for such linguistic functions as vocabulary, grammar, and logic, but there are also the underpinnings of such poetic functions as metaphor (the imputing of figurative meanings and abstract concepts); synesthesia (the exchange of imagery between the various senses); and the classifying of words by their sound and shape, in memory, which can be drawn on for meter and rhyme. H. Gene Blocker has proposed that poetic possibilities are always present but are suppressed during the instrumental use of language for conversation. When I open my mouth to speak, a certain limited program is put into place, as it were, but if I were in the situation of composing verse, other aspects would come to the fore. Blocker says, "In esthetic experience the conventions associated with art allow us to release this rich source of extra significance." (Maxwell, 1984, p. 128)

Poetry has long been associated with hypnosis (Edmonston, 1986). Vivid language and complex word structures within a rhythmic pattern combine to make the individual images singularly compelling but the entire meaning open-ended. In addition, the story of the poem may capture and absorb attention while the regular rhythm of the standard three-second line provides a natural patterning for the central nervous system (Snyder, 1983). The aspects of poetry that have made it an important mnemonic and educational device for oral cultures lend increased capacity for it to function as one of the social variables encouraging trance development in a culturally specific way (Rouget, 1985).

Various forms of socially countenanced altered states of consciousness are found in virtually every culture. Hypnotic skills are valued and cultivated long before literacy becomes general throughout a society. Typically they are used in a variety of ways to supplement conscious behavior. They can be employed for physical healing, dispute arbitration, or marking rites of passage. As we shall see, they are also important in defining and adjusting social roles. Through all this they are deeply involving, closely connected with communal celebration in dance and music (Bourguignon, 1973). These uses are related to the intrinsic daily rhythm of alterations in consciousness (the "common everyday trance"), on the one hand, and the socially sanctioned use of dissociation to redefine the self, on the other. Despite literacy, the human brain continues to construct a spoken world.

Oral skills are peripheral neither to human culture nor to human cognition. Until the advent of widespread literacy, oral skills were not merely central; they were the only methods of cultural and personal evolution. The underlying structure of poetry is simply an elaboration of everyday "practical" thought. In their study of the relationship between the poetic use of metaphor and ordinary cognition, Lakoff and Turner (1989) conclude that poetry is an elaboration of basic cognition made more dense and vivid by the skill of the poet:

It is commonly thought that poetic language is beyond ordinary language—that it is something essentially different, special, higher, with extraordinary tools and techniques like metaphor and metonymy, instruments beyond the reach of someone who just talks. But great poets, as master craftsmen, use basically the same tools we use; what makes them different is their talent for using these tools, and their skill in using them, which they acquire from sustained attention, study, and practice. (p. xi)

The oral poet used verbal skills much like the modern hypnotherapist. Elaborating on basic metaphors shared by all, the poet provided a method for the learning of shared social values from one generation to the next. Our literate bias may obscure the importance of these skills as well as blind us to their persistence today. This form of poetry is in a real sense hypnotic in that if it were not "entrancing," it would not be effective. Functional communication and aesthetic appeal are dependent on one another in oral communication.

PART TWO
ABILITIES

Hypnotherapy can be conceptualized as the interaction
between two fundamental brain functions. The first is the
rhythmic alteration in level of consciousness the brain
undergoes throughout the course of the day. Associated
with changes in the relation between the two hemispheres,
attention follows a path from alert and active external
orientation to a more quiescent internally focused state
and then back again in a recurrent cycle. Hypnosis
appears to be a socially sanctioned and defined means of
developing and utilizing this basic rhythm.

The second fundamental ability is the capacity to
comprehend and create metaphor. Our understanding of
ourselves and the world both emotionally and intellectually

is fashioned from metaphor. The brain uses a process of imagery and analogy to create meaning. Our understanding is a story that is continually being shaped for new circumstances.

5 THE COMMON EVERYDAY TRANCE

Everyone carries within him his somnambulist of whom he is the mesmerizer. When the reverie is good, when it has the continuum of good things, it is the somnambulist in us who imperceptibly commands the action of his mesmerizer.

Gaston Bachelard, 1971

One of the most important issues in hypnosis research is the nature of the relationship of hypnotic phenomena and everyday behavior. By extension, we are also concerned with the way in which brain function in hypnosis may relate to function outside of formal hypnosis. As a consequence of his observations of the clinical work of Milton Erickson, Ernest Rossi proposed an "ultradian rhythm theory of hypnosis." He demonstrated that the changes in cognition, affect, and behavior that occur as part of the ultradian cycle ("the common everyday trance") are similar to the changes that occur during hypnosis. The common mechanism underlying both of these processes is reputed to be a change in hemispheric dominance with a relative increase in right hemispheric activity. A review of studies of hemispheric function suggests that ultradian changes do parallel the changes found in hypnosis. Hemispheric function in hypnosis, however, is also a function of both individual differences and of the nature of the task presented. Moreover, these changes are complex and are not limited to the cortex but involve the whole brain. Cerebral function in hypnosis appears to be the result of both intrinsic temporal rhythms and extrinsic contextual demands.

In 1982, Ernest Rossi proposed a relationship between hypnosis and ultradian cycles (recurrent rhythms of less than twenty-four hours) as a result of his observations of Milton Erickson's hypnotherapeutic work. Rossi noted that Erickson's sessions were often lengthy and varied greatly as to when a hypnotic induction would be initiated. He describes his observations as follows:

Sometime or other during those leisurely interviews with their traded memories and anecdotes, it would suddenly become apparent that the patient was quietly nodding his head in a slow and rhythmical fashion—with lids closing over faraway-looking eyes. A hypnotherapeutic trance was being induced in an indirect manner that once again had escaped the author's attention.

It soon became apparent that the author was missing the initial moments of hypnotic induction because he was focusing his attention on MHE rather than the patient. MHE was continuously observing the patient with a careful and highly focused attention: he would monitor the patient's heart rate (by observing pulsations in the face, throat, legs, or hands), the speed of reflexes (eyeblink, swallowing, respiration), and the degree of overall body movement. In his later years, MHE would usually wait for the patient's physical and mental processes to "quiet down" before he induced trance, explaining that he was waiting to utilize those "natural" periods of quietness and receptivity. We soon began to call these quiet periods the "common everyday trance" . . . because it seemed they were part of natural everyday life. The housewife staring vacantly over a cup of coffee, the student with a faraway look in his eyes during the middle of a lecture, and the driver who automatically reaches his destination with no memory of the details of his route, are all varieties of the common everyday trance. . . . Trance readiness, or the common everyday trance, may be understood as highly individual and variable but behaviorally recognizable portions of the ultradian cycle. Hypnotherapists can learn to recognize the behavioral characteristics of this naturally occurring cycle and facilitate hypnotherapeutic trance at this time by utilizing Erickson's naturalistic approaches. Hypnotherapy may be conceptualized as a facilitation of these naturally occurring ultradian cycles, during which parasympathetic and right-hemispheric processes can be maximized to facilitate healing. (Rossi, 1982, pp. 21–22, 30)

Following on these observations, Rossi noted parallels between features of trance and a number of different ultradian cycles that seem to recur at approximately 90- to 120-minute intervals. These cycles include phasic changes in a wide range of psychophysiologic, motor, cognitive, perceptual, and more complex social behavior. The changes correspond to what Erickson characterized in clinical work as "a state of response attentiveness" (1979, p. 2), which he utilized in his hypnotic inductions. Rossi suggests that in doing so, Erickson was choosing the time when the subject would be most likely to respond to suggestion with manifestations of trance. In other words, by using engrossing stories, intriguing verbal ploys, and paradox, Erickson tacitly encouraged the individual to respond more fully as this state unfolded. Thus, in a very real sense, Rossi is postulating a truly "permissive" technique designed to enhance and facilitate intrinsic biologic rhythms.

The features of ultradian quieting are very similar to the features seen in traditional hypnotic states (Rossi, 1986b). These changes suggest a general trend toward increased parasympathetic activity and an associated relative increase in right hemisphere function compared to the alert waking state (Bakan, 1978; Kripke, 1982). The subject's respiratory rate slows and deepens; this is often accompanied by yawns or sighs. The pulse will slow and the skin may blush and warm. Eye blinking becomes less frequent; the eyeballs move less, the upper eyelids droop, and the pupils dilate. The sclera reddens and tears may be obvious. Body movements and muscle tone are reduced, and there is a general slowing of reflexes and the startle response. These features are together the features of a relaxed and faraway expression. There are fewer facial movements, and there may be an increase in asymmetry between the two sides of the face. Subjects report perceptual alterations with changes in the subjective experience of hearing, seeing, and touch. They tend to engage in fantasy and personal thoughts. Emotional intensity increases despite the relative lack of external expression. Rossi (1986b) describes the period as a combination of increased internal sensitivity combined with a nondemanding form of increased interpersonal sensitivity.

Consideration of Rossi's theory leads to an examination of three specific areas: first, the ultradian changes in mood, cognition, and behavior and how they parallel those that occur in trance; second, the extent to which both these changes (ultradian and/or hypnotic) are accompanied by a shift in hemispheric dominance, specifically an increase in right hemisphere activity; and, third, the nature of brain function in hypnosis, particularly the role of subcortical attentional, emotional, and motivational systems.

ADAPTATION IN TIME

Time is an environment as "real" as the one in space. The biologic imperative for evolutionary fit is just as great for both. Temporal organization allows for the efficient use of available resources. This presupposes a sort of biologic clock or system that synchronizes the organism with the time of day. Time is not a thing but a dimension, a relationship between events. Timekeeping is the sequencing of events so that they occur in the same order, maintaining their relationship in a consistent pattern. Biological clocks function to preserve the relationship between certain biochemical processes and either the external world or other physiologic rhythms.

The term *biologic clock* conjures up the image of an immutable internal timepiece that moves at an equal rate and in an arbitrary fashion through a preordained course. The reality is quite different. Temporal organization in living organisms results from the synchronization of a multitude of metabolic processes (Winfree, 1980, 1987). Although these processes generally appear to be related to a twenty-four-hour day (or some part of it), the time course of the various cycles is variable. The rhythms seem to function in the form of what is known as a "relaxation oscillator" (Moore-Ede, 1982)—that is, the cycle is made up of components that, though they function in sequence, typically do so at a very uneven rate. Each of these cycles has an intrinsic rhythm, but it is highly sensitive to external conditions as well as the other associated physical and psychological rhythms. It represents a compromise between its own individual beat and the need to harmonize with the other elements.

The rhythmic quality of human life persists even in the absence of any external schedule (Moore-Ede, 1982). Studies of humans living for extended periods in isolation, away from any external time cues, consistently reveal the existence of an internal circadian rhythm that very closely approximates the twenty-four-hour day. The synchronization of the various cycles that make up the rhythm is not regulated by a single mechanism. For example, falling asleep and waking up (which one might suppose would be closely related) are in fact regulated by two separate mechanisms (Winfree, 1980). These cycles coordinate and collaborate, not like a precise atomic clock but more like a community of individuals working together. The result is a system of impressive regularity that nevertheless remains flexible and responsive.

The rhythms of the brain are governed by neural pacemakers that derive their rhythmicity from the inherent firing rate of the cells making up their circuit (Connor, 1985). The primary biologic clock for many of the major rhythms of brain and body appears to be a small circuit of neurons called the suprachiasmatic nuclei (scn) of the hypothalamus (Moore-Ede, 1982). The hypothalamus is part of the older part of the brain below the cortex, and it is the site of hormonal and autonomic nervous system coordination. It also has close connections with the emotional centers of the limbic system. But the scn is not a clock in our sense, providing a rigid timetable for the other parts of the brain. Rather, it serves to modulate and coordinate the existing rhythms of the various components. Brain processes possess an inherent rhythmicity of their own. Each of these rhythms is built with its own inherent structure and temporal limits. The scn serves to give a cue or downbeat periodically so that the rhythms may be synchronized.

Body time is a multicomponent, multimedia affair. It is put together from a conglomerate of clocks, some clearly important, others not so important and still others occupying an ambiguous rung on the ladder of temporal status. But the clocks are not isolated units, each one responsible for driving a particular rhythm independently of all the rest; clocks interact, influence and are influenced, modulate, entrain, couple and uncouple, in a highly mobile set of relationships, which are mediated by messages encoded as chemistry and as electrical impulses in the nervous system. (Campbell, 1986, p. 113)

Circadian rhythms that organize bodily functions around the twenty-four-hour day derive from the need of the organism to coordinate with the daily shifts from day to night. By contrast, the more fluid, less predictable ultradian rhythms serve to coordinate us more closely with our psychological environment, with the context of our world and the meaning we assign to it (Campbell, 1986). Most animals show alternating bouts of activity and rest, usually associated with feeding, across the course of a single day (Moore-Ede, 1982). Laboratory animals show significant ultradian rhythm of reward-seeking behavior with a tight temporal correlation between feeding and self-stimulation in an environment without external time cues (Katz, 1980). This suggests an integrated phasic response that results in learning being most sensitive when it will be most useful for the animal. These shorter activity-rest rhythms do not appear to correspond to the light-dark cycle of the day as does the circadian wake-sleep rhythm. They are highly variable despite their rhythmic nature. The animal evidence supports the notion of at least two separate regulatory centers. Lesions in the brain stem of the cat can, depending on location, produce either increased or reduced frequency and amplitude of the cycles (Sterman, 1985). A similar cycle is prominent in the human fetus and newborn but gradually becomes less prominent with age.

Dreaming as an Altered State

The notion of temporal organization serves to remind us of the continuous nature of what are usually considered discrete mental states. By convention we emphasize distinctions between different states of consciousness as if the boundaries were clearly fixed and immutable. But these distinctions are to a large measure arbitrary. Certainly, the barrier between waking conscious thought and dreaming is far more fluid than has been supposed. Indeed, Kripke (1978) has suggested that the most distinctive phase of sleep, the repeating rapid eye movement (REM) cycle (or at least the underlying mechanism), continues to operate during the waking state as represented by ultradian cycles. Rebound from REM (following REM deprivation) is substantially reduced if subjects experience waking fantasy (Hartse, 1982). Narcoleptic subjects, who suffer from spontaneous REM sleep episodes during the waking course of the day, typically show clusters of these episodes not in a random way but according to a ninety-minute cycle (Sterman, 1985). Finally, LaBerge (1985) has presented electrophysiologic evidence of the phenomenon of "lucid dreaming"; the experience of conscious awareness in the middle of a dream. Thus there is evidence for the notion that there is a rhythmic fluctuation in waking consciousness similar to the alternation between REM and non-REM states during sleep.

Researchers have noticed the similarities between cognition in dreaming and trance states for over a hundred years (Hobson, 1988). Both are characteristically distinct from the normal waking state with an increase in the intensity and fluidity of emotions, a structure and content that does not always correspond to how we understand external reality, vivid and often bizarre sensory impressions that are uncritically accepted, and the difficulty of retaining details of the experiences once we are back in the waking state (Hobson, 1988). Similarly, both dreams and ultradian rhythms of consciousness are a regular and predictable part of our everyday lives, whether we notice them or not. In a human life span of seventy years, an individual will devote at least six full years to dreaming (Hobson, 1988).

This evidence stimulated Hobson and McCarley to put forward an activation-synthesis hypothesis on the biologic basis of dreaming (1977). The increase in brain activity during REM sleep is the result of the removal of inhibitory control of systems that are usually active in the waking state (hence the activation). When the noradrenergic neurons' modulatory effect is suddenly released, other brain circuits that have been under inhibitory control suddenly become active. Moreover, there are qualitative as well as quantitative changes. "Not only are they more active, but the 'mode' of their activity is changed: they run free of restraint from both external stimuli and internal inhibition. By such a mechanism, we may not only explain how the mind may be turned on during sleep but also account for its unusual operating properties during dreaming" (Hobson, 1988, p. 206).

Simultaneously, information from the external world is inhibited. This involves two processes: in the first, the systems are kept so busy with internal processes that they are unable to receive external stimuli; second, activity in the reticular formation of the brain stem (which also coordinates eye movements) actively inhibits input.

The brain also disconnects the motor system so that, with the exception of the eye movements, there is a state of voluntary muscle paralysis. This prevents the body from acting out any of the experiences that are generated during the dream (Pompeiano, 1979). The evidence suggests that in REM sleep the circuits controlling motor function are in fact highly sensitized and ready for action but are simultaneously blanketed by a strong inhibitory process (Chase, 1983). Strong pulses of activity go from the brain stem to the thalamus as well as the visual cortex. These waves occur in coordination with the rapid eye movements. The structure and rhythm of these movements are associated with the specific eye movements of the dreamer and the content of the dream. In the absence of external input, the brain interprets the signals generated to the visual system as if they were external events. Thus, the brain is activated to process information while excluding external information and actively inhibiting motor responses (Hobson, 1988).

Cortical activation and heightened sensory thresholds appear to account for the specific patterns of brain activity found in dreaming (Antrobus, 1986). Thus, the brain, while in a highly activated state, receives a barrage of what it takes to be external sensory input and which it creatively synthesizes according to its past experiences, present needs and wishes, and the inherent patterning of the rhythmic discharges. Simultaneously, the activation of the limbic system and the hypothalamus autonomic system in the brain stem intensifies the emotional involvement of the dreamer in the dream experience.

McCarley and Massaquoi (1985) have proposed a limit cycle model of REM sleep that involves the alternating discharge of two different sets of neurons originating in the brain stem. The first is a group of cholinergic neurons in the pontine reticular formation, which seem to initiate the REM period. The second group is composed of noradrenergic neurons in the locus coeruleus and dorsal raphe nucleus, which have a peak discharge activity at the end of the REM cycle. In effect, the alternation between non-REM and REM sleep is a reciprocal balance between these two sets of neurons, with the noradrenergic system generally predominating during waking states and the cholinergic predominating during REM sleep. The two achieve a dynamic balance, alternating in control in a rhythmic dance.

This balance relates to the underlying biologic function that dreaming may serve. Whereas biogenic amine neuron systems are capable of neurotransmitter depletion, other brain systems are capable of functioning continuously without exhaustion (Hobson, 1988). On the whole, the brain is somewhat more active during REM sleep than during the normal waking state, but there appears to be a specific decrease in the activity of noradrenergic neurons (Steriade, 1976). Thus, while the rest of the brain continues to work, the noradrenergic system, which is essential for modulating alert consciousness, appears to temporarily go "off-line."

One of the most attractive aspects of this theory is its positive aspect. It looks at a night of sleep as much as preparation for the subsequent day's activity as recovery from that of the previous day. This change in emphasis may seem slight or even trivial, but it is not: in calling attention to the preparatory action of sleep, we shift our thinking from a catabolic or excretory model to an anabolic or storage model. . . .

REM sleep would thus guarantee rest for those neurons most sensitive to fatigue—the small ones that are critically necessary for efficacious arousal; simultaneously, there is stereotyped, high-level activation of non-fatiguable brain circuits, assuring their daily use in a safe setting. . . . According to this view, REM sleep is an active maintenance program. (Hobson, 1988, pp. 290–291)

Thus the states of REM sleep and dreaming are fundamentally a creative brain process. There is evidence of a summing up and a restoring process from previous activity and an anticipation and preparation for subsequent behavior. At the same time, while certain processes are rehearsed and stored in memory, other information that would destabilize the system may in fact be eliminated (Crick, 1983).

Our dreams tell us clearly that the repertoires for these "instinctual" acts are indeed represented within the central nervous system. The extraordinary plasticity of the dream experience includes a rich overrepresentation of significant behaviors: fear, aggression, defense, and attack; approach-avoidance; and sex. At the level of our psychological experience, we find evidence of the whole repertoire. By the principle of isomorphism, this denotes a substrate for behavior at the level of neural programming. (Hobson, 1988, p. 295)

The REM cycle is closely related to mood regulation. In depression, patients have changes in ultradian cycles with increased REM density and a shortening of the REM latency (the period of time between the start of sleep and the onset of the first REM cycle at night). The ultradian disturbances reveal significantly slower ultradian periodicities when compared with normal controls (Lange, 1982). Furthermore, depressed patients show an increased sensitivity to cholinergic drugs that is associated both with their sleep changes and their mood state (Sitaram, 1976). The generation of depressive states not only involves the same anatomical structures as does REM sleep, but there are characteristic REM disturbances found in depression (McCarley, 1982).

The link between ultradian rhythms and REM sleep also underlines the important issue that the entire brain is actively involved in generating these states. The left hemisphere, usually associated with waking consciousness, is also actively involved in dreaming. Dreaming appears to be lateralized to the left hemisphere (Greenberg, 1986). Patients with left hemisphere lesions are more likely to report a loss of dreaming (Epstein, 1983). Although the right hemisphere plays an important role in generating some of the visual features of dreaming, the left hemisphere seems to be involved in synthesizing the associated meaning (Antrobus, 1987). Both the verbal report of a dream and the dream experience itself are mediated predominantly through the left hemisphere (Antrobus, 1987). This is true despite the fact that the right hemisphere is relatively more active in REM sleep than it is in non-REM sleep (Gordon, 1982). A similar involvement of the whole brain in producing a flexible but recurrent alternate form of processing is found in the waking cycle.

The BRAC

Kleitman suggested in 1961 that many ultradian rhythms were synchronized on a single ninety-minute cycle. He termed this the "basic rest activity cycle" (BRAC). Since that time over fifty studies have further outlined the nature of this cycle (Kleitman, 1982). These studies, however, have also shown that the ninety-minute ultradian rhythm represents a loosely organized group of rhythms rather than a single biologic oscillation (Lavie, 1985; Hobson, 1986). These rhythms involve virtually every facet of physiologic function including cortical function, hormonal secretion, and renal, gastric, and immunologic regulation (Rasmussen, 1986).

ULTRADIAN RHYTHMS IN BRAIN FUNCTION

The clearest evidence for ultradian rhythms comes from studies of sustained performance. In an extended study of eleven young male subjects involved in a complex vigilance task, an ultradian rhythm in both heart rate and performance measures was identified over a period of up to forty-four hours. The rhythm became progressively more distinctive as the task continued, and the pattern was found in over three-fourths of the analyses (Orr, 1974). Similarly, a study of sixteen subjects involved in order tasks requiring auditory and proprioceptive feedback demonstrated a clear periodicity of around a hundred minutes with a marked rhythmic modulation in the efficiency of motor control (Gopher, 1980).

In addition to a wide variety of physiologic alterations that follow an ultradian pattern, there are a number of alterations in cognition, mood, and behavior that are of particular significance in hypnosis (Rossi and Cheek, 1988). There is evidence for a marked ultradian rhythm in vigilance (Okawa, 1984) with associated changes in peripheral blood flow (Romano, 1980), respiratory amplitude (Horne, 1976), and visual evoked potentials (Zimmerman, 1983) as well as changes in pupillary diameter, stability and reactivity to light, and saccadic eye movements (Lavie, 1981). Time series analyses show a significant associated recurring increase in daydream and fantasy, with associated increases of visual imagery (Kripke, 1978). These daydreams are more intense when they occur in an eyes-closed, drowsy state (Kripke, 1978; Orr, 1974). There is also evidence for a parallel recurring cognitive and emotional cycle with increased emotional responsiveness and a more subjective cognitive processing of information (Evans, 1972; Holloway, 1978; Overton, 1978; Thayer, 1987). Subjects appear to repeat the cycle approximately sixteen times per day, every 70 to 120 minutes. Kripke (1978, 1982) noted that the subjects were personally unaware of any repeating cycle in their mental lives.

The daily pattern of daydream or reverie appears to follow the structure of the ultradian rhythm. The evidence suggests that they are of significant adaptive value not only for relaxation but for problem-solving, distraction from unpleasant stimuli, the maintenance of vigilance, or detailed memorization (Caughey, 1984; Luria, 1976). Judging by the content, daydream is apparently a workshop of unfinished intellectual, emotional, and social concerns. The vast majority of daydreams involve the reworking and restructuring of previous experience that was in some way unsatisfying or unfinished (Caughey, 1984; Kripke, 1978). In addition, Hoyt (1989) reported a positive association between measures of positive-constructive daydreaming and measures of absorption and hypnotizability, suggesting a connection between the two states.

Investigators have found evidence for a parallel recurring emotional cycle with increased emotional responsiveness and a more subjective cognitive processing of information (Evans, 1972; Holloway, 1978; Overton, 1978; Thayer, 1987). Thayer (1987) conducted a pair of experiments that demonstrated a daily rhythm of moods that was associated with particular cognitive patterns. The subjects' perceptions of the difficulty of personal problems correlated with their feelings of low energy and sadness.

Just as there are characteristic interactional rhythms within a conversation, so too a number of repeating cycles can be shown to occur over a twenty-four-hour period. Hayes and Cobb studied the activity of a couple kept isolated in a "free-running" environment (1982) and found regularly recurring cycles of conversational activity. The most significant of these occurred sixteen times per circadian day, or about every ninety minutes. Again, the cycle was not rigid but responded to a variety of social and environmental cues.

There is an ultradian rhythm demonstrated in EEG alpha activity (Kripke, 1978; Manseau, 1984), EEG delta activity (Kripke, 1972), and auditory EEG-evoked potentials (Ornitz, 1973). Globus and his coworkers (1970) demonstrated that performance in vigilance tasks fluctuated in wakened subjects in parallel with the predicted changes from REM to non-REM states if their sleep was interrupted. Alpha rhythm frequency is positively correlated with body temperature, cerebral blood flow, and rate of brain energy metabolism (Gundel, 1984). Peaks for the other EEG rhythms, though much more variable from individual to individual, are also periodic and are associated with relatively greater right hemisphere activity (Gordon, 1982; Gundel, 1983).

A careful study of nine subjects revealed two ultradian components of daytime arousal (Tsuji, 1988). The shorter of the two had a period of about a hundred minutes and seemed to reflect an oscillation in focus of vigilance between external and internal activities. The longer component had a period of between three and eight hours and appeared to reflect a variation in level of consciousness between full wakefulness and drowsiness. Tsuji and Kobayashi (1988) suggest that the shorter component is superimposed upon the longer one and that its appearance may be submerged by changes in the longer one. In other words, degree of daytime sleepiness or other changes in the overall level of arousal may obscure the cycles.

Ultradian variations in EEG activity appear to reflect periodic oscillations in the brain stem arousal systems. In a study of eight subjects kept in an isolation chamber, Manseau and Broughton (1984) found a significant cycle of EEG activity in each hemisphere occurring every 70 to 120 minutes. The rhythms occurred simultaneously in the two hemispheres. The only specific differences were a slight overall increase in alpha activity and a slight increase in theta activity in the right hemisphere. The ultradian periodicity, however, was evident in the overall frequency and amplitude of the EEG rather than in one specific rhythm. There was marked interindividual variation in the individual rhythms. Manseau and Broughton concluded that these findings suggest that the oscillations reflect changes in subcortical arousal systems regulating the overall activity of the cortex rather than being the result of a single rhythm arising within the cortex.

As one would expect, the ultradian rhythm is readily modifiable by both physiologic and contextual priorities. Strong motivation, continuous high performance demands, and chronic stress resulting in high arousal levels tend to mask the relatively weak endogenous rhythm (Broughton, 1985). In tasks involving continuous sustained performance under conditions demanding extreme vigilance, the ultradian rhythm may disappear temporarily (Kripke, 1978; Orr, 1974). Subjects who are actively involved in complex, continuous external tasks for which they are highly motivated show little evidence of phasic alterations in their cortical function (Broughton, 1985). In contrast, ultradian rhythms are more easily detected under conditions of increased sleep need, reduced external performance demand, and lowered motivation to focus externally (Broughton, 1985).

Sterman (1985) has reported pervasive changes in the EEG that follow an ultradian rhythm; they are most marked in the resting state and disappear when the individual is performing complex visuomotor tasks. Sterman also noted the similarity between the characteristic EEG ultradian changes and sensorimotor patterns related to movement suppression that are typically enhanced in the performance of complex visuomotor tasks. These patterns are associated with increased practice and subsequent improved task performance.

These similarities are intriguing from two perspectives. In the first place, they tend to support the notion of two forms of attention, one underlying focused awareness and the other a more generalized vigilance. The former, whether directed inwardly or outwardly, has typically been associated with the induction of the trance state. The latter is reduced in hypnosis (see below). Second, the changes are consistent with the increased internal absorption associated with visual imagery that occurs with the ultradian changes in consciousness. Both of these features are seen as part of the EEG changes of the trance state and strongly suggest a link between ultradian rhythms and trance.

Hypnotic susceptibility does appear to change over the course of the day. Aldrich and Bernstein (1987) reported a bimodal distribution of Harvard Group Scale Hypnotic Susceptibility (HGSHS) scores when they are done at different times. This is the first direct evidence that changes in hypnotic responsiveness parallel the circadian pattern of physiologic rhythms.

Further support for Rossi's hypothesis comes from some highly original work involving breathing rhythms. Although nasal airflow may seem an unlikely marker of brain function, a connection between breathing and altered states of consciousness is part of the traditional lore of most meditative practices. In fact, the relationship apparently is a strong one. There are cyclic alterations in relative airflow between the left and right nostrils that can be measured quite precisely (Hasegawa, 1977). The average period is about two to three hours, but it can vary widely. The alteration in airflow is the result of alternating cycles of sympathetic and parasympathetic autonomic nervous system function regulated by the hypothalamus (Levin, 1979; Eccles, 1981). Sympathetic activity constricts blood vessels in the nasal mucosa and increases airflow; parasympathetic activity produces vasodilation in the mucosa and reduced airflow.

This nasal ultradian rhythm is correlated with an increase in contralateral cerebral hemispheric activity (Werntz, 1981, 1983; R. Klein et al., 1986). The shift in nostril dominance is reflective of a generalized shift of autonomic nervous system activity (Kennedy, 1986). The alterations in hemispheric function are related to changes both in the style of cognition, particularly in an increase in vivid visual imagery, and in performance on specific tasks. Thus these studies support the notion of an ultradian rhythm of cerebral function associated with characteristic physical manifestations mediated by the autonomic nervous system. Whether or not these changes are directly related to the findings reported by Aldrich and Bernstein is yet to be established. Efficiency on verbal and spatial tasks alternates in cycles of around ninety minutes, supporting the notion of alternating hemispheric dominance (Klein, 1979). This pattern of changing performance is also related to the pattern of nasal airflow (R. Klein et al., 1986). Thus there is a tendency for subjects to do better on verbal tasks when there is increased airflow in the right nostril, but left nostril airflow is associated with better spatial performance. This suggests that asymmetries in autonomic nervous system function are related to asymmetries in hemispheric activation and, as a result, changes in cognitive style. Moreover, there is evidence that the system is a two-way street. Both groups were able to show that forced uninostril breathing could precipitate the anticipated hemispheric changes (R. Klein et al., 1986).

Thus the ultradian rhythm mediates between external circumstances and the internal metabolic rhythm of the brain. Lavie (1985) calls the ultradian variations in wakefulness the "gates of sleep," as the transition from wakefulness to sleep occurs most easily at these times. It is significantly easier to fall asleep during the BRAC than at any other time during the day. Conversely, far more awakenings at night (approximately 80 percent of spontaneous awakenings) occur during REM sleep. Thus, these phases of relative ease of transition from waking to sleeping provide a structure by which constant small adjustments can be made with the larger circadian rhythm to allow it to remain synchronized with a day-night cycle that alters gradually but progressively with the seasons.

It is this transitional role that suggests that these gates can be used for changes to other states of consciousness as well. This model also serves to underline the fluid nature of the ultradian rhythm. In this sense, referring to biologic clocks as if they are rigid mechanical devices can be misleading (Winfree, 1980). By contrast, the ultradian rhythm is a loosely organized collection of diverse functions without a single regulator and extremely sensitive to external conditions (Colquhoun, 1981; Webb, 1981). In this sense, the ultradian rhythm is a gate, or opportunity, that permits the transition to occur more easily but that can be overridden if necessary (Colquhoun, 1981).

Recurring rhythms serve to adapt physiologic processes and environmental constraints. An important implication for hypnosis is the idea of phase or state dependency (Fischer, 1972). In other words, the response to particular environmental cues, such as hypnotic induction, depends upon the phase into which the individual is entering at the time. Access to cognitions, memories, and emotions does show a significant ultradian pattern (Evans, 1972; Overton, 1978; Holloway, 1978). An induction occurring at the beginning of a phase of quiescence is likely to produce much more dramatic refocusing of attention than one that occurs at the beginning of a dramatic increase in outward activity. As William James suggested:

You need only suggest an idea which the mind itself takes hold of. But the subject's mind can only be hypnotized in its passage from the waking to the sleeping state. All persons go through this hypnotic [hypnagogic] state twice a day. A good subject is one who can be caught on the road to sleep and suspended—that is, prevented from deep sleep. If the mind of the subject is caught at just this point and given a suggestion, it immediately acts upon the idea. Everything depends on the subject allowing himself to be entranced, and hardly anything on the operator, except that he must engender the subject's trust and be able to fix attention on the relaxed condition. (James, quoted in Taylor, 1983, p. 25)

Perhaps we can consider hypnosis not as a single entity but as one culturally defined context of a rhythmic biologic opportunity to enter into a number of different states of consciousness. There do not appear to be any reliable psychological or physiologic concomitants of trance that are unique to hypnosis (Sarbin, 1979). The nature of the process and the suggestions made, the expectations of the individual, previous experience, and current goals will all play a role in determining the nature of the experience as will the individual's own biologic propensities (Spanos, 1986).

When all the factors are taken together, it is clear that there is no complete ultradian model that accounts for all the current data. In humans, an ultradian rhythm exists, but the components are inconstant and highly sensitive to context. This is not to say that they are unimportant, however. The study of the rhythmic organization of the brain is an account of its temporal order, the equivalent in the time dimension of the importance of neuroanatomy in the spatial order.

Initially, the concept of a biologic rhythm in dreaming may have seemed mystical, especially when it was proposed that such a rhythm could influence our waking lives. Stage REM and the rhythm of dreaming are quite real, and we now know that the waking oscillations are quite real. Whether the REM-dream oscillator in particular is at work during wakefulness remains to be seen, but careful experimental observations are certainly demonstrating that when we are awake, there is a multiform cyclic regulation of our bodies, our behavior, and our minds. (Kripke, 1982, p. 337)

Ultradian rhythms of cerebral function can be identified, and they are highly sensitive to external influence. They are blunted by high-vigilance external tasks and enhanced by quiet internal absorption and the associated physiologic changes. These conclusions underline the need to examine the specific changes in cerebral function in hypnosis in order to determine how they relate to the ultradian rhythms.

HEMISPHERIC FUNCTION IN HYPNOSIS

Much of our awareness of the dual nature of cerebral functioning comes by way of the observations made by neurologists on changes in function in brain-damaged patients. Following Broca's demonstration that the loss of comprehensible speech was typically associated with lesions in a particular area in the left hemisphere, it was natural for investigators to look for other specific functions that could be localized in one hemisphere or the other. The scientific study of the divisions of function between the two hemispheres reached a new level with the work of Sperry and others (Sperry, 1982). These studies involved patients in whom the corpus callosum had been severed in an attempt to control severe and intractible epilepsy. As a result, the cerebral hemispheres in these patients functioned relatively independently. The basic strategy of the studies was to present tasks to one hemisphere at a time and compare performance. This work has since been extended, using sophisticated and often highly ingenious techniques, to normal individuals as well. Although there is a great deal of methodological difficulty and theoretical controversy in the field, the bulk of the evidence in right-handed subjects suggests a

left hemisphere superiority in tasks involving grammatically organized word sequences, mathematics, analysis, logic, sequences over time, and motor coordination. Right hemisphere function seems dominant in tasks involving imagery, certain visual and constructive activities such as drawing, copying, assembling block designs, perception and manipulation of spatial relations of and between objects or configurations, and the simultaneous grasping of fragments or particulars as a meaningful whole. Various descriptions of the two modes of thought mediated by the two hemispheres have been suggested. The left hemisphere mode is described as symbolic, abstract, linear, rational, focal, conceptual, propositional, secondary process, digital, logical, active, and analytic. The right hemisphere mode is described as iconic, concrete, diffuse, perceptual, appositional, primary process, analogue, passive, and holistic. The two modes are antagonistic and complementary, suggesting that a unity and struggle of opposites is characteristic of mental functioning. (Bakan, 1978, p. 163)

In addition to different information-processing styles, there is increasing evidence of a difference in the relationships of the two hemispheres to the rest of the brain. Their cellular architecture is different. The left hemisphere has many more connections within itself, whereas the right has many more connections with subcortical structures (Geschwind, 1987).

The differences between the two hemispheres are not as rigid as was initially believed, however. For example, there is a circadian rhythm of hemispheric function for some tasks (Zimmerman, 1983). Whereas the original studies were interested in establishing the differences between functions of the two hemispheres, more recent studies have stressed the close cooperation that occurs between them in normal individuals (Gazzaniga, 1985). The two hemispheres are specialized separately for some specific tasks, but they also show a close collaborative integration of functions. The question becomes not which hemisphere is dominant but how both reorganize in response to a given task.

Complex tasks involving rapid alternation between left and right hemispheric tasks show that hemispheric dominance can change dramatically in sequence with the tasks (Gevins, 1983). Thus, hemispheric dominance is highly sensitive to contextual demands. Similarly, employing different strategies for the same task will involve different hemispheric activities. For example, when performing a musical task, musicians who use written musical notation predominantly use their left hemisphere, whereas individuals who do not read music will use their right hemisphere (Davidson, 1977). Stimuli are processed differently in each hemisphere, but they are equally available in both. Relative hemispheric predominance for a particular task can alternate very rapidly or slowly depending on how the hemispheres are activated by the contextual interpretations of the "upstream" subcortical processing system (Gevins, 1983; Kissin, 1986). Nevertheless, the extensive communication between the hemispheres allows for the full exchange of processed information (Popper, 1977).

Thus, though the hemispheres are specialized for different aspects, complex brain function ultimately involves the integration of those aspects. For complex tasks, using both hemispheres provides results that are superior to those achieved by using either hemisphere alone (Liederman, 1985). Although the right hemisphere has an advantage in processing aspects of emotional communication (Underwood, 1985) and simple imagery tasks (Gur, 1982), the left hemisphere also plays a significant role. For example, elementary organization of visual imagery is a role for the right hemisphere, but its organization into a complex whole and the interpretation of its significance seem to be tasks involving predominantly the left hemisphere (Farah, 1985; Antrobus, 1987).

The importance of not associating particular psychological styles exclusively with one hemisphere or another extends to the work in imagery. In studies of split-brain patients, Farah and her coworkers (1985) showed, contrary to expectations, a far more significant role for the left hemisphere than for the right in some forms of visual processing. The left hemisphere also plays a critical role in constructing complex visual imagery (Antrobus, 1987).

Hemispheric differences in sequencing information processing may be as important as differences in the type of processing. Recent studies have identified different types of attentional demands for the two hemispheres. The interactions of task with hemisphere are more marked for tasks not requiring attention to the environment (Ray, 1985). Tasks requiring internal focus were associated with significant increases in parietal alpha rhythms. There was marked hemispheric differentiation for beta rhythms in the temporal areas for emotional tasks and in the parietal areas for cognitive tasks. The two types of tasks also elicited different patterns of cardiovascular response. This suggests that we need to distinguish between attentional tasks that require external orientation and those that require internal orientation as well as the degree of emotional involvement.

Most significantly, Ray also noted that with lengthier, more complex tasks, hemispheric dominance changed over time. This may account for some of the equivocal findings reported in the literature. For example, visual discrimination tasks, which initially show a right hemisphere advantage, show a progressive left hemisphere advantage over time (Kinsbourne, 1987). Thus, when measured at different times the same task may demonstrate two different sets of lateralized effects. Consequently, depending on the length of time studied, a single task could be interpreted as showing a left hemisphere dominance, a right hemisphere dominance, or no overall asymmetry. The findings to date suggest not a sharp discrimination between two completely different sets of functions but a flexible and dynamic organization and reorganization of available resources according to the nature of the ongoing needs. This suggests a model of modular function with the brain performing tasks by dividing up information according to salient features for maximum efficiency. Holtzman and Gazzaniga suggest that the data

reflects competition between the hemispheres for a shared pool of resources— resources that can be utilized by either hemisphere and, to the extent that the hemispheres do not have access to a common data base, that are not specialized for individual processing structures. In addition, these resources must either reside in subcortical structures or be transferred between the hemispheres via subcortical pathways. . . . Although our findings imply that processing resources can be distributed among different processing structures, it remains to be determined whether competition between tasks for a common structure is a consequence of time-sharing processing structures, or whether it reflects the limits in dedicated resources that subserve specific cognitive operations. (Holtzman, 1982, p. 1327)

All of these concerns relate to the role of the two hemispheres during hypnosis. There is a modest, time-limited, and task-related relationship between EEG hemispheric activity and contralateral eye movements (Neubauer, 1988). Highly susceptible hypnotic subjects were reported to have increased amounts of right hemisphere alpha rhythms and a greater tendency to left lateral conjugate eye movements, suggesting a relative increase in right hemispheric activity (Bakan, 1969; Gur, 1973). Other studies, however, failed to replicate these findings (Spanos, 1978), and conjugate eye movements are the subject of methodological controversy (Gur, 1975). On balance, the evidence seems to suggest a moderate association between hypnotic susceptibility and left lateral conjugate gaze (DeWitt, 1976; Smith, 1980; Warren, 1981).

A variety of further evidence supports the notion of increased right hemisphere activity in hypnosis (Gabel, 1988). In a single case study, Chen (1983) reported that during oral surgery in which hypnosis was employed as the anaesthetic, both right and left hemispheres showed a reduced cortical power spectrum, but that this reduction was significant only on the left-hand side. The left side of the body may be more responsive to hypnotic suggestion, and conversion symptoms more commonly involve the left side (Fleminger, 1980; Sackeim, 1982; D. B. Stern, 1977).

Frumkin and her coworkers (1978) reported that high and moderate hypnotizables showed a significant decrease in right ear (left hemisphere) advantage following a hypnotic induction, but Crawford and her coworkers (1983b) reported the opposite results. In their study, only less hypnotizable subjects showed a significant change in cerebral laterality during hypnosis while the high and medium subjects did not. A shift to left ear dominance during hypnosis for highly susceptible subjects has been shown for musical stimuli but not for verbal stimuli (Levine, 1984). Subjects with low susceptibility do not show this alteration (Spellacy, 1987).

Highly susceptible subjects made a more significant shift to the use of a holistic problem-solving strategy and a greater use of visual imagery during hypnosis than did less susceptible subjects (Crawford, 1983a). Highly hypnotizable subjects also seem to use either their right or their left hemisphere more specifically for particular tasks than do subjects with less hypnotic ability. Using ratios of alpha amplitude between left and right hemispheres, MacLeod-Morgan and Lack (1982) have demonstrated that this ratio changes in hypnosis from left to right or from right to left, depending on the nature of the task involved. Furthermore, the two reported that highly susceptible subjects showed more dramatic change in the ratios between the two hemispheres regardless of the direction of the task.

Similarly, other investigators have found that tasks that involve the hemispheres differentially (verbal versus imagery tasks) tend to produce differences that are more marked in the hypnotic state (Mészáros, 1985). Mészáros also demonstrated a significant preference for right hemisphere activity among hypnotized subjects. MacLeod-Morgan (1985) replicated earlier work and showed that highly hypnotizable subjects show more specific lateralization during right and left hemisphere tasks, as measured by the change in alpha ratio, than do low hypnotizables. But other elaborate studies of right hemisphere function have not demonstrated a consistent relationship between hypnotizability and right hemisphere specificity for particular tasks (De-Pascalis, 1988). LaBriola and her coworkers (1987) demonstrated that highly hypnotizable subjects show an increase in right hemisphere activity, whereas subjects with low scores do not. They also noted, however, that task effects predominated, with all subjects showing significantly greater left hemisphere activity during verbal tasks. These controversies are difficult to resolve because of methodological differences between the studies. Changes in the relationship between the hemispheres over time may also explain part of the conflicting results. This may reflect changes in ultradian phases (Zimmerman, 1983), situational demands, or emotional states (Crawford, 1988; Ray, 1985). All these features influence the way in which attention is focused in hypnosis.

Attentional Processes

Electrophysiologic techniques allow us to study the way in which stimuli are processed by the brain. Changes in cortical electrical activity, known as the evoked potentials, which occur in response to various sensory stimuli, can tell us both how information is processed in time and how it is assimilated into the ongoing activity of the brain (Hillyard, 1979). Studies of sensory processing reveal that "the overall shape of the evoked potential is a function of the relative activities of different centers in the brain, as a consequence of which different configurations of electrical activity in the brain produce differently shaped evoked potentials" (Kissin, 1986, p. 59).

In order to focus attention, stimuli must be recognized as important, and cerebral resources, in the form of the attention process, must be directed toward those items. Attention seems to involve two distinct phases: an early passive phase and a second, more active and specific attentional process (Broadbent, 1977). Early elements of the evoked potential appear to be related to the passive phase of attention, whereas the later elements, particularly the P_3 element, is indicative of the second (Hink, 1978; Parasuraman, 1980).

The P_3 (P indicating a positive electrical charge) occurs at about 300 milliseconds after the stimulus is first presented. It is regarded as evidence that the stimulus has been processed by the major brain centers. The P_3 appears to originate in the amygdaloid-hippocampal complex and represents the integration of motivational and emotional input with the cortical processes (Kissin, 1986).

Highly susceptible subjects have been reported to show a greater degree of polymodality in the distribution of EEG amplitudes (Karlin, 1981). Draguitinovich (1986) has reported that hypnotic susceptibility is correlated with a greater peak amplitude of the P_2 sensory potential. Other workers (Sabourin, 1982; DeBenedittis, 1988) have demonstrated a significant association between theta activity and hypnotic phenomena (see below).

There is evidence of cerebral changes with specific hypnotic phenomena. Children who were given suggestions of temporary hypnotic deafness (they were told that the volume of the sound was about to be turned down) showed significantly decreased brain stem auditory evoked responses in both the hypnotic and the normal waking state (Hogan, 1982). The children who were the most hypnotizable had the most marked changes in both states. Similarly, adult subjects were asked to visualize a cardboard box blocking a television monitor they had been watching. Highly susceptible subjects demonstrated significant suppression of the later components of the evoked response (P_3) during hypnotic "obstructive" hallucinations (Spiegel, 1985a). These changes were significantly greater in the right than in the left occipital regions. This effect held true when the subjects were compared both with a low susceptibility group and with controls.

In a similar study by Barabasz and Lonsdale (1983), when strong odors were presented to subjects who had been given hypnotic suggestions of not being able to smell ("negative hallucinations"), they showed enhanced evoked potentials (P_3). The P_3 component is associated with "downstream" information processing for novel and relevant information. Hence the changes in the P_3 were consistent with the changes that would be expected to follow from the hypnotic task. Thus, this study and one by Spiegel and his colleagues showed evidence of specific changes in evoked potentials that were related to the way in which hypnotic suggestion influenced information processing (Spiegel, 1988b).

Spiegel has also reported significant increases in the P_1 amplitude during hypnotic attention and decreases in the P_1 and P_3 amplitudes during the obstructive hallucination task. The highly hypnotizable subjects had consistently lower P_1 amplitudes than did less hypnotizable subjects, whether in hypnosis or during the normal waking state (1988a). The P_1 is related to early ("upstream") components of the attentional process (Hillyard, 1979). These studies suggest that hypnotic ability is a complex skill involving cortical and subcortical structures.

Studies of electrodermal activity in hypnotic subjects have shown similar results. In one, there was a reversal in the asymmetries of the electrodermal activity, suggesting a shift to right hemisphere predominance (Gruzelier, 1985). Highly susceptible subjects showed a lower baseline level of electrodermal activity, a more rapid habituation to the presentation of an auditory stimulus tone, and a reduction in the number of nonspecific responses. Less susceptible subjects showed changes in the opposite direction—higher baseline, slower habituation, and an increase in nonspecific responses. Nonspecific responses are indicators of general level of arousal and are found in states of sustained broad attention. These differences were specific to the hypnotic state and were not found under conditions of quiet relaxation or listening to a story. Gruzelier and Brow suggest

that the increase in orienting responses in unsusceptible subjects under hypnosis represented a broadening of attention and perhaps a resistance to hypnosis along with an increase in anxiety; delayed habituation is often an accompaniment of anxiety. Thus unsusceptibility may not be a passive state of indifference to the hypnotic process but may involve active and possibly defensive changes.

In summary, susceptibility to hypnosis involved a narrowing of attention revealed by a loss of sensitization, . . . involved faster habituation and lowered levels of arousal, . . . and involved a shift in hemispheric influences (Gruzelier, 1985, p. 299)

There were decreased left-sided electrodermal responses during hypnosis for subjects who were susceptible to hypnotic induction (Gruzelier, 1988). In the same study, without hypnosis the susceptible subjects showed a diminished response on the right side. This again suggests the notion of increased flexibility of processing strategies in hypnotically susceptible individuals. Subjects who were not susceptible to hypnosis showed no consistent asymmetries. Gruzelier and his co-workers also found that the degree of change in processing times was highly correlated to the degree of hypnotic susceptibility.

Similarly, susceptible subjects showed a consistent pattern of habituation to extraneous stimuli, whereas unsusceptible subjects showed an increased responsiveness (Gruzelier, 1987a). The susceptible subjects showed a significantly faster habituation than did subjects who were simulating hypnosis (Gruzelier, 1988). Stressful recall situations increased left hemispheric responses, but suggestions of relaxation and increased hypnotic depth decreased these responses (Freeman, 1986; Gruzelier, 1988). The evoked potential studies during hypnosis suggest a consistent decrease in left hemispheric responses for susceptible subjects (Gruzelier, 1988).

This evidence supports the notion that the functions of the two hemispheres are associated with the two different types of attention noted in Sterman's observations (1985). Dimond has suggested that the left hemisphere is active in selective attention, which is associated with fast habituation, and that the right hemisphere is involved in a state of more general vigilance, which habituates more slowly (Dimond, 1979; Gruzelier, 1985). Inhibition of the left hemisphere activity rather than increased right hemisphere activity may be a more accurate description of the EEG changes observed in hypnosis (Harrist, 1988).

Hypnotic induction requires the narrowing of attention through engagement of left hemisphere selective attention processes. Suggestions of sleepiness and inducement of mild sensory fatigue by fixation on objects slightly strenuous to look at facilitates an increase in central inhibition which in turn underlies the loss of a critical attitude. Inhibition is predominantly lateralized to the left hemisphere as shown by the combination of left and not right hemisphere haptic processing time with susceptibility and the "depth" of hypnosis. Left hemisphere control of the right hemisphere also becomes attenuated and permits a release of those right hemisphere functions which have been popularly ascribed to the hypnotic experience. (Gruzelier, 1985, p. 300)

Gruzelier (1988) has proposed a multistage process of brain function during hypnosis. In the first stage of sustained focused attention, there is a relative increase in left hemisphere activity in susceptible subjects. The second stage of "letting go" involves a gradual inhibition of left hemisphere function followed by an increase in right hemisphere activity in the third stage. Gruzelier underlines the need for appreciating the nature of the task demands as well as the ongoing changes in relationship over time in brain function.

The further stages in hypnosis are dependent on the aims of the hypnotic induction, and the nature of posterior hemispheric involvement will reflect the demands of the hypnotist's instructions to the subject; perceptual sensitivity may be diminished as in the case of the suggestion of tunnel vision. Cognitive flexibility is also observed in the allocation of processing resources (MacLeod-

Morgan and Lack, 1982; Crawford, 1982b), a feature which may reflect a trait component of susceptibility to hypnosis. (Gruzelier, 1988, p. 74)

The data also underline the variety of individual differences. Even the most standardized hypnotic induction will produce dramatically different experiential effects from person to person (Sheehan, 1982; Pekala, 1986a, 1986b). In fact, even simple alpha wave biofeedback results in a wide variety of individual and context-dependent differences in both the generation of alpha and the subjective experience of the trainees (Plotkin, 1979, 1980).

The studies of hemispheric function in hypnosis are complex and the results are conflicting. Study design, including the duration and complexity of the task and the indexes of hemispheric laterality used, is particularly critical. Taken together, the studies suggest that changes in lateralization of hemispheric activity do occur in hypnosis and that these changes generally result in increased right hemisphere activity relative to the left. These responses are highly variable, however. The studies further suggest that hypnosis is not a unitary state but a reorganization of ongoing cerebral relationships. The pattern of such changes depends both on the nature of the task and on differences in the way each individual interprets the context in which the task is performed. By implication these conclusions point toward examining total brain function, including the underlying subcortical structures, in hypnosis.

SUBCORTICAL FUNCTION IN HYPNOSIS

Although most of the research to date has focused on hemispheric function, increasing attention is being paid to the role of subcortical structures. The limbic system, with its close connections with the cortex and the rest of the body, is in a central position for integrating psychologic and physiological processes. Thus the limbic system is active in the generation of altered states of consciousness. Two structures with competing effects, but forming a single complex, appear to be principally involved. The hippocampus is active in the onset of the hypnotic state and in generating the ultradian rhythm, whereas the amygdala is active in the termination of trance (Kissin, 1986; DeBenedittis, 1988). It is worthwhile reviewing the structure of the attentional process and particularly the role of the amygdaloid-hippocampal complex.

The system that regulates attention and maintains a state of consciousness consists of three components: a general awareness system, which deals with information from the environment; a self-awareness system, which relates the information to the ongoing sense of self; and an activating system, which modulates the level of arousal.

Increased parasympathetic activity modulated by the anterior hypothalamus blocks RAS activity and stimulates cholinergic cells in the brain stem, which initiated REM sleep (Sakai, 1980). Close to the locus coeruleus are a group of large reticular neurons (FTG) that have a reciprocal relationship with the noradrenergic neurons. They become particularly active in REM sleep. This process gradually intensifies during sleep, resulting in inhibition of the RAS and progressive activation of the medial thalamus and septal hippocampal circuits (Kissin, 1986).

The general awareness system involves the thalamus and basal ganglia—portions of the limbic system (Kissin, 1986). The early phase of attention mediated by the thalamic-basal gangliar system is responsible for coordinating responses to nonverbal communication and synchronizing interactional rhythms. These processes must be an early component of the attentional process so that its rhythms can be anticipated and attention can be refined according to what seems most pertinent. Similarly, emotional and motivational factors come into play at this level (Kunst-Wilson, 1980). The thalamic-basal gangliar complex also appears to be the major subcortical center for differential hemispheric channeling of perceptual stimuli. This system, which determines which hemisphere will be preferentially activated by input ("upstream processing"), has a downward arm that helps focus attentional processes and an upward projection to differentially activate the hemispheres (Kissin, 1986).

The self-awareness system involves limbic and posterior inferior parietal components as well as the posterior inferior parietal lobe where the majority of the sensory input from the body converges. Integrating as it does emotional and somatosensory input, this area modulates the range of activities we refer to broadly as "feeling" (Kissin, 1986). This is a wider and more pervasive sense of self than the self-awareness that comes through normal consciousness. This system is involved in the generation of a continuing sense of self (Mesulam, 1985), which suggests that alterations in the state of awareness will produce corresponding alterations in the experience of the self. Lesions in this area produce marked distortions in self-awareness (Mesulam, 1978).

There appear to be three possible activation systems available to alert consciousness, and each will result in a unique state (Kissin, 1986). The reticular activating system (RAS) is primarily responsible for normal alert consciousness (Vanderwolf, 1981). It appears that the RAS's connections are relatively more activating for the left hemisphere (Geschwind, 1987). This would account for the general association of the left hemisphere with normal waking consciousness and the substantial changes in self-awareness that occur in altered states of consciousness (Kissin, 1986). Inhibition of the noradrenergic RAS results in different activating systems modulating consciousness: the cholinergic neurons of the pons (for REM sleep) or the dopaminergic neurons of the thalamus (for altered consciousness in the waking state). This latter system and the circuits that regulate its function are of particular interest in hypnosis (Hassler, 1978; Kissin, 1986).

The EEG in the alert state is characterized predominantly by beta and gamma wave activity stimulated by the RAS. The medial thalamic nuclei can inhibit normal RAS activity and produce the lower frequency alpha waves that are typically seen in relaxed awake states. Thus there is a reciprocal relationship between alpha and beta activity. Sustained medial thalamic inhibition of the RAS appears to be the critical feature in altered states of consciousness (Hassler, 1978). Alpha activity generated by the thalamus also stimulates increased theta wave activity produced by the septal-hippocampal complex (Kissin, 1986). Hypnosis thus appears to involve a change from the alert beta-driven state of consciousness to a predominantly alpha-theta-driven altered state of consciousness.

These reactivities reflect the inverse relationship between alpha and beta rhythms. In the normal state of alert arousal, the left hemisphere has a high level of beta waves and a low level of alpha waves. Under the same condition, the right hemisphere has a somewhat lower level of beta waves and a moderate level of alpha waves. The overall effect of these activities as measured by power spectrum techniques would be greater activity in the left hemisphere than in the right, i.e., left-hemispheric dominance.

There are relative changes in these relationships and in power spectral balance during periods of high emotional arousal. Under those conditions, both the left hemisphere and right hemisphere would show high levels of beta activity and almost no alpha activity (alpha blockade). Consequently, in emotional arousal, particularly that associated with negative valence where more energy is directed to the right hemisphere (Davidson, 1974), the two hemispheres would either show essentially equal power spectral levels of activity or the right might actually show slightly greater activity. However, even in the first instance of equality, the experimental data would show a shift to the right because of the change from left-hemispheric dominance in a normal alert condition.

There are still other imbalances during states of low arousal (stage 2 sleep, hypnosis, altered states of consciousness). The left hemisphere would be characterized by the low levels of beta and moderate levels of alpha activity. The right hemisphere would show low levels of beta wave activity and high levels of high-amplitude alpha activity. The overall power spectral effects would show a relative shift to the left hemisphere even though the actual activity of the left hemisphere is markedly decreased. . . .

It appears then that under normal or low arousal conditions, the left hemisphere may tend to be driven more by RAS beta activity and the right hemisphere probably more by thalamic alpha activity. The thesis is suggested here that at low levels of arousal, the right hemisphere has greater activation through thalamic alpha control and thus experiences a different type of awareness than that of the left hemisphere under RAS beta stimulation. On the other hand, with very high arousal levels, the right hemisphere appears to be more directly activated by the RAS beta-wave system and assumes an equal or even greater level of excitability than the left hemisphere. (Kissin, 1986, pp. 228–230)

Most of the electrophysiologic studies of hypnosis have focused on changes in hemispheric function, typically alpha and beta wave activity as monitored by scalp recordings. By contrast, Kissin (1986) has proposed that the major neurophysiologic mechanisms underlying altered states of consciousness involve three major effects: a strong excitation of the reward system of the brain, a relative decrease in RAS-driven beta activity to a thalamic alpha-theta wave activity, and a shift from left hemispheric dominance to right hemispheric dominance. He also proposes that these states are activated through the inhibitory effect of the septal-hippocampal circuit, resulting in a suppression of noradrenergic RAS beta activity and a release of thalamic alpha and theta wave activity. In this process, alpha activity represents an intermediate state between predominantly beta and predominantly theta states (Banquet, 1973; Schuman, 1980; Sabourin, 1982). Thus, though there is strong evidence for a continuum between normal waking states through relaxed states, which are predominantly alpha driven, and profound hypnotic states, in which theta activity is more common, it would appear that measures of theta activity may be critical in identifying characteristics that are unique to the hypnotic state.

Theta Activity in Hypnosis

In animal studies, theta activity has long been associated with consolidating learning (Stumpf, 1965). In a recent review, Winson (1990) demonstrates that theta activity is seen in most mammals during REM sleep and when they are actively engaged in critical behavior. In particular, theta appears to be associated with exploring the environment with regard to its most critical elements and consolidating that information for later use (for example, exploration in the rat, prey behavior in the rabbit, and predatory behavior in the cat are all associated with increased theta activity but more automatic behaviors such as eating and sexual activity are not).

Attentional processes shape the way a task is performed in a number of different ways. The overall level of arousal must be balanced with the importance and difficulty, while irrelevant sensory input is filtered out (Eason, 1984; Oakley, 1990) and specific cognitive resources are allocated (Josiassen, 1990). The presence of theta activity (4–8 Hz) appears to reflect at least two types of changes in attentional processes (Schacter, 1977). Vogel and his coworkers (1968) described two types of theta. Theta occurring in Class I inhibition is seen most commonly in a relaxed, drowsy state, whereas theta occurring in Class II inhibition is associated with efficient, automatic, and sustained mental performance. Class I inhibition is related to a low voltage irregular theta that is spread diffusely over the cortex (Schacter, 1977). During Class I inhibition, sensory stimulation will induce alpha activity, an increase in motor reaction time, and a later decrease in recall of stimuli presented during this phase. In rested subjects, presentation of a stimulus blocks alpha activity. In contrast, drowsy or sleep-deprived subjects typically respond to the presentation of a stimulus with an increase in alpha activity (Schacter, 1977). Also, drowsy or sleep-deprived subjects typically make far more errors whenever Class I theta activity is seen on the EEG.

In contrast, Class II theta appears to reflect a selective inattention that increases efficiency in the solving of problems, perceptual processing, and memory retention (Mundy-Castle, 1951; Ford, 1954; Volavka, 1967; Vogel, 1968; Legewie, 1969; Ishihara, 1972, 1973; Yamaguchi, 1973; Dolce, 1974; Brown, 1971). In contrast to the low voltage irregular and diffuse theta activity that is associated with drowsiness, theta activity seen during problem solving is more commonly focal, and of a higher amplitude and greater regularity, and appears to shift to different areas depending on the nature of the task (Legewie, 1969; Schacter, 1977). Alert subjects who are solving complex problems or being required to make complex perceptual discriminations are more successful when they exhibit an increase in Class II theta activity (Gale, 1971a, 1971b, 1975; Walter, 1967; Daniel, 1967; Adey, 1967; Haslum, 1973; Beatty, 1974). This form of theta, seen in the later stages of hypnosis or meditation, indicates an active, highly focused form of cognitive processing.

Sabourin (1982) has shown a significant relationship between hypnotizability and the low-voltage theta waves both in the trance state and in normal waking states. These findings have been replicated by Delmonte (1984a, 1984b). Interestingly, theta in the trance state occurred predominantly in the frontal and central areas, whereas in the normal waking state it occurred in the occipital (posterior) area. Sabourin has also suggested that theta rhythms are associated with a high frequency of mental imagery.

Increases in theta activity may not be limited to the hypnotic state. Tebēcis (1975b) has suggested that there are greater differences in theta activity between groups than between states. Experienced hypnotic subjects and experienced meditators were shown to demonstrate higher levels of theta activity both during the waking state and during trance or meditation than did inexperienced controls (1975a, 1975b). Theta density was also significantly higher in the hypnosis group than in the meditation group (1975a). These differences were demonstrated in both the eyes-opened and eyes-closed normal waking conditions. There were no significant differences between the groups for alpha, beta, or delta activity. (The occurrence of the increased theta activity in nonhypnotic and open-eyed trance activity together with the differences that theta waves in trance demonstrate electrophysiologically from those that occur in the onset of sleep make it unlikely that this change in theta activity is simply related to drowsiness [Banquet, 1973; Tebēcis, 1975a; Ikemi, 1988].) Thus, experienced hypnotic subjects showed increased theta activity in normal waking and in hypnotized conditions when compared to controls, without showing any significant differences in the level of theta between the two states themselves (Tebēcis, 1975b).

Crawford and her coworkers (1990) examined the relationship between theta activity during hypnotic analgesia. Highly hypnotizable subjects demonstrated significantly greater power in the theta range than did subjects with lower hypnotizability scores. In addition, there was a significant shift of theta activity for the highly hypnotizable subjects during the testing. While experiencing the cold pressor test without hypnosis, the highs had significantly more theta activity in the left hemisphere. When hypnosis was introduced during the pain experience, however, there was a marked decrease in left hemisphere activity and a marked increase in the right frontal and temporal areas.

Further support comes from Japanese studies of a state similar to hypnosis. Increased theta activity and decreased CNV responses have been reported by Ikemi (1986, 1988) during the practice of the "self-regulation method" (SRM), which uses a series of instructions similar to those found in self-hypnosis. Ikemi reported a significant increase in theta and a significant decrease in beta activity during SRM. The changes included increased theta in all areas of the brain and decreases in beta in the central parietal and temporal areas.

A general increase in theta activity in hypnotically susceptible subjects may also be associated with changes in brain responses to stimuli, such as the contingent negative variation (CNV) (Rizzo, 1980). The changes appear to be related to the focused attention found in hypnosis, which minimizes the impact of distracting stimuli. Ikemi's group found similar changes in the CNV (1986, 1988). The reduction in CNV amplitude was most prominent in the central areas—an average 25 percent reduction from controls. Ikemi also reports a significant reduction in the number of errors in a task to evoke the CNV. In other words, the subjects were able to focus attention both during and immediately after the SRM technique far more effectively.

A measure of overall arousal related to anticipation or anxiety concerning a potential stimulus is CNV amplitude. The CNV is also reduced by hypnotic and sedative drugs, but this is typically associated with an increase in errors (Shagass, 1978). In contrast, while the SRM technique produced a reduction of CNV amplitude, at the same time the performance of the subjects improved. Ikemi's interpretation of this finding is that attention was focused on the task at hand and generalized arousal was significantly reduced. This suggests a state of focused awareness typically associated with hypnosis.

The potential confusion between drowsiness and meditative states or hypnosis is less marked in experienced subjects utilizing an active technique. Whereas controls who have been instructed simply to relax show a gradual transition to the early stages of sleep, yoga meditators show little evidence of EEG-defined sleep but do demonstrate stable patterns of alpha and theta EEG activity despite evidence of physiologic relaxation (Elson, 1977; Corby, 1978). Discrete bursts of high voltage theta are more common in experienced meditators (Hebert, 1977) and appear to be related to problem-solving ability (Vogel, 1964) and to hypnotic susceptibility (Galbraith, 1970). The characteristic EEG changes of trance occur in an active-alert hypnotic induction, suggesting that these changes are not a product of simple relaxation (Cikurel, 1990).

It would appear that hypnotic inductions or meditation techniques that emphasize relaxation and comfort (such as TM) may be more likely to produce Class I theta as the subjects relax and become drowsy. In contrast, hypnotic procedures or meditative techniques that emphasize selective attention or performance of a particular task appear to be more likely to produce Class II theta (Schacter, 1977). In meditation, drowsiness is associated with low voltage irregular theta but the alert, relaxed stage is associated with active mental processing and rhythmic theta trains (Taneli, 1987).

The Amygdala and Hippocampus

In contrast to the large number of studies that use scalp recordings there are relatively few that utilize depth recordings. Studies of the amygdaloid-hippocampal complex during hypnosis have been made using depth electrodes implanted in patients with intractable epilepsy who are being considered for neurosurgical procedures. De-Benedittis and Sironi (1986, 1988) have demonstrated that stimulation of the amygdala reliably produces arousal from the hypnotic state, whereas stimulation of the surrounding area is ineffective. Thus, entry into hypnosis is associated with increased hippocampal activity, but increased amygdaloid activity produces a return to the normal waking state. These findings strongly support the role of this complex in the hypnotic state and the notion of an excitatory-inhibitory balance between these two structures.

Their activity in hypnosis is consistent with what we know about their general function. The evidence suggests that the hippocampus is not responsible for a particular psychological function. Rather, its activity plays a pervasive role in a wide variety of "computational-representational activity" (Schmajuk, 1984). The sophisticated functions of the cortex in humankind require an increasingly sensitive mechanism for their orientation to the environment (Sarter, 1985).

The amygdala (the word comes from the Greek for "almond") receives extensive input from the association areas of the cortex and the hippocampus and has extensive two-way connections with the hypothalamus. The amygdala plays a critical role in coordinating emotional states with the appropriate external objects. Combined with the association areas, the amygdala is also essential for the interpretation and expression of the emotional component of language. Because of these functions, it is actively involved in a wide range of behavior that relates to emotional and motivational states.

The amygdala is one of the areas that underwent the most extensive changes in the brain through the evolutionary process. With its close connection to modality-specific association areas, coupled with its connections with the hypothalamic areas that regulate internal states, the amygdala plays an important role in associating emotional states with sensory patterns (Sarter, 1985). The amygdala has extensive connections with three general areas: critical memory circuits, all the modality-specific association areas, and the hypothalamic areas that regulate internal bodily states. "In essence, it is argued that the human amygdala is responsible for activating or reactivating those mnemonic events which are of an emotional significance for the subjects' life history and that this (re-)activation is performed by charging sensory information with appropriate emotional cues" (Sarter, 1985, p. 19).

The hippocampus (which comes from the Greek for "seahorse") has connections similar to those of the amygdala. The hippocampus is responsible for the registration and retrieval of emotionally important memories, making sure they are available for comparison with the external world. The cells of the hippocampus are involved in complex attentional processes that involve chunking the information that is being attended to into relevant segments (Wickelgren, 1979). O'Keefe and Black have theorized that the hippocampus is a complex map of the self and the relevant environment against which incoming sensory input can be compared (1978). This map is critical in maintaining the attentional balance by focusing on stimuli that are considered important and inhibiting attention from being directed elsewhere (Devenport, 1981).

The coordination of all these activities by the amygdaloid-hippocampal complex is inextricably tied in with its attentional functions. Full focused attention is mediated through the complex. Whereas the thalamic basal gangliar complex screens information on its way up to the cortex, the major portion of amygdaloid-hippocampal complex activity occurs during the downstream phase of information processing after information has passed through the cortex (Moscovitch, 1979; Kissin, 1986). This is in keeping with the functions of the cells of the two systems. Cells in the upstream basal ganglia respond to more basic elemental qualities of input, whereas downstream hippocampal cells respond to more complex chunks of information (Edelman, 1987; Wickelgren, 1979).

The amygdaloid-hippocampal complex thus plays a pivotal role in determining the appropriate level of consciousness for the integration of cognitive performance (Edelman, 1989; Murray, 1985). This activity is associated with the presence of the slow theta rhythm that occurs in the hippocampus during altered states of consciousness (Sterman, 1985; DeBenedittis, 1988).

Winson (1977, 1985) has demonstrated that increases in the theta rhythm in the hippocampus are indicative of a specific type of intense neuronal processing that is associated with both a cyclic modulation of input signals and a change in the mode of information processing that corresponds to behavioral changes.

In functional terms, there was a switching of the path of information flow through the hippocampus during each of several behavioral states. Information was passed from the entorhinal cortex through the hippocampus to the limbic system target structures that were different for each behavioral state. This rerouting of information is most readily interpreted as a change from one scheme (or, in computer terms, program) of information processing to another. (Winson, 1985, p. 208)

Thus the amygdala is predominantly excitatory, stimulating externally oriented behavior, and the hippocampus is predominantly inhibitory, stimulating processing of information and comparing it with existing knowledge. Thus, through its connections with the association areas, the amygdaloid-hippocampal complex can compare and integrate new input with existing cognitive models. Together they have extensive connections with the hypothalamus through which they influence the functioning of the autonomic nervous system and hormonal secretion to regulate physical states and level of arousal. With access to the full resources of the association cortex and their role in regulating autonomic and hormonal balance through the hypothalamus, the complex is critical in altering the states of consciousness and in synchronizing face-to-face communication.

It appears that increased theta-wave activity in hypnagogic states is indicative of increased activity of the inhibitory septal-hippocampal circuit, with a corresponding depressant effect on the posterior hypothalamus and a reduction in the activity of the noradrenergic locus coeruleus-driven RAS alert consciousness system. We previously described theta activity in the hippocampus as indicative of increased attentional activity. . . . Attention is of all activities the most selective, and consequently requires the greatest level of inhibition of irrelevant material. Increased hippocampal activity in attention presumably indicates not so much the stimulatory effects of attending, but rather the active inhibitory effect of screening out all irrelevant matter. The actual level of excitation during attention is set by the amygdala. . . .

These reflections on attentional mechanisms help us to reassert the basic formulation of the amygdaloid-hippocampal complex as an excitatory-inhibitory balance control center. In attention both elements, the excitatory amygdala and the inhibitory septal-hippocampal circuit, are coactive, both under the driving influence of the locus coeruleus-driven noradrenergic RAS. In altered states of consciousness, the major energy center has shifted from the locus coeruleus to the thalamus and a dopaminergic alpha-wave pattern now drives the amygdaloid-hippocampal complex. Under the conditions of a dominant thalamic-driven alpha rhythm, septal hippocampal circuit activity becomes pre-eminent, theta-wave activity creeps into the EEG, there is further slowing of the alpha-wave activity, and an altered state of consciousness ensues. (Kissin, 1986, pp. 330–331)

The conjunction of memory, internal regulation, and sensory association functions permits the fine-tuning of the focus of attention with a combination of relative precision and flexibility. The amygdaloid-hippocampal complex may primarily function by selecting the state of consciousness appropriate for the perceived or remembered material, with the amygdala being responsible for excitatory input and the hippocampus (and the related septal complex) for inhibitory processes (Kissin, 1986). The amygdaloid-hippocampal structures in essence determine the noteworthiness of both internal and external stimuli (Margulies, 1985), coordinating focused, or selective, attention, as it takes over from a more generalized, or distributed, attention when important events are identified. The evidence suggests that these hippocampal functions operate in a phasic and rhythmic manner, providing support for the ultradian model (Margulies, 1985).

It is also important to note that the system can be activated by strong emotional experiences, whether intensely pleasurable or intensely painful. Thus, this complex appears to be related to the formation of state-dependent learning and memory (Rossi and Cheek, 1988). This would tend to support the relationship between hypnosis and ecstatic altered states of consciousness, on one hand, and the connection between dissociation and various types of traumatic experience, on the other (Mandell, 1980; Kissin, 1986; Rossi and Cheek, 1988).

The amygdaloid-hippocampal processes can also be activated in the absence of external stimuli. Focused internal attention and absorption produce an expectancy that will produce activation with a significant P_3 wave even in the absence of a stimulus (Picton, 1974). Hypnotic ability might therefore be conceptualized as an increased facility in enhancing amygdaloid-hippocampal activity, resulting in increased theta wave production. By focusing attention during an hypnotic induction, the able hypnotic subject appears to be initiating a change in subcortical function that alters the relationship between the hemispheres.

Thus, though incomplete, the evidence suggests that the changes in hemispheric activity in hypnosis are related to qualitative shifts in amygdaloid-hippocampal information processing and are associated with an increase in alpha theta activity. These shifts may also occur as part of an endogenous rhythm, both in the waking state in the ultradian rhythm and during the REM phase of sleep. The evidence would further suggest that individuals may be able to elicit them deliberately in altered states of consciousness such as hypnosis (Mandell, 1980). For example, experienced meditators have been reported to show higher susceptibility scores and greater amounts of EEG alpha theta than do controls (Delmonte, 1984a, 1984b). They have a greater capacity for relaxed, absorbed attention and are psychologically more open than controls. They also have stronger orienting and recovery responses to stimuli during meditation (Delmonte, 1984a). Thus, subcortical structures may play a critical role both in maintaining the ultradian rhythm and in mediating the effects of past learning and present contextual demands upon hypnotic responsiveness.

The rhythms of behavior reflect intrinsic rhythms of the brain itself. Rossi (1982, 1987) has pointed out the manner in which Erickson utilized minimal cues of spontaneous trance behavior in the form of characteristic alterations in behavior, cognition, and affect, which characteristically follow a ninety-minute ultradian rhythm. What is of particular significance is that these rhythms of the brain are generated by areas in the limbic system that regulate emotional and physiologic states and attentional processes, and that help provide the frame of meaning for personal experiences (Rossi and Cheek, 1988). It would appear that the brain uses these rhythms to weave experiences into our personal structure.

Many questions remain unanswered. Our understanding of cerebral ultradian rhythms has changed as they have been shown to be remarkably responsive to external influences. There is no single ultradian rhythm; rather, there is a group of rhythms that entrain together. The role of brain stem and limbic-hypothalamic clocks is to coordinate these intrinsic rhythms of body and mind (Rasmussen, 1986). There do appear to be striking similarities between the cognitive, behavioral, and electrophysiologic features of the trance state and those observed in the quiescent phase of the ultradian cycle.

Further examination of the link between the ultradian rhythm and hypnosis is indicated with careful consideration of methodological requirements. Particular attention must be paid to the features that synchronize both states. As ultradian rhythms may mark the gates of sleep with reduced sleep latency (Lavie, 1985), they may also indicate changes in the relative care of hypnotic induction over time.

Investigators made significant strides in the field of neurology in the last decades of the nineteenth century by identifying anatomic and functional relationships. Perhaps the last decades of the twentieth century will witness similar progress in psychiatry when corresponding temporal functional patterns are identified.

If it can be established . . . that most classical hypnotic phenomena are more readily experienced during those periods of the ultradian rhythms when they are most available (primarily during the common everyday trance), we may have a resolution of the state-nonstate controversy. The state theorists would be correct in part with the validation that there are real alterations in a broad range of psychophysiological processes relevant for experiencing what has been traditionally called "hypnosis." The nonstate theorists would be correct in part with the validation that there is nothing really unique about the "hypnotic state": it does not have a separate and discrete reality outside the normal range of psychophysiological fluctuations in ultradian rhythms we all experience throughout the 24-hour day. Hypnosis (or trance) does not exist as a mysterious special state. Rather, the experience we have traditionally called "hypnosis" is a ritually induced way of enhancing and vivifying certain naturally occurring ultradian behaviors. (Rossi, 1986a, pp. 105–106)

Further studies that control for some of the methodological differences seen in the existing literature are also required to enlarge our understanding of hemispheric function in hypnosis. Although studies of brain function in hypnosis have not yielded a simple coherent model, they have outlined some important features that require further investigation. These include the notion that though right hemisphere activity is of significance, left hemisphere dynamics are equally in play, particularly in the early stages of hypnosis; the importance of training and repeated studies over time differentiating between naive and trained subjects as well as between those who score well and poorly on hypnotic susceptibility scales; and, perhaps most important, the differences in task demands and context. Researchers should also pay attention to phasic EEG changes over time and the significance of frontal and central alpha theta activity. Early theories emphasized a sort of neophrenology, "localizing" hypnotic phenomena in the right hemisphere. That hemisphere does show an advantage in specific forms of visuospatial, emotional, and attentional functions (Heilman, 1986), which are critical in synchronizing interactional rhythms and interpreting contextual input (see chapter 3). Some studies of subjects with low hypnotic ability suggest not an absence of response but a very active and effective interference with the expected changes by the left hemisphere (Gruzelier, 1985). Thus, the right hemisphere may play a special role in the hypnotic state, but full involvement appears to require the active participation of both hemispheres.

Gruzelier and his coworkers (1987b) used a variety of electrodermal, haptic, electrocortical, and divided visual field evidence to chart the relative activity of the two hemispheres during hypnosis. They demonstrated that an initial left hemisphere bias followed by an inhibition of left hemispheric processing was critical for hypnotic induction. Simultaneously, a gradual increase of right hemispheric activity (which also increases left hemisphere inhibition) coincides with the emergence of increased visual imagery, sensitivity to contextual cues, and focused attention. They postulate that a fourth stage arises when a specific task is introduced. In this stage, hemispheric activity is contingent upon the nature of the task and involves a more efficient use of cerebral resources. This supports the suggestion put forward by Crawford (1983a) that hypnotic ability is based upon not only cognitive but psychophysiologic flexibility.

Hypnotic ability appears to be correlated with absorptive capacity and the use of vivid imagery both during hypnosis and at other times (Telegen, 1974; Crawford, 1989a). This ability appears to be associated with a greater intensity of affect (Crawford, 1989b, 1989c). Instructive and vivid daydreaming is associated with hypnotic ability both in adults and in children (Crawford, 1982a; Allen, 1985). Observing this mounting evidence for a psychological flexibility, Crawford (1990) has proposed that these abilities are associated with greater physiologic flexibility: an enhanced ability to change the focus of attention, an efficient distribution of resources in response to problems, and a higher degree of laterality (the ability to use either the right or the left hemisphere according to the demands of the situation). In support of this hypothesis she cites the mounting evidence of greater EEG hemispheric specificity and greater degrees of right or left hemisphere activity according to task in highly hypnotizable subjects (MacLeod-Morgan, 1979, 1982; Karlin, 1980; Mészáros, 1985; DePascalis, 1986, 1988). In further support of this view, Crawford and her coworkers have presented evidence for significantly greater differences in hemispheric activity in both alpha and beta activity at rest, in hypnosis following suggestion, and during suggested emotional states (Crawford, 1989c, 1990; Mészáros, 1989; Sabourin, 1991).

The evidence suggests that hypnotic flexibility involves not an absolute shift but a cooperative reorganization of total cerebral function. This reorganization seems to be driven by the activity of subcortical structures, particularly the amygdaloid-hippocampal complex and the medial thalamus. These limbic structures modulate cognitive, emotional, motivational, and attentional processes to ensure the appropriate state of consciousness. In hypnosis this involves inhibition of generalized awareness and an increase in alpha and theta activity. Cerebral function in hypnosis represents a balance between intrinsic cerebral rhythms and extrinsic contextual demands.

The brain has a structure in time as well as in space. There is growing evidence for the importance of a number of internal rhythms, including the ultradian, for emotion, perception, cognition, and behavior. These rhythms involve the whole brain and are reflected in transitions in the type and focus of attention, the selection of cognitive strategies, and the relative amounts of hemispheric activity. These rhythms, however, are not rigid but extremely sensitive to context, serving an adaptive function in helping to synchronize the individual with the environment. Rhythms modulate input so that learning can be efficient and pertinent to ongoing concerns. In this sense, these rhythms are partially shaped by context while also shaping the way in which that context is perceived. Hypnosis can thus be conceptualized not as an exotic state but as a socially mediated process that arises from the everyday information processing of human cognition. Later chapters will examine the ways in which these states can be utilized, either in a social context to create meaning and identity (chapter 7) or in a medical context to enhance self-regulation of a disease process (chapter 8).

6 A STORY IN MIND

Though analogy is often misleading, it is the least misleading thing we have.

Samuel Butler, 1912

Part of the biologic heritage of the human facility for face-to-face communication is the way in which the brain organizes information. That organization appears to be fundamentally metaphoric in nature. Cognitive organization develops by our matching new or complex experiences with what we already know. Repetition of what we understand with gradual alterations leads to the extension of our knowledge through both conscious and unconscious learning. All learning, in a real sense, depends on having a story in mind.

PROSPERO'S SPELL

Absorbing attention has always been the first task of the oral poet, who used language and story to entrance an audience, both for entertainment and for instruction. Standing as he did in the Elizabethan world, halfway in the transition from the oral world to literacy, Shakespeare was the master of these verbal techniques. He understood the need not only for comprehension, the intellectual understanding of events, but also for apprehension, which includes a more sensual and emotional involvement (Barton, 1984). One of the best examples of this form of "hypnotic" involvement comes at the beginning of *The Tempest*.

The play opens with that symbol of surprise and impending doom: a shipwreck in a great storm. Not only were the thunder and lightning and other special effects likely to quiet the audience and get them quickly to their seats, the subject matter would also have had a compelling effect, for virtually everyone in Elizabethan London was involved in some form of maritime venture. Shipwreck was a form of personal and financial disaster that touched the lives of everyone in one way or other.

In the next scene, Shakespeare abruptly shifts gears. The tempest has vanished, and we are back on dry land observing a conversation between Prospero and his daughter, Miranda. Prospero reveals that the storm and shipwreck are the product of his magic and that the ship's crew is in no danger. He tells her to sit comfortably and listen intently, and he will reveal to her the significance of the wreck and its connection with their own arrival on the island when she was a small girl. While Miranda is entranced with the story, so is the audience. We participate in her anxiety and its relief and her absorption in this complex and mysterious tale. As he finishes, Prospero concludes:

Here cease more questions:
Thou art inclined to sleep: 'tis a good dulness,
And give it way: I know thou canst not choose.

[*Miranda sleeps*]

Come away, servant, come. I am ready now.
Approach, my Ariel, come.

With this hypnotic induction, the real action of the play begins and, with it, a process of psychological transformation that will involve all the characters. The story is as absorbing and moving today as it was nearly four hundred years ago. It illustrates not only Shakespeare's mastery of language and verbal rhythm but also the power of story and metaphor to communicate the most complex and subtle of human truths. It demonstrates our inherent capacity both to comprehend and to apprehend the language of metaphor.

But the use of metaphor is not restricted to poetry and drama. Everyday language, too, is rich and varied. Even in our most mundane conversations, we play with meaning to express ourselves. Metaphor pervades our normal conceptual system. Most of human experience and communication is open-ended and ambiguous. Metaphor enables us to understand these experiences in terms of what we already know. Meaning is defined by social convention and direct personal experience. It is this combination that defines "the meaning of meaning" (Putnam, 1975). The "basic domain of experience," the route for metaphorical constructions, is shared by all members of a culture. These experiences include our bodily awareness and our interactions with the physical environment and with other people.

Listen closely to anything anyone says, and soon you'll hear analogies. We speak of time in terms of space, as like a fluid that's *running out;* we talk of our friends in physical terms, as in *"Mary and John are very close."* All of our language is riddled and stitched with curious ways of portraying things as though they belonged to alien realms.

We sometimes call these "metaphors," our ways to transport thoughts between the various mental realms. Some metaphors seem utterly pedestrian, as when we speak of "taking steps" to cause or prevent some happening. Other metaphors seem more miraculous, when unexpected images lead to astonishing insights—as when a scientist solves a problem by conceiving of a fluid as made of tubes or of a wave as an array of overlapping, expanding spheres. When such conceptions play important roles in our most productive forms of thought, we find it natural to ask, *"What is a metaphor?"* But we rarely notice how frequently we use the same techniques in ordinary thought.

What, then, *is* a metaphor? It might be easy to agree on functional definitions like *"A metaphor is that which allows us to replace one kind of thought with another."* But when we ask for a structural definition of "metaphor," we find no unity, only an endless variety of processes and strategies. (Minsky, 1986, p. 299)

Lakoff and Johnson have mounted a detailed critique of the traditional view of human reasoning they label "objectivism" (1980). According to the old model, metaphor was part of the world of "primary process" thinking, the magical and fantastic inner world of the primitive, the child, and the psychotic. Maturation consisted of the development toward "secondary process" thinking in which rational analysis is learned and then applied independent of current personal experience. By contrast, the new model suggests that "metaphor is pervasive in everyday life, not just in language but in thought and action. Our ordinary conceptual system, in terms of which we both think and act, is fundamentally metaphorical in nature" (Lakoff and Johnson, 1980, p. 3).

The cognitive patterns used to organize information are not objective but personal and metaphorical (Lakoff, 1987; Johnson, 1987). "Furthermore, their structures typically depend on the nature of the human body, especially on our perceptual capacities and motor skills" (Johnson, 1987, p. xi). Perceptual processes pervade cognition. Meaning derives from experience with regard to its content and to structure.

In this view, imagination is not restricted to fantasy or creativity. Instead, it underlies day-to-day thinking and decision making by providing the format through which we make sense of our world. Metaphor, then, is not a fanciful elaboration but, rather, expresses the dynamic interaction between language and direct experience.

On the traditional view, reason is abstract and disembodied. On the new view, reason has a bodily basis. The traditional view sees reason as literal, as primarily about propositions that can be objectively either true or false. The new view takes imaginative aspects of reason—metaphor, metonymy, and mental imagery—as central to reason, rather than as a peripheral and inconsequential adjunct to the literal.

. . . In the new view, meaning is a matter of what is meaningful to thinking, functioning beings. The nature of the thinking organism and the way it functions in its environment are of central concern to the study of reason. (Lakoff, 1987, p. xi)

THE IMAGE SCHEMA

Johnson (1987) proposes two major types of imaginative structure that are central to all forms of cognition. The first is the *image schema,* "a recurring, dynamic pattern of our perceptual interactions and motor programs that gives coherence and structure to our experience" (p. xiv). Image schemata are the core of our conceptual systems and are grounded in perception, bodily movement, and experience. For example, because of our lifetime experience of gravity, we have an up-down orientation that provides us with a schema that can be applied to any concept describing continuous change—for example, a person may go "down" into trance or go "up" into a more alert state of consciousness. In this way, cognition is "embodied"—that is, it grows out of physical experience. Further, though these structures are preconceptual and nonpropositional, they can be used to elaborate metaphor and provide meaning. In fact, because of their fundamental and automatic nature, they are even more powerful than abstract propositional thinking.

Cognitive models represent the physical world as perceived by our senses with a high degree of reliability and consistency. Cognition involves, among other things, the creation of a mental space for the manipulation of concepts that is modeled on our understanding of physical space (Fauconnier, 1985). Visual patterns, geometric shapes, and the time taken to study and manipulate these patterns, parallel actual experiences very closely (Shepard, 1984; Kosslyn, 1987).

For example, the nature of mental space affects our ability to use visual imagery. Altering cognitive strategies alters the imagery and the experience. It is possible to increase the representational capacity of spatial imagery by encouraging subjects to use a three-dimensional rather than two-dimensional representation (Kerr, 1987). Moreover, specific mental images are associated with specific spontaneous eye movements, patterns of face and arm muscle movements, and the alpha activity of the right occipital area of the EEG (Lusebrink, 1987).

The way in which the stimulus is evaluated and processed is more important than the stimulus itself. Psychophysiologic changes appear to follow the pattern of emotional response or the nature of the internal imagery rather than the object per se (Carroll, 1982). Some subjects may show the same kind of response to many different stimuli (in terms of either intensity or direction), whereas others may have a wider degree of discrimination. Similarly, subjects may group stimuli quite differently, and these differences will reflect both contextual demands and individual variation (Kosslyn, 1987). Subjects who use vivid visual imagery as a memory strategy tend to do better on tests of creative thinking (Shaw, 1987).

The image schema emerges from the continuous interaction between perceptual and motor programs (Neisser, 1976; Jeannerod, 1985), which involve components at virtually every level of the central nervous system. Thus though originating in sensory awareness, they are not limited to a single sensory modality but contain components of all the modalities (Brooks, 1968).

"Experience," then, is to be understood in a very rich, broad sense as including basic perceptual, motor-program, emotional, historical, social, and linguistic dimensions . . . rejecting the classical empiricist notion of experience as reducible to passively received sense impressions, which are combined to form atomic experiences. By contrast, experience involves everything that makes us human—our bodily, social, linguistic, and intellectual being combined in complex interactions that make up our understanding of our world. (Johnson, 1987, p. xvi)

The basic image schemata structures appear to be strict analogues of the various sensory modalities. Our ability for cross-modal transfer of information allows us to use these structures in novel contexts (Marks, 1987a, 1987b). Thus, we can be aware of a physical sense of balance or "balance" in the composition of a painting. In fact, this type of metaphor functions as a form of creative synesthesia in which we can also talk about the "bright" sound of a trumpet or the "loud" colors in a painting. Thus, though direct physical experience serves as a basis, metaphoric elaboration is very much an active psychological process. We do not passively accept patterns imposed on us from outside but actively work to structure and restructure our perceptual basis. It is in this sense that the brain is fundamentally creative. This type of cognitive process is highly goal-directed and not the result of the application of disembodied and abstract principles. The goal-directedness of these processes also implies that they are heavily context-dependent: we decide on what constitutes meaning on the basis of what is meaningful in a particular situation.

These basic-level categories are not constructed of atomic units but are perceived as functioning wholes. This involves elements of our basic physical experience and our memory of past experiences with similarly structured situations and personal and social constructs (Beck, 1987). Image schemata are gestalt structures that emerge from repeated exposure to these patterns of experience. These are gestalt structures in that meaning is derived from its distinction between figure and background, a meaning that cannot be reduced to specific elements but emerges from their relationships. Thus they are preconceptual and nonpropositional structures of that experience. But though image schemata are not propositional, they are essential for formal logic. They function by representing to us the kinds of connections that may be made. Johnson (1987) and Turner (1987) demonstrate that the operations of formal language, including our understanding of causation, arise from our experience of the world around us. The image schema constrains understanding both of a basic experience and of metaphorical extensions by limiting the number of possible connections and the forms in which these connections can be made. Johnson describes the identification of the image schematic structures as "putting the body back into the mind" (Johnson, 1987, p. xxxvi).

In actual use, human reasoning need not be consistent with the canons of formal logic. As Nisbett and Ross (1980) have shown, we have no difficulty comprehending and accepting as meaningful patterns that violate the strictures of logic provided that they tally with the structure of our experience. This means that, in actual practice, meaning takes on a much richer sense than the narrow one imposed by the older model. In this context, the meaning of traditional logic is a subset of a broader notion of what is meaningful to human beings. *"Propositional content is possible only by virtue of a complex web of nonpropositional schematic structures that emerge from our bodily experience.* Once meaning is understood in this broader, enriched manner, it will become evident that the structure of rationality is much richer than any set of abstract logical patterns completely independent of the patterns of our physical interactions in and with our environment" (Johnson, 1987, p. 5).

Central, or basic-level, categories determine the possible extensions because of their connection to real-life experience. In other words, basic-level categories are the easiest concepts for people to recognize and share, and the further one gets away from them, the more idiosyncratic and arbitrary are likely to be the connections. This use of basic-level structure is also found in semantic studies (Zubin, 1986) and is borne out by cross-cultural experimental evidence (Berlin, 1974; Hunn, 1977).

The notion that there are central cognitive processes that are based on our experience of the physical world and from which other models are then elaborated is also supported by the evidence of language acquisition and cognitive development in children (Karmiloff-Smith, 1986; Scholnick, 1987). The image schemata begin to develop in infancy with the ability to orient in space around auditory, kinesthetic, or visual cues, long before the development of complex linguistic and analytic abilities. These skills combine with the basic schemata to allow for the development of metaphoric thinking (Haskell, 1989).

METAPHOR

The second imaginative structure listed by Johnson is *metaphor*

conceived as a pervasive mode of understanding by which we project patterns from one domain of experience in order to structure another domain of a different kind. So conceived, metaphor is not merely a linguistic mode of expression; rather, it is one of the chief cognitive structures by which we are able to have coherent, ordered experiences that we can reason about and make sense of. Through metaphor, we make use of patterns that obtain in our physical experience to organize our more abstract understanding. Understanding via metaphorical projection from the concrete to the abstract makes use of physical experience in two ways. First, our bodily movements and interactions in various physical domains of experience are structured, . . . and that structure can be projected by metaphor onto abstract domains. Second, metaphorical understanding is not merely a matter of arbitrary fanciful projection from anything to anything with no constraints. Concrete bodily experience not only constrains the "input" to the metaphorical projections but also the nature of the projections themselves, that is, the kinds of mappings that can occur across domains. (Johnson, 1987, pp. xiv–xv)

Metaphor, the description of one thing in terms of another, is a personal and social process for elaboration from image schemata. Metaphors are not random fantasies but are highly structured in parallel with the schema on which they are based (Haskell, 1988). Although the image schemata that form the root metaphors for our understanding of the world come from our common physical experiences, the manner in which they are used is highly contextually bound. Comparative studies of other cultures have shown that the conceptions of space and time, and even the basic categories of visual and auditory perception, are defined by cultural and personal variables as much as by our neurologic capacities (Johnson, 1987). This ecological structure constrains the types of elaborations that will work effectively. Metaphor is powerful because of these analogical parallels with the personal structure of experience.

According to this view, thinking proceeds not in a linear fashion but in several directions simultaneously via a cluster of associations. Rather than comprising linear propositional arguments, our conceptual thinking is arranged in multidimensional gestalts that are defined by categories that emerge from our natural experience. These gestalt properties resist reduction but facilitate linking. Consequently, similarly structured language is more compelling (easier to assimilate) than a series of formal propositions.

According to this model, analytical and analogical approaches to understanding are simply end points along the continuum. Propositional thinking is a particular subset of human thinking that has been formalized and structured by the development of literacy. Literacy first allowed the development of an idea of a logic that was independent of any situational needs. Metaphor will be the more useful of the two for understanding open-ended, complex, or contextually varying experiences.

The process of problem solving usually is not "logical"; insight follows when a person suddenly sees the logical connections between various aspects of a problem that were previously opaque. Logic is not really a very useful process when we are confronted with a new problem. The logical connections are apparent only when we have solved the problem. Insight is the process wherein we consider the various parameters of a problem and then abruptly see the logical connections that we previously were not aware of. In a sense insight is akin to the process of artistic creation. It does not involve the principles of formal logic, though we usually can provide a formal logical analysis of the problem after we have had the flash of insight that allows us to solve the problem. (Lieberman, 1984, p. 327)

Metaphor is highly goal-directed. The purpose of metaphor is communication, particularly in situations where new meanings are being developed (Gerrig, 1988). Furthermore, its use is systematic. Studies of reaction time show that subjects move systematically from familiar metaphors to more complex ones when the simpler ones are inadequate (Blank, 1988). These extensions occur automatically; they are attempts to extend meaning in the face of uncertainty.

The analogical reasoning used in metaphorical thinking has been the subject of considerable recent study. Investigators have appreciated that in areas of uncertainty, such as ongoing research or technological development, the lack of clear-cut data makes traditional analytic methods inappropriate. Analogical reasoning, therefore, is important in prediction, design, transmission of new concepts, and decision making (G. A. Klein, 1987).

Klein makes the important point that traditional studies of decision making (of how people translate their concepts into behavior) have been concerned about the question of bias, of how people deviate systematically from an analytic ideal. He suggests that these should be viewed not as traits to be eradicated but as part of the architecture of human thought. For example, people will predictably reason by analogy with previous experiences when faced with uncertainty. Furthermore, they are likely to work from one or two examples rather than checking through all the logical possibilities. In fact, the best decision makers are skilled precisely because they quickly identify useful options rather than devoting time to identifying a whole list of possible alternatives (Ebbesen, 1980; Woods, 1984; Hammond, 1984; Rasmussen, 1985; G. A. Klein, 1986). Klein further suggests that the characteristics central to the effective use of analogical reasoning in decision making include a heightened situational awareness, flexibility, and the ability to identify and stick with the most effective strategy.

Metaphor is a quick, informal way of envisioning a situation in which there are many variable or interacting causes, making for ambiguity and uncertainty (Townsend, 1988). We can use metaphor to form flexible models that reflect a complex situation in a way that allows us to identify critical features. This allows for the clarification of goals and increased situational awareness; we can apply information from a wide variety of sources that may not be obviously connected to the problem at hand. Metaphor is memorable, allowing for easy memory formation and retrieval. It can also be open-ended, allowing for the generation of new understandings and for the evolution of concepts and behavior. "This may suggest a model of memory as an 'analogy bank.' This may differ from semantic models that treat memory as organized files of abstracted features. An episodic model of memory may be better able to account for how concrete experiences are stored, including contextual and emotional cues, that allow for the retrieval of those experiences in a variety of demand situations" (G. A. Klein, 1987, p. 214).

The use of metaphor underlines the creative, context-dependent nature of memory. McCabe (1988) has shown that metaphor structure influences what we recall in a variety of ways. The relationship is a fluid one and reflects the individual's interpretation of demand characteristics of the context, the vividness of the imagery, and the nature of the central concept. The strength of the imagery, the quality of the relation between image and object, and the structural similarity all increase both the level of recall and the perceived quality of the metaphor.

McCabe (1988) performed a series of experiments using both written and tape-recorded metaphors found in spontaneous speech. She found that quality, similarity (isomorphism), and vividness of imagery of the metaphor resulted in greater learning and retention.

In summary, every aspect of context studied had an impact on judging, imaging, and remembering metaphor. Elsewhere (McCabe, 1980, 1983) the length of context was found to affect the relationship between perceived quality and similarity. Here, mode of presentation affected levels of recall and perceived quality. The types of materials found in different contexts occasioned different relationships between memory and three attributes: imagery, similarity and quality. (McCabe, 1988, p. 130)

More complicated issues will be described not by a single metaphor but by a group of metaphors that usually fit together in a coherent fashion (Lakoff and Johnson, 1980). The various metaphors will highlight different aspects. They are connected in related clusters that are not logically driven but formed on the basis of primary experience. The universal nature of such experience implies that the same types of connections will be valid for most individuals.

What may at first appear to be random, isolated metaphorical expressions . . . turn out to be not random at all. Rather, they are part of whole metaphorical systems that together serve the complex purpose of characterizing the concept of an argument in all of its aspects, as we conceive them. Though such metaphors do not provide us with a single consistent concrete image, they are nonetheless coherent and do fit together when there are overlapping entailments, though not otherwise. The metaphors come out of our clearly delineated and concrete experiences that allow us to construct highly abstract and elaborate concepts. (Lakoff and Johnson, 1980, p. 105)

The tendency of metaphorical structures to be linked in families is a product of the way that information is organized in the brain (Marks, 1987c). Memory units, or engrams, are linked by associative learning into more complex structures, which tend to share many of their simpler constituent elements. Hence, activation of one complex will tend to activate other complexes if a sufficient number of the simpler units are common property. Both auditory and visual information appears to be processed in this way (Oden, 1977).

We structure the less concrete and more ambiguous concepts in terms of a larger number of more concrete concepts. This means that the larger domains of personal experience can be both described and, ultimately, transformed by the number of potential metaphors. The implication is that a concept cannot be broken down into discrete elements and still be understandable. Our overall understanding of a concept comes from the interaction of the various metaphorical concepts. This is the paradox of metaphorical thinking; a recombination and novel juxtaposition of previously understood concepts can be used to obtain new understanding.

Thus, as with image schemata, some of the central qualities of the metaphorical concept are not discrete properties but gestalts, products of interactions and context. Understanding is achieved by our perceptual, emotional, motor, and cognitive associations with the image and not from some external logic. These are the parameters of the interactional properties. We can alter the boundaries of metaphors by either extending them or narrowing them. Metaphors are in this sense, again, open-ended, responding fluidly to contextual needs.

The limitations of metaphorical thinking are also obvious: the boundaries may be extremely vague and hard to define; the process is often not immediately available for verification; and the results may be imprecise. To emphasize the central role of metaphor does not constitute an endorsement for the illiterate or the illogical. Literacy and its consequence, propositional logic, are important cultural tools that, despite limitations, have generated concepts such as science, art, social justice, and personal freedom. My argument is that they supplement as well as alter the underlying oral and metaphorical inheritance.

As Nicholas Humphrey (1984) has suggested, social interaction is as fundamental a human experience as gravity. Other people and their behavior shape our preconceptual structures as surely as do physical experiences. Cognition is embodied by experience with others, and this experience is as important for key metaphors as are physical forces. Humphrey has suggested that our conceptual structures evolved as a way of flexibly tuning and synchronizing our social interactions. In oral (nonliterate) societies, thinking is predominantly social thinking. These cultures see the universe surrounding them as alive and personal, and they treat their world accordingly (Luria, 1976; Ong, 1982). Social interactions are a major pressure in human evolution. Thought follows social structure.

In this light Mark Turner (1987) has demonstrated the central role of kinship as a powerful metaphor in human thinking. We know from anthropological studies that kinship structures are important in defining social structure, personal roles in society, and the systems of obligations and responsibilities as well as rights that pertain to each individual. Turner demonstrates that kinship can be extended metaphorically to account for a complex system of analogical reasoning that underlies our notions of causality, similarity, and human creativity.

Examples from the physical world can provide us with an image schema for basic intellectual operations, but at more complex levels kinship analogies are particularly powerful. In fact, notions of kinship and family resemblance provide us with our basic metaphor for describing metaphor. As the title of Turner's book, *Death Is the Mother of Beauty*, suggests, kinship patterns are used metaphorically to reflect a causation that is somewhat mysterious and ambiguous and that generates consequences that are similar but not identical.

William James described consciousness as a flowing stream, most distinctive in its preservation of a continuity while remaining in flux. Turner demonstrates, with a wealth of examples from literature and science, that the notion of a general flow that maintains similarity but incorporates change finds a natural link with our understanding of biological inheritance. He also shows that there is a limited number of inference patterns that the kinship model will allow. (For example, "Isolation is a cause of anxiety" is more limited and less fertile than "Solitude is the mother of anxieties.") Complex situations (and this includes virtually everything that human beings think, feel, and do) will always require metaphors that are both vivid and flexible.

Metaphor is central to cognition, whether conscious or unconscious. As Putnam (1981) has shown, unless abstract symbols are mediated through personal experience they have no meaning, and metaphor has been described as providing this mediation: it is a bridge between semantics and pragmatics (Townsend, 1988). It functions to transduce information and integrate behavior by mediating between our cognitive models and our interpretation of the context, between what we think and what we do.

Lakoff and Johnson suggest that the use of language and its development is an example of the functioning of this structure. Sweetser has demonstrated the extensive role of metaphoric understanding in the developmental changes of the semantic structure of Indo-European languages (1990). The way that linguistic categories are used in different cultures serves to reflect the way in which those cultures emphasize what is important. These concerns in turn influence not only cognition but basic perception (Kay, 1978; Berlin, 1974; Smith, 1981). Knowledge cannot be dissociated from human minds and the contexts in which they find themselves. The use of metaphor is not simply a passive recognition of similarities between two situations but an active structuring that allows the brain to observe similarity in the processes of different mental models (Johnson, 1987). Indeed, there is evidence that this form of manipulation of cognitive models is critical for scientific thinking (Gentner, 1982). Dennett (1984) uses the term "intuition pump" to describe this process.

The objectivist model sought to establish truth by attempting to describe an abstract system that exists outside of human minds. By contrast, Lakoff and Johnson emphasize that our logical structures emerge from the interaction of our subjective experiences and our imaginative processes. The new model, which they call experientialism, emphasizes that our concepts are understood within the framework of a wider conceptual network based on human experience. At the base of all of our cognitive processes, including language and formal logic, is the ability to use and understand metaphor. Similarly, metaphor is a vehicle that can cross the boundary between conscious and unconscious processes.

UNCONSCIOUS LEARNING

Unconscious cerebral activity is implicit in the creative function of metaphor. Once considered impossible by definition, unconscious learning has been the subject of considerable recent research (Kihlstrom, 1987; Libet, 1985). Carefully designed studies, using a variety of methodologies, have demonstrated learning effects for both auditory and visual sensory input that has been processed outside of conscious awareness (Bowers, 1986; Lewicki, 1987; Kihlstrom, 1987).

Not only can stimuli in any sensory modality influence behavior without conscious awareness, but the types of information are also extremely variable. These include: "subliminal" stimuli that occur too quickly for conscious awareness (Lewicki, 1987); state-dependent stimuli that are associated with one particular state of consciousness or pattern of physiologic responses (Rossi, 1986a); simultaneous stimuli that compete for attention, as in the dichotic listening task (Lewicki, 1986); and stimuli for which conscious memory has been lost (Bowers, 1987). Such learning can have distinctive effects on emotional states without being recognized (Robles, 1987). Moreover, the boundary between consciously and unconsciously registered information appears to be fluid with such factors as cognitive style (Sheehan, 1982), individual differences in absorptive capacity (Hilgard, 1977), social expectations (Spanos, 1986a), and developmental stage (Karmiloff-Smith, 1986) playing a role in which the boundaries may be settled.

Karmiloff-Smith (1986) has approached the relation between conscious and unconscious meaning from the perspective of childhood development. She argues that cognitive development requires a recursive three-phase model that depends on basic-level image schemata and multiple levels of metaphoric representation in which conscious awareness is only the final stage. Thus, in this view, conscious access emerges from the interaction of metaphoric structures at multiple levels.

Lewicki (1986) outlined three criteria for a nonconscious process: (1) the individual has no conscious control over the operation of the process, which appears to occur outside of awareness and in automatic fashion; (2) we can infer the process only by seeing its results, not by any direct knowledge of how it's constituted; and (3) the format that regulates the function (the "nonconscious cognitive algorithm") is not consciously learned but generalized from a number of separate experiences. Lewicki hypothesizes that these processes may go unnoticed or undervalued by the conscious mind. He suggests:

Cognitive algorithms seem to be responsible for much more than performing highly specialized cognitive operations maintaining the consciously controlled processes ("housekeeping operations"), like installing new information in memory or scanning the memory in search of desired information. They seem to be ubiquitous and directly responsible for outcomes of various "high level" cognitive processes traditionally attributed to a conscious level of processing, like judgments, inferences, or evaluations. (Lewicki, 1986, p. 11)

To account for nonconscious acquisition of information, Lewicki (1986) has proposed the term "internal processing algorithm" (IPA). Explicit in his hypothesis is the idea that the IPA is not only a body of knowledge but a strategy for selecting perceptions, processing data, and initiating appropriate responses. The research to date supports the IPA model, demonstrating that the unconscious processing of information does not occur in an impersonal "objective" fashion but is linked in categories based on individual relevance. These studies suggest that the information thus obtained is crucial in the modulation of interpersonal relationships and personality development.

Lewicki reviews an extensive body of literature suggesting that much information that affects our performance is processed on a level below conscious awareness. A wide variety of brief or subtle auditory and visual inputs can be shown to be registered physiologically even though they occur below the threshold of our conscious awareness. These stimuli also influence subsequent behavior, altering strategies used in solving complex tasks and affecting judgment and emotional responses to other people. Moreover, there is a growing body of evidence that such information can be stored in long-term memory (and consequently has the potential for the long-term influence of behavior) without the need for conscious mediation. Lewicki concludes:

The results demonstrate that people acquire more information than they are aware of, that this nonconsciously acquired information is stored in long-term memory in a form not available at the level of conscious awareness, and that this information nonconsciously influences subsequent relevant cognitive processes. . . .

Nonconsciously acquired information (even if it pertains to a single, concrete instance) can bias the process of encoding subsequently encountered stimuli, thereby promoting the self-perpetuation of internal cognitive algorithms. (Lewicki, 1986, p. 220)

Implicit learning of auditory information has been studied using the dichotic listening method. In this task, subjects wearing headphones receive different information simultaneously in each ear. They are required to repeat what they hear coming from one ear and to try to ignore the other. (The right ear usually has an advantage in right-handed subjects.) Words being heard by the neglected ear rarely enter conscious awareness. Words coming via the unattended channel, however, have been shown to alter autonomic nervous system responses (Corteen, 1972, 1974; von Wright, 1975) and to influence semantic processing of the attended words (Lewis, 1970; Treisman, 1974). In addition, words on the unattended channel that have particular individual significance have a much greater impact (Nielsen, 1981; Bargh, 1982). This may reflect a greater activation of the right hemisphere for salient stimuli. This hemisphere, EEG studies have shown, is much more actively involved in listening to stories than it is in processing technical material (Ornstein, 1979).

Studies using visual stimuli have shown the same sorts of results. Words presented on a screen so quickly that they are below our perceptual ability to recognize that they were there at all could be reliably shown to influence subsequent word association tasks (Marcel, 1980, 1983; Fowler, 1981). In other words, visual data of which the subject was consciously unaware clearly influenced subsequent behavior.

More important for our purposes, these effects are not simply related to linguistic tasks. Bargh (1982), Czyzewska (1984), and Lewicki (1986) have all demonstrated that such information can change the subject's emotional state, critically affect the way they evaluate other people, and change preexisting attitudes concerning social interactions. Hasher and Zacks (1984) have shown that much basic information about the environment is learned unconsciously. And Reber (1976, 1985) concluded that "complex structures, such as those underlying language, socialization, perception and sophisticated games are acquired implicitly and unconsciously" (1976).

Moreover, not only are these processes out of conscious awareness, but the conscious mind quickly denies their existence. In a study by Nisbett and Wilson (1977), when subjects were confronted with the suggestion that their behavior had been influenced in a subliminal fashion, "virtually all subjects denied it, usually with a worried glance at the interviewer suggesting that they felt either that they had misunderstood the question or were dealing with a madman" (p. 244).

The IPA does not have to be consistent with consciously processed knowledge or attitudes and may use either formal logic (Reber, 1985) or a more synthetic approach (Brooks, 1978), or both. The issue is a critical one. Brooks has proposed that these processes are unavailable to conscious, verbal, analytic modes of thought and that they operate by a nonanalytic analogical system of information processing. This may in part explain the discrepancies between the learning the subjects demonstrated and their verbal rationales. The hypothesis that the rules under which unconscious cognitive algorithms work are different in those processes used in conscious cognitive strategies is an appealing one. If there is not a single common verbal or symbolic language, it would explain why these processes are inherently unavailable to conscious awareness. Moreover, it would explain the astonishing ability of these processes to form complex visual, auditory, and motor strategies on the basis of what consciously seems to be either insufficient or trivial information (Runeson, 1983; Beair, 1984; Lewicki, 1986).

The relative strength of the various schemata may be determined by their positioning either anatomically or in timing. The brain achieves stability by combining spatial organization (the linking of particular anatomical structures) and temporal organization (repeating cycles of activity produce a resonance that preserves the integrity of the system). The connecting step is the process of synaptic facilitation (Kandel, 1982). The temporal processes and their resonance facilitate information transduction through the synaptic channels (Kissin, 1986). In this way, structural and temporal integrity can be maintained while learning is incorporated into the system. Changes in the temporal patterning change the synaptic connections, which, as a result, changes the temporal organization and resonance of the module (Bateson, 1987).

In addition, the role of emotion in governing competition between schemata is critical. The intensity of emotional accompaniment for any particular state of mind serves to stabilize it and prevent its being supplanted by another. Autonomic nervous system arousal increases when individuals attempt to assimilate new information into existing schemata, and that arousal will have an emotional evaluation (Fiske, 1981, 1982; Mandler, 1982). These emotional evaluations are based both on previous experience and on how much the new perception differs from our expectations (Kahneman, 1982). The intensity of the emotional reaction is the focal point in a process that interrupts habitual cognitive processing and redirects priorities by assigning more cerebral resources to solving the problem (Bower, 1981; Clark, 1982). Although a portion of this information does intrude into consciousness, much of the cognitive and emotional evaluation of novel data is procedural and therefore largely outside of conscious awareness (Zajonc, 1984; Kihlstrom, 1987).

Emotion colors cognition. Strong affect reduces the complexity of verbal descriptions. Strong negative emotion greatly simplifies the representations we make of people we don't like (Sypher, 1987). Depressed mood increases the availability of negative and unpleasant memories while increasing the difficulty of retrieving positive memories (Teasdale, 1983). These emotional responses are largely organized around our perception of other people, particularly those who are significant to us (Young, 1978).

Evoked potential studies suggest that this learning is associated with psychophysiologic changes indicating involvement of both cortical and limbic structures (Lacey, 1980). The pattern of autonomic response of heart rate, respiration, and skin conductance supports this contention (Lang, 1980). What we do involves not only what we think but how we feel, and that process involves all the parts of the brain (Donohew, 1988).

The pattern of unconscious learning, the modulation of social behavior by brief and subtle auditory and visual stimuli, is just what we would anticipate from our review of face-to-face communication. Facial expression and the prosodic elements of speech provide a continuous, rhythmic shaping of human interaction, usually below the level of conscious awareness. Moreover, this process requires ongoing adjustment on the part of both sender and receiver. Ease of learning depends critically on the phase of the interaction in which the information is introduced (Coles, 1982). Thus unconscious learning does not imply passive brainwashing but rather requires active personal involvement.

THERAPEUTIC METAPHOR

Metaphor and unconscious learning are directly relevant to our model of hypnotherapy. Many of these insights are implicit in the clinical work of Milton Erickson. Over the course of his career, Erickson moved from traditionally structured, explicitly defined uses of hypnotic techniques to a more informal storytelling approach. His work was instrumental in generating interest in the use of metaphor in the clinical setting (Zeig, 1980, 1988). Erickson integrated story, strategic interventions, and a flexible use of trance phenomena to allow the patient to deal with conflict in a dynamic fashion (Erickson and Rossi, 1976, 1979, 1981). The stories, ostensibly about experiences from the life of Erickson's family, his own childhood, or other seemingly innocuous material, typically involved a structure that was analogous to that of the presenting problem and life situation of the patient.

The seemingly casual, naturalistic style of hypnotic communication he used may be particularly powerful in stimulating unconscious learning. The techniques of oral poetry are precisely those that are most suited for transmitting complicated information in the way it can be most easily utilized (Porush, 1987). Unexpected combinations of information and indirect approaches to a goal are most effective in eliciting a search for meaning (Weiner, 1985). Unconscious presentation of material necessary for problem solving may be more effective and generate a greater utilization of the total available resources than simple presentation of the information on a conscious level (Yaniv, 1987). This is particularly true when the material presented is high in imagery value and presents many related elaborations (Clement, 1986). These kinds of approaches are more effective than "logical" statements in stimulating alternative solutions that are more personal and elaborate. Such analogical structures are also more effective in integrating relevant information from short-term to long-term memory (Kosslyn, 1981).

Because he [Erickson] did not encourage patient responsiveness and working-through, the primary effect of such interpretations tended to be teaching and influencing behavior. In this way, Erickson functioned in a manner similar to that of the creative artist or writer in relationship with society at large. Just as these use metaphors to teach, to move, and to influence their audiences and spectators, the Ericksonian approach produces similar effects with individual patients or families.

An important difference from the artistic production, however, lies in the particularity of Erickson's metaphorical constructions. He developed metaphors from the patient's own words and from his meticulously keen observations of patients' behavior and reactions. In this manner, his metaphors appear to result from a creative homospatial process arising from a particular therapeutic context in each case. . . . Erickson's metaphors are new and unique. Although less extensively derived from verbal interaction than is usual in psychoanalytic psychotherapy, they seem to result from superimposition of mental imagery derived from Erickson's highly developed observational skills.

. . . Choice of an appropriate scene, then, would likely depend on the therapist's ability to superimpose a concrete image on to what he senses or believes is the source of a patient's conflict. (Rothenberg, 1988, pp. 52–53)

Rothenberg has reviewed the relationship between creativity and psychotherapy. He suggests that particular creative processes are important in generating the metaphoric structure required for change. The first he refers to as the "homospatial" process that consists of "actively conceiving two or more discrete entities occupying the same space, a conception leading to the articulation of new identities" (Rothenberg, 1988, p. 7). The result is a new metaphor that combines elements of each. Presentation of homospatial stimuli (in his studies, Rothenberg superimposed two different slides) resulted in significantly higher levels of creative response as compared to when the images were shown either separately or side by side. "Creation of effective metaphors is one of the prime functions of the homospatial process. Multiple discrete entities are brought together into the same mentally represented space and the resulting conception is articulated into metaphorical phrases, e.g., 'the road was a ribbon of moonlight'" (Rothenberg, 1988, p. 38).

Rothenberg also describes what he terms the "janusian" process of "actively conceiving two or more opposites or antitheses simultaneously" (p. 11). He demonstrated a significantly higher use of rapid opposites responding on word association tasks for subjects who were rated as more creative (including Nobel laureates in science) when compared to controls. Rothenberg cites this as evidence for a predisposition to use this particular cognitive process when presented with novel stimuli. The janusian process is a transitional stage that is unstable and is usually not seen in the final product. He proposes that this process serves a generative function during the formative stages of the creative process. By identifying elements in a particular situation that appear to be contradictory, the process begins to make a transition toward a more complete and satisfying model. Once these conflicting elements are defined antithetically, cognitive processes that seek out symmetry, balance, and integration can begin to operate.

In Erickson's model, the unconscious is viewed as a source of a lifetime's accumulation of skills, automatic processes that may be used to bypass the restrictions of consciously learned limitations. These processes function as a loose confederacy, their only obvious common feature being that they operate on a level that is not available to conscious awareness. "I have viewed much of what I have done as expediting the currents of change already seething within the person and family—but currents that need the 'unexpected,' the 'illogical,' and the 'sudden' move to lead them into tangible fruition" (Erickson, quoted in Watzlawick, 1974, p. ix).

In its most potent form, metaphor includes significance (must have structural equivalents for both conscious and unconscious aspects), vividness (to involve a full intellectual and emotional as well as perceptual involvement), and a drive toward resolution. The components that combine to create an effective metaphor are thus contextual and in practice are formed by the elements that have always produced a good story.

The context of a word always plays a part in specifying its meaning. Words and sentences are almost always ambiguous; they are never precise unless we take into account the context of the communication. This lack of precision is not a deficiency of language; it rather is an aspect of language that mirrors human thought. As Cassirer (1944) and Bronowski (1971) note, the inherent imprecision of any linguistic statement keeps the frontier of human language open. We must always creatively interpret an utterance: the new interpretation always has the potential of achieving a new insight. (Lieberman, 1984, p. 82)

Erickson did not develop any form of systematic theory but maintained a resolute focus on the process of therapy, an approach for which Jay Haley coined the term "strategic therapy." The key to Erickson's work lies in his selection of metaphor. Rather than creating metaphors arbitrarily, he emphasized that his communication was based on the patient's own metaphors, that is, in the description of the presenting problem, in the language the patient used to describe both the situation and himself. Erickson's choice of metaphor content was also guided by his perception of the psychological task the individual faced. This included an implicit life stage model which individuals in particular points in their lives in a particular culture all experience (Haley, 1973). As with the other components of the therapeutic interaction, the therapeutic metaphors are best understood within the context of a chain of therapeutic stories moving from general to more personal themes but always provided by both the spoken and the nonverbal cues of the patient.

Metaphor encourages experiential participation rather than restricted intellectual understanding. Metaphor can encourage affective change (by the emotional tone of the story), behavioral change (by suggesting the next step in a particular sequence), perceptual change (by encouraging a response attentiveness and absorption focused on immediate experience), and cognitive change (by changing the frame of reference). Thus, though a patient may be more aware of one particular aspect or may have some particular facility with one element, change involves metaphoric extension through all these levels.

Erickson's Stories

There are numerous examples of Erickson's use of storytelling techniques in his hypnotic inductions and therapeutic interventions. A fascinating example is presented in detail in a pair of papers concerning a case dating from the mid-1930s (Erickson, 1980b, 3:320–335, 336–355). In these papers, he describes the treatment of a case of premature ejaculation using a hypnotic story that, though ostensibly about a mildly embarrassing social situation, significantly paralleled the patient's personal experience. Erickson describes this process as the development of an experimental neurosis, the resolution of which simultaneously resulted in the resolution of the patient's symptom. As Erickson wrote,

This complex had been formulated to symbolize or to parallel his actual neurosis. In consequence of this procedure there appeared to result an identification of the induced conflict with his original neurosis and a fusing of their affective reactions. After the patient had been forced to relive, abreact, and gain insight into the suggested conflict, it was discovered that he had made a clinical recovery from his original neurosis and that he was still able to function normally a year later. (3:335)

In great detail, Erickson provides a commentary on the wording of his metaphor and the precise effect each element was designed to achieve. The seemingly "irrelevant" story was clearly a highly developed creation that was of great significance to the patient despite the lack of obvious connection. The metaphoric structure itself was enough to provide a powerful connection.

The procedure employed was that of fabricating a story which would parallel and symbolize the patient's actual neurosis in terms of an ordinary, credible, but unpleasant instance of social behavior. . . .

In considering how to devise or formulate a suitable complex applicable to the subject, the task seemed to be essentially a problem of, "It is not only what you say, but how you say it." Under the proposed experimental conditions "what" was to be said had to be a seemingly innocuous and credible but fictitious story of a past forgotten social error by the subject. . . .

The "how" of telling this story seemed primarily to be a task of so relating the fictitious account that it would become superimposed upon his actual experiential past in a manner that would cause him to react appropriately to it emotionally, to incorporate it into his real memories, and thus to transform it into a vital part of his psychic life.

This could be done, it was reasoned, by taking the objective items contained in the essential content of the story and so weaving a narrative about them that they would stimulate a wealth and a variety of emotions, memories, and associations that would in turn give the story a second and much greater significance and validity than could its apparent content.

To do this would require a careful choice and use of words which would carry multiple meanings, or which would have various associations, connotations, and nuances of meaning which would serve to build up in a gradual unrecognized, cumulative fashion a second more extensive but unrealized meaningfulness for the story.

Also, the words, by their arrangement into phrases, clauses, and sentences, and even their introductory, transitional, and repetitive uses could be made to serve special purposes for building up emphasis or cutting it short, for establishing contrasts, similarities, parallelisms, identifications, and equations of one idea to another, all of which would build up a series of associations and emotional responses stimulated, but not aroused directly, by the actual content of the complex. Additionally, sharp transitions from one idea to another, sequential relationships of various ideas and objects, shifts of responsibility and action

from one character to another, the use of words that threatened, challenged,
distracted, or served only to delay the development of the narrative were all
employed to formulate a story possessing a significance beyond its formal content. . . .

Essentially, the task, as worked out, was comparable to that of composing
music intended to produce a certain effect upon the listener. Words and ideas,
rather than notes of music, were employed in selected sequences, patterns,
rhythms, and other relationships, and by this composition it was hoped to evoke
profound responses in the subject. These responses were to be of a type not only
hoped for in terms of what the story could mean but which would be in accord
with the established patterns of behavior deriving from the patient's experiential past. (3:336–338)

Metaphors are associations of ideas elaborated by the personal interpretation of experience. Experiences will be associated because of
their perceived overall structural similarity rather than by the connections of formal logic. The evidence supports the notion that therapeutic
metaphor, in order to be effective, must be "isomorphic"—have an
overall structural correspondence with that of the patient's presenting
problem (Gordon, 1978; Lankton and Lankton, 1983)—or "coherent"—have a relationship through a common basic metaphor with
the patient's belief system (Lakoff and Johnson, 1980). Elaborations are
limited by the constraints of perceptual experience, constraints composed of biologic, social, and personal variables. In therapeutic terms,
associations that fit these restrictions will be accumulated; those that do
not, will not.

An important feature of Lakoff and Johnson's model is that it demonstrates how the structure of language can influence behavior. It is
often difficult to step back far enough to see how language does this.
Although our physical experience shapes basic preconceptual structures, the elaboration produced by metaphor also allows for flexible
transitions to models that are more useful when the situation changes.
Metaphor is the structure by which psychological change and growth
can occur.

In their study of Erickson's work, the Lanktons (1983) suggest that
metaphor in therapy can be structured by a formula that considers each
of these elements as a possible dramatic theme, using the patient's
responsiveness as a clue for which elements to select and then pursue.
The successful completion of certain hypnotic phenomena can be
linked to the therapeutic goal (for example, storytelling might be used
as an introduction to clinical trance). Similarly, the development of a

transient hypnotic anaesthesia of the hand can be used as a stepping-stone in the development of anaesthesia as a clinical pain control method.

The Lanktons recognize the hybrid nature of metaphor: the blend of the individual patient's experience of a situation and of some desired state. The hybrid functions as a bridge to allow transition from one to the other.

While conducting a massive mental search for related associations, the mind brings together the common symbols and elements of a new perceptual framework by entertaining the metaphoric theme. The blending of the original perceptual framework and the metaphoric framework only increase the number of associations that seem relevant. The presence of so many possible associations creates the same effect on the mind as that produced by unconditioned stimuli: heightened attentiveness. (Lankton, 1983, p. 80)

An individualized embedded metaphor structure is employed involving metaphors that (1) match the presenting problem, (2) describe and encourage the emotional, cognitive, and behavioral "resources" that would be useful in dealing with the problem, and (3) link the application of these resources to the problem situation. This results in a "nested" structure, rather like a set of Chinese puzzle boxes, in which a "linking" metaphor is embedded in a "resource" metaphor, which is embedded in a "matching" metaphor, which is embedded in the hypnotic trance (Lankton, 1983, p. 127). "It is construction of such interlocking networks of associations that gives 'body' or substance to trance as an altered state of consciousness with its own guideposts, rules, and 'reality' " (Erickson, 1980a, 1:464).

The initial matching metaphor offers a dramatic theme parallel to the client's presenting problem. Its purpose is to absorb conscious attention and stimulate a search for meaning at an unconscious level. Metaphors to retrieve resources are aimed at encouraging the individual to use abilities from other contexts within the therapeutic setting. These are often associated with trance phenomena, which can serve as "convincers" of an increased range of possible responses.

The final step involves metaphors that link the presenting problem with the newly recovered resources. For example, each repeated hypnotic age regression may be used to relive past traumatic experiences in a progressively more positive way. The embedded structure is closed by ending the matching metaphor in a way that is dramatically coherent, emotionally satisfying, and personally and socially acceptable. The dramatic structure of tension followed by resolution promotes a sense of closure around a problem issue. Just as with other narratives, the resolution may be settled or ambiguous. What is critical is that it be satisfying within the given context. Erickson's stories were sufficiently open-ended to encourage the patient to generate his or her own unique response rather than being a simple covert prescription for a specific behavior.

The Lanktons also emphasize the value of linking metaphor to posthypnotic suggestion and to the social context of the individual. This serves to encourage state-dependent learning by associating the metaphoric development with the applications for which it is required in the context in which it will be needed. This introduces the notion of generative change—that is, a therapeutic response that offers the patient the ability to go beyond a resolution of the present context. This is a more explicit version of what Spiegel (1979) has referred to as the "ripple effect" of hypnotherapy.

Of course, the structure of therapy itself can provide a metaphor for other relationships. The relationship in therapy can be considered a rehearsal, a playground, or a laboratory in which new strategies can be tried out and the consequences of failure minimized. Both problems and solutions can be explored in a way that is not possible in other relationships and without the consequences that they might have in other situations. Rothenberg describes this as the "critical paradox of the therapeutic situation" (1988, p. 29).

A primary value of the therapeutic use of metaphor is the stimulation and subsequent understanding it provides for the therapist and the modeling it offers for the patient. The therapist is challenged to loosen up, be spontaneous, and to use his highest intuitive powers in order to create metaphors. While allowing himself to think freely and intuitively about the patient, he must also listen quite carefully in order to base the metaphors on what the patient brings to him. Particularly effective metaphors are often those that are based on something in the patient's experience. . . . Appreciating the therapist's willingness to take risks, the patient can also loosen up, tap his own intuition, and take some daring risks at reformulation of his understanding of himself. (p. 47)

Metaphor functions to build rapport (a common language), to build structure and coherence (provide meaning and sense), and to suggest possible outcomes both by suggesting that a resolution is possible and by stimulating a search for the appropriate resolution. Metaphors are associations of ideas elaborated by the personal interpretation of experience. Experiences will be associated because of their perceived overall structural similarity rather than by the connections of formal logic.

Therapeutic metaphor requires an active involvement on the part of both individuals. This model implies a two-way interaction between behavior and cognition with changes in one producing corresponding changes in the other. The analogies must connect with the individual's experience: evoke an emotional response and be relevant to the existing situation. The metaphor is not measured by some arbitrary aesthetic values but is useful or fitting depending on its ability to stimulate alterations in behavior. It is because of the systematic structure of metaphor that the concepts can grow and develop, be elaborated like a musical theme and variations.

The role of metaphor in therapy is central to the question of how the mind can transform itself. In the classic *Mind: An Essay on Human Feeling* (1970), Langer reviewed neurophysiologic, linguistic, and aesthetic evidence of the nature of metaphor. She contends that metaphor plays a central role mediating among feeling, thinking, perception, and behavior. Metaphor has the "symbolic equivalence of sensations"—it motivates behavior as powerfully as do direct perceptions. This equivalence stems from metaphor's use of vivid sensory-based language and its foundation in subjective feelings and values. Without this crucial link, feeling is blocked and thinking is dry and ineffective. In this sense, the primary goal of therapy is to produce an experience that simultaneously evokes intellectual, emotional, and imaginative processes.

We tend to think of a story as a closed entity complete with beginning, middle, and ending. As Langer (1970) points out, however, no work of art (indeed, no human communication) is ever self-contained. It was part of Erickson's unique contribution to demonstrate that telling a story of necessity evokes participation in the listener. His approach is inherently collaborative. Thus his stories are truly open-ended, requiring completion through those metaphoric processes that are particularly relevant within that context. In a literal sense, Erickson's stories continue to be told.

The Biologic Basis of Metaphor

Metaphor may have been critical in the evolution of human consciousness. Gregory Bateson (1987) suggested that metaphor is the mental equivalent of biological information transduction. He compared the way in which metaphor encodes meaning to the way in which information is processed in the biologic world. Structuring information in terms of similarity and differences is the fundamental biologic organization. Evolutionary processes have depended upon it.

They managed to organize themselves in their embryology to have two eyes, one on each side of a nose. They managed to organize themselves in their evolution so there were shared predicates between the horse and the man, which zoologists today call homology. It becomes evident that metaphor is not just pretty poetry, it is not either good or bad logic, but it is in fact the logic upon which the biological world has been built, the main characteristic and organizing glue of this world of mental process. (Bateson, 1987, p. 30)

The wisdom of metaphor is the wisdom of evolution, a search for similarities and differences, a pursuit of pattern and its disruption. Bateson described this as the process of "learning to learn," the development of adaptive action. This is the process found throughout biology of self-organization through communication of information at different levels. The fundamental matrix of the human brain is metaphoric.

In contrast, logical processes are a created set of rules, a technique or tool developed by humankind. Bateson suggests that formal logic is a result of the interaction of this metaphoric communication with our verbal abilities, the use of language to make abstract structures. He explains,

All verbal communication necessarily contains metaphor. And metaphor when it is dressed in words has added to it those characteristics that verbalism can achieve: the possibility of simple negation (there is no *not* at the preverbal level), the possibility of classification, of subject-predicate differentiation, and the possibility of explicit context marking.

Finally, there is the possibility with words, of jumping right out of the metaphoric and poetic mode into *simile.* What Vaihinger called the *as if* mode of communication becomes something else when the *as if* is added. In a word, it becomes *prose,* and then all the limitations of the syllogisms that logicians prefer . . . must be precisely obeyed. (1987, pp. 28–29)

The traditional view of conceptual thinking involves our progressive abstraction or movement from concrete examples to "pure" thought. In contrast, the experientialist viewpoint suggests that conceptual thinking consists of systematic families of metaphors, with varying degrees of overlap, that fit together not by a logical imperative but by their usefulness in covering an area and in their structural similarity. The traditional view of abstract thinking, with its emphasis on logical connections, cannot account for this kind of association. The use of metaphor, as in the case of play therapy with children, allows for the expression and recognition of aspects of a problem when the whole may be too painful, complex, or pervasive to be dealt with consciously. We have often neglected the therapeutic value of metaphor because of a prejudice that associates vividness, mental imagery, and emotional power with primary process, or primitive, thinking.

The old model was plagued with a Cartesian dualism between conscious and unconscious, rational and irrational. The new model asserts that logic and language emerge from a larger cognitive structure, the continuous tip of a metaphoric iceberg. Propositional language is, in fact, a distillation of metaphoric thinking from an analogical to a digital representation. Lakoff and Johnson (1980) suggest that the attempt to understand metaphor by reducing it to its literal meaning ignores the fact that we can understand that meaning only in the light of another metaphor. They suggest that a more useful metaphor for metaphor is to conceive of it as a sense like hearing, seeing, or feeling. Perhaps metaphor is a sixth sense, an added perceptual dimension.

Metaphor is the basis for a generative understanding. We first attempt to structure what is ambiguous on the basis of what we already know. As the context or our needs change, the open-ended nature of metaphor allows for an ongoing attempt to achieve a better fit; it allows for extension and growth of understanding, for a revision of existing beliefs. This makes metaphor the ideal tool for psychological or interpersonal experience. Each person's collection of self-images will in this way have an ongoing ability to develop and elaborate. This model of human thinking fits the evolutionary pattern of being inherently conservative and yet capable of organic change. Thus, literally, the extension of understanding is metaphoric, altering existing knowledge in terms of a slightly modified version that incorporates both stability and change.

HYPNOTIC STORIES

Meaning in face-to-face communication derives from context, and we sort out the meaning by two methods. The first is what the social psychologists refer to as the frame: the ongoing information provided by nonverbal and prosodic cues. The second method is from comparisons with a preexisting cognitive structure or schema (Tannen, 1987). Both of these steps involve conscious and unconscious learning. Metaphor is the process by which new learning is integrated so that a schema may be altered. With its unique relationship to context, metaphor also provides a means by which an existing schema can be compared with current reality (Gibbs, 1989).

The use of metaphor can be seen as a natural problem-solving strategy that is pervasive and effective (Helstrup, 1988); it reveals the process of change on both the theoretic and technical levels (Evans, 1988).

Metaphor involves a method of changing concepts by providing a tool for dealing with complex or abstract structures (Engel, 1988). The study of metaphor can reveal the hidden aspects of the interaction between brain function and social context (Lakoff, 1989). Metaphor is also essential for collaborative learning. A recent study of therapeutic metaphor suggested that metaphor that evolved from a collaborative, creative process enhanced mutual understanding, whereas noncollaborative metaphor led to pervasive misunderstanding (Angus, 1988). Similarly, McMullen (1989) has demonstrated that in psychotherapy successful cases are much more likely to demonstrate metaphoric treatment of central therapeutic themes than are unsuccessful cases.

As a means for dealing with complex or uncertain issues, metaphor will always play a critical role in all forms of psychotherapy (Evans, 1988). As Erickson's work suggests, the ability to integrate uncertainty and novelty in a metaphoric structure is a basic hypnotic skill. Moreover, metaphor is critically important in developing and changing social roles. We use metaphor in the way that we define ourselves as well as others. As we shall see in chapter 8, that ability to alter a self-concept through metaphor is an important aspect of dissociation and provides ways of dealing creatively with self and others.

PART THREE
USES

———————————————————————————————

This part deals with some of the clinical uses to which hypnotic abilities can be applied. Although the evidence is preliminary, hypnotherapy has been shown to modify physiologic function and thus can help in the treatment of a wide range of medical disorders. This evidence has both significant theoretic implications and practical clinical applications. Hypnotherapy also allows us to understand multiple personality disorder. This disorder can be conceptualized as the patient's spontaneous use of hypnotic abilities as a means of coping with mental or physical trauma. Hypnosis can be part of the socially sanctioned bridge that helps the patient achieve psychological and cultural reintegration.

The final chapter explores the work of Milton Erickson, who emphasized the naturalistic and collaborative nature of the hypnotic process. At its best, his legacy is itself a strong hypnotic suggestion to conceptualize hypnotherapy as a creative partnership.

7 SIGMUND FREUD MAKES A HOUSE CALL: HYPNOSIS AND MEDICAL DISORDERS

Anyone who desires to rejoice at the truth of something without evidence must also learn to survive without experience.

Roger Bacon

One of the most intriguing claims made about hypnosis is that it has the capacity to alter various psychophysiologic functions. Until very recently these claims were largely unsubstantiated, but a growing number of well-designed studies have suggested a potentially useful role for hypnosis in a number of medical disorders. Hypnosis has been shown to be effective in controlling pain, ameliorating gastrointestinal and respiratory dysfunction, and operating as an adjunct in other disorders. A great deal of work remains to be done, however, particularly in the area of differentiating the effects of hypnosis from those of such approaches as biofeedback or other cognitive techniques.

THE HOUSE CALL

In 1893, a case report was published of a house call made by a young neurologist by the name of Sigmund Freud. His colleagues had brought him in to consult on the case of a distraught mother who was unable to feed her newborn child. The conventional medical treatments of the time had failed, and the physicians hoped that Freud, recently returned from studies with the great professor Jean-Martin Charcot of Paris, would be able to use his hypnotic training to help the patient.

Freud had long been a friend of the family and knew the patient personally. He described the woman, who was in her twenties, as a person of "quiet common sense" and "naturalness." He regarded her marriage as a happy one. The child was their second infant. Although the patient had been unable to breast-feed her first child, she was eager to do so with the second baby. It was at this point that the difficulties began. She produced little milk, and her breasts were painful when she attempted to nurse. She was agitated and sleepless, severely nauseated and unwilling to eat. After four days, her weight loss began to alarm the physicians. At that point they called on Freud.

When he arrived, Freud noticed that the patient was obviously furious and that his reception was less than warm: "Far from being welcomed as a saviour in the hour of need, it was obvious that I was being received with a bad grace and that I could not count on the patient having much confidence in me" (Freud, 1893, p. 36). Despite these misgivings, after completing the examination, Freud began to induce hypnosis. Within three minutes, the patient appeared to be in a profound hypnotic state. "I made use of suggestion to contradict all her fears and the feelings on which those fears were based: 'Do not be afraid. You will make an excellent nurse and the baby will thrive. Your stomach is perfectly quiet, your appetite is excellent, you are looking forward to your next meal, etc.'" (p. 36). When she was reawakened, she felt well and was amnesic for the hypnotic suggestions.

When Freud called on his patient the next day, the reception was even cooler than before. The patient's appetite had returned and she had slept well throughout the night, but the sight of a large lunch had brought a return of the symptoms and the patient, her husband, and family were openly hostile. Once again inducing hypnosis, Freud decided to change his tack:

I acted with greater energy and confidence. I told the patient that five minutes after my departure she would break out against her family with some acrimony: what had happened to her dinner? did they mean to let her starve? how could she feed the baby if she had nothing to eat herself? and so on.

When I returned on the third evening the patient refused to have any further treatment. There was nothing more wrong with her, she said: she had an excellent appetite and plenty of milk for the baby, there was not the slightest difficulty when it was put to her breast, and so on. Her husband found it rather queer, however, that after my departure the evening before she had clamoured violently for food and had remonstrated with her mother in a way quite unlike herself. But since then, he added, everything had gone all right.

There was nothing more for me to do. The mother fed her child for eight months; and I had many opportunities of satisfying myself in a friendly way that they were both doing well. I found it hard to understand, however, as well as annoying, that no reference was ever made to my remarkable achievement. (p. 37)

Of all the aspects of hypnosis, none is more dramatic than its use in altering physiologic function. Although always controversial, hypnosis was actively used in medicine in the latter part of the nineteenth century, but its use gradually died out (Ellenberger, 1970). After a half century of relative obscurity, hypnosis is once again finding a place in the treatment of physical illness. The past two decades have witnessed a resurgence of interest in the use of cognitive, emotional, or physiologic strategies to alter disease processes. If the place of hypnosis is to be legitimate, we must accumulate scientifically acceptable evidence of its value.

Studies of the hypnotic alteration of physiologic function in the clinical setting have lagged drastically behind laboratory studies in experimental sophistication. Many of the early studies of the efficacy of hypnosis in treating medical disorders were too methodologically flawed to be of any significant value (Wadden, 1982; Brown, 1986; Barber, 1984). Most lacked control groups, standardized protocols, adequate sample size, and other basic requirements. Although many are of historical or technical interest, no conclusions can be drawn from studies that do not meet current criteria for what constitutes an adequate scientific report (Glantz, 1980; Sackett, 1980; Hayden, 1982; Oxman, 1988). But recent studies using rigorous experimental designs are beginning to tell a more convincing story.

THE CONTROL OF PAIN

Of the various hypnotic alterations of psychophysiologic function, the most dramatic, as well as the most extensively investigated, is the control of pain. Ernest Hilgard (1977) and his coworkers have been among the leaders in the systematic study of hypnotic analgesia in the laboratory setting. In extensive investigations, using experimental paradigms to induce pain (typically either a tourniquet cutting off the circulation to a limb or plunging the limb into cold water), they have demonstrated that various types of pain can be reduced by hypnotically induced analgesia (but not by hypnosis alone). Further, Hilgard has reported a relatively strong correlation between hypnotic susceptibility, as measured by the Stanford Hypnotic Susceptibility Scale (SHSS), and hypnotic analgesia in the laboratory.

In these studies, two-thirds of the high susceptibility group, but only 13 percent of the lower and 17 percent of the medium susceptibility groups, were able to reduce their pain by one-third or more. Twenty-six percent of the high, 57 percent of the medium, and 31 percent of the low susceptibility groups were able to reduce their pain by 10 to 32 percent when compared to controls. The remaining subjects—7 percent of the high, 26 percent of the medium, and 56 percent of the low susceptibility groups—reduced their pain by less than 10 percent (Hilgard, 1977).

Hilgard also observed that though there is a strong association between hypnotic ability and the ability to control pain, it does not account for all of each subject's ability to reduce pain. Approximately 30 percent of the subjects who did not score highly on the hypnotizability scales still achieved significant pain reduction. Conversely, Hilgard notes that even in the high susceptibility group only two-thirds could reduce their pain by a third or more in the experimental situation (Hilgard, 1977, p. 171). Those who were successful often went beyond the hypnotist's direct suggestions and elaborated their own imagery to counteract the pain, whereas the low susceptibility subjects demonstrated little ability in learning pain control using these methods. Further, many susceptible hypnotic subjects could markedly improve their performance with practice. Pain reduction was not related to any measures of depth of trance, but could occur quite satisfactorily at any level.

The relationship between standardized measures of hypnotic ability and pain relief has come under further scrutiny. Some studies support Hilgard's findings (DeBenedittis, 1989), but others suggest that other cognitive approaches can be equally effective with patients of low susceptibility (Miller, 1986; Nolan, 1987; Spanos, 1986a, 1986c). There is also evidence that the relationship between hypnotic susceptibility and clinical pain reduction is nonlinear (Price, 1987). Price and Barber (1987) found that the relationship was strongest at the extreme of the pain experience for sensory responses, but that the important clinical variable of emotional responses to pain did not correlate with hypnotic susceptibility.

Experimentally induced pain, while undeniably noxious, is different from the experience of patients in the clinical setting. Whereas experimental pain is brief, undergone voluntarily, and can be terminated at any time by the subject, in the clinical setting, pain is often long term, comes against the wishes of the individual, and is usually experienced as being outside of personal control. Moreover, it is part of a disease process that directly alters both physical and mental functioning. The associated illness or injury may be extremely debilitating or even potentially fatal.

Whether the pain is acute or chronic will also influence the value of hypnosis for pain control. Patients undergoing head and neck surgery who were trained with preoperative hypnosis had significantly shorter postoperative hospitalizations than did matched controls (Rapkin, 1988). In contrast, in a sample of patients with a diagnosis of chronic pain without an identified physical illness, Edelson and Fitzpatrick (1989) found that subjects trained in hypnosis did not experience significant pain relief after a one-month follow-up.

Traditionally, medicine has attempted to distinguish between "functional" and "organic" (that is, "real") pain. It has become increasingly clear that this distinction is too simplistic (Melzack, 1982). Current research into the experience of pain tends to divide pain into two types: "sensory" pain, which correlates reasonably well with the intensity of pain stimuli, and "psychological" pain, which involves the cognitive and emotional responses and attributions of the individual to the context of the pain (Rachlin, 1985). Expectation plays a significant role in influencing the emotional response to pain (Price, 1980). Patients with pain experience a significant amount of distress with increased levels of depression, anxiety, and feelings of alienation, regardless of the cause of the pain (Trief, 1987). Conversely, anxiety and depression, unpredictability and uncertainty about the meaning of the pain, all significantly increase pain experience (Turk, 1981).

Current thinking attempts to categorize pain by measuring behavioral, physiological, and cognitive-affective response systems (Rachlin, 1985; Brown, 1987). Multimodal approaches recognize the heterogeneity of the pain experience. Thus pain, which may originally be the result of irritation or damage to tissue, can also be enhanced and then maintained by initial or later contextual cues (Jay, 1986). Chronic pain patients are much more likely to exhibit symptom-specific stress-related psychophysiologic responses, showing a tighter relationship between stress and severity of their symptoms than do other patients (Flor, 1989). Swanson has suggested that chronic pain be considered as a separate emotion—as separate but related to anxiety and depression (1984). He suggests that we look on the distinction between acute and chronic pain as having the same relationship as fear and anxiety or grief and depression.

In an attempt to integrate the various approaches, Grau has suggested a "working memory hypothesis" of brain analgesic systems (1987). According to this model, pain experience activates both opioid and nonopioid analgesic systems. Alterations of memory of pain experience can alter subsequent responses to pain. This model suggests a specific way in which contextual cues, both at the time of the initial experience and subsequently, can affect the intensity of pain experience and its associated meaning. Thus, pain in the clinical setting is influenced by a number of cognitive and social factors.

Generally speaking, reviews of the literature have supported the value of hypnosis in analgesia and stress reduction in a number of disorders, whether following the dissociative formulation (Miller, 1986) or a social psychology approach (Nolan, 1987). The suggestion, however, that hypnotic pain relief can be explained as simple anxiety reduction is demonstrably not the case. Although pain reduction is correlated with hypnotic susceptibility scores, it is not correlated with anxiety reduction (DeBenedittis, 1989). There is a relationship between anxiety and pain experienced, but it is a fluid and subtle one that varies with a number of factors including pain intensity, contextual variables, and the relevance of the anxiety to the pain (Hilgard, 1975; Weisenberg, 1984; Schumacher, 1984; Rachlin, 1985). Pain reduction involves a decrease in both the amount of sensory pain and the suffering experienced, and it is not attributable simply to reduction of anxiety. There is a curvilinear relationship between the emotional state and the amount of pain experienced (Price, 1987). Some forms of anxiety (those that are not related directly to the pain) may in fact lead to a reduction in the pain experienced (Weisenberg, 1984).

Strategies for Pain Control

Studies of clinical populations also tend to support the notion of significant individual variation in pain management. Two-thirds of patients spontaneously use some form of pain control or coping strategy, whereas one-third "catastrophize" or experience a worsening of pain (Chaves, 1987). Hypnotic pain reduction techniques typically involve both physical relaxation and cognitive training (including imagery). Both relaxation with deep breathing exercises and verbal suggestion using pain relief imagery are effective at reducing objective and subjective measures of distress during painful medical procedures (Holmes, 1983; Kaplan, 1983). Relaxation techniques also tend to stimulate positive cognitions (Kaplan, 1983). Thus, physical relaxation and cognitive training cannot be considered as two entirely separate procedures.

Similarly, a variety of cognitive approaches may be effective in different circumstances. A focus on cognitive skill learning rather than on pain reduction significantly reduces reported pain (Weisenberg, 1984). Both distraction and redefinition of pain are effective techniques (McCaul, 1984), although distraction may be more effective for acute pain or chronic pain of low intensity, and redefinition of the pain may be more effective for intense chronic pain (McCaul, 1984). Similarly, imagery training reduces pain, but imagery that is more psychologically personalized is significantly more effective (Raft, 1986). Such imagery can be developed spontaneously or enhanced through an active collaboration between therapist and patient (Raft, 1986).

The cognitive skills needed to relieve pain may be more varied than was originally assumed. Highly susceptible subjects are much more likely to use different cognitive strategies spontaneously in an attempt to reduce pain than are subjects with low hypnotic ability (Spanos 1986a, 1986c). Both high and low hypnotically susceptible subjects can significantly reduce pain if they are given different methods of approaching the problem. The high susceptibility group did best if given instructions when under hypnosis, but the low susceptibility group did equally well if they were given the instructions in the waking state. Approaches that emphasize the contextual aspects of hypnosis and pain relief can be highly effective in teaching effective pain control techniques even to those patients who are initially rated as being less hypnotically susceptible (Kroger, 1988; Stam, 1987). In addition, some strategies may be more effective for catastrophizers, and others more effective for subjects who do not catastrophize (Heyneman, 1990). These findings underline the difficulty in sharply defining the distinction between hypnotic and nonhypnotic skills. Similarly, they point out a possible relationship between hypnotic skills and the placebo response in pain control.

The relationship between hypnotic ability and placebo analgesic response is complex. Early reports suggested that there is no relationship between magnitude of placebo effect and hypnotic susceptibility (McGlashan, 1969; J. A. Stern, 1977). More recently it has been suggested that although "hypnotic" analgesia and "placebo" analgesia may be mediated by different mechanisms, both can be influenced by contextual variables (Stam, 1987). This suggests that subjects with both high and low hypnotic susceptibility scores could benefit from a combination of the approaches. Highly susceptible subjects, however, achieved significantly more pain relief with hypnosis than they did with placebo. The results would appear to support the contention that though subjects with high hypnotic ability tend to have greater pain relief than do other subjects, all subjects can have their responses to hypnotic or placebo analgesia enhanced by contextual variables (Stewart, 1990).

The Mechanisms of Hypnotic Pain Control

Mechanisms of hypnotic pain control are as poorly understood as they are fascinating. Successful hypnotic analgesia appears to be related to EEG measures of hemispheric coherence (Chen, 1981). Using a particular approach—the restricted environmental stimulation technique (REST)—Barabasz (1989) was able to show an enhanced response on the SHCS as well as an increased pain tolerance that was associated with increased EEG alpha density during the initial hypnotic session.

Neurochemical studies of hypnotic control of pain are few. In one study, patients suffering arthritic pain showed a correlation among levels of pain, anxiety, and depression. Anxiety and depression were inversely related to plasma norepinephrine levels. Depression was correlated with dopamine levels and negatively correlated with levels of serotonin and beta endorphin. Following hypnotherapy there were clinically and statistically significant decreases in depression, anxiety, and pain, and increases in beta endorphin–like substances (Domangue, 1985). Hypnotic analgesia is not affected by cholinergic agents (Sternbach, 1982).

The relationship between pain and endorphins is a complicated one and the role of endogenous opiates in hypnotic relief of pain remains controversial (Barker, 1977). Naloxone, an opiate antagonist, blocks the analgesia produced by brain stem electrical stimulation and by acupuncture (Mayer, 1976; Fields, 1981). Naloxone can partially, but not totally, reduce or block the analgesia produced by placebos (Grevert, 1983). But hypnotic relief of experimental (Goldstein, 1975) and chronic clinical pain is not affected by opiate blockade (Spiegel, 1983a). A series of careful studies by Finer suggests that endorphins are not primarily involved in reduction of pain by hypnosis (1982). Others have suggested that only particular forms of the beta endorphins found in peripheral blood during painful experiences unaltered by hypnotic suggestion are associated with the hypnotic response (Guerra, 1982). But DeBenedittis (1989) found that hypnotic analgesia was unrelated to beta endorphin or ACTH plasma levels.

Specific Pain Conditions

Headache. Over 90 percent of headaches are due to either muscle contraction or vascular causes (of which migraine is the most commonly known) or both (Diamond, 1982). Muscle contractions in the face, head, and neck, and vasomotor responses are thus central to this common pain syndrome. Even for the migraine patient, muscle contraction plays a significant role in the syndrome, with most headaches being of a mixed type (R. A. Cohen, 1983). In fact, migraine patients may have even higher levels of cranial muscle tension than do tension headache patients (Bakal, 1982). Also, the muscles of their head and neck have chronically high levels of activity even in the absence of a headache (Vaughn, 1977) and may show particular trigger areas (Travell, 1976).

Longitudinal studies of migraine patients show that the onset of headaches correlates with mood states, both during the headache and for periods of about twelve to thirty-six hours prior to the headache (Harrigan, 1984). In particular, feelings of constraint and fatigue produced the highest correlations with headaches. There is evidence that for all forms of headaches of a recurrent severe type, only treatment of the underlying psychological stress or psychiatric disorder is effective (Weatherhead, 1980).

Psychophysiologic measures (heart rate, frontal EMG, skin conductance potential, skin temperature) differentiate both migraine and tension headache patients from normal controls (R. A. Cohen, 1983). Individuals who are prone to repeated headaches have psychophysiologic evidence of increased sensitivity of their autonomic nervous system, so that they tend to respond to stimuli more dramatically and in a more stereotyped fashion than do normal controls (Price, 1979; Rickes, 1977; Bruyn, 1980). Headache subjects tend to show greater degrees of arousal both under stress and during relaxation. The migraine patients differed from tension headache patients in that they showed greater vascular responses to stress.

The evidence accumulated to date suggests that a number of hypnotherapeutic and biofeedback approaches can be highly effective in the treatment of some patients with chronic migraine. Although no one technique has been demonstrated to be most effective, all the methods appear to be superior to a standard treatment relying on pharmacological approaches alone.

In one study, migraine patients treated with hypnosis had a significant reduction in the number of attacks and in their severity compared to a control group who were treated with traditional medications (Anderson, 1975). This difference did not become statistically significant until the second six-month follow-up period. In addition, at the end of one year the number of patients in the hypnosis group who had experienced no headaches for over three months was significantly larger. A later controlled trial (Olness, 1987) showed that self-hypnosis was significantly more effective than either propranolol or placebo in reducing the frequency (but not the severity) of migraine headaches in children between the ages of six and twelve.

A number of studies have compared hypnosis with biofeedback in the treatment of migraine headache (Andreychuk, 1975; Friedman, 1984). Similarly, both treatments have also been compared in the relief of tension headache (Schlutter, 1980). In all these studies, both hypnosis and biofeedback relaxation were found to be effective in relieving headache symptoms, but neither modality was shown to be superior. Similarly, some reports have shown a correlation between hypnotic susceptibility and therapeutic response (for example, Andreychuk, 1975), but other studies have shown a lack of correlation (for example, Friedman, 1984).

The literature on hypnosis also supports the notion that a number of different approaches may be equally effective in the relief of headache. Fully a dozen different hypnotic techniques have been reported in the treatment of chronic migraine (Alladin, 1988). Of these, hypnotic training emphasizing relaxation, hand warming, and direct suggestions of symptom removal have all been shown to be effective in reducing the duration, intensity, and frequency of migraine attacks during a ten-week treatment course and at thirteen-month follow-up when compared either to controls or to a hypnotic treatment involving suggestions of glove anesthesia imagery (Alladin, 1988). Similarly, the similarities between hypnotic and nonhypnotic treatment may outweigh the differences (Spinhoven, 1988a).

Alteration in hand skin temperature correlates with hemispheric and regional cerebral blood flow changes as measured by xenon inhalation techniques (Mathew, 1982). Patients with migraines demonstrated a greater general cerebral blood flow response than did normal controls. The changes tended to differ in direction and/or magnitude depending on whether the hands were warmed or cooled. This supports the notion that patients with migraines have an excessive vasomotor responsiveness that differs in pattern and magnitude from normal subjects. Both warming and cooling the hands reduced the frequency and severity of the headaches, but warming was somewhat better in achieving these results (Claghorn, 1981).

Hand warming appears to be the simplest method of establishing increased voluntary control of the sensitive vasomotor system (Anderson, 1975; Brown, 1987). Suggestions for hand warming are more effective at relieving migraine symptoms than are other types of suggestion (Alladin, 1988). Therapeutic suggestion significantly increases subjects' ability to increase or decrease skin temperature control (Bregman, 1981). Both biofeedback and relaxation training have also been shown to be effective methods for learning hand warming (Bregman, 1981). The changes produced tend to be short-lived (lasting around ten minutes for most subjects), with the temperature gradually returning to baseline thereafter for normal controls. In addition to these techniques, a multimodal approach can be employed, which includes stress reduction, improved interpersonal communication, general ego strengthening, and other preventive measures as well as hypnotic analgesia during headache.

Studies of various cognitive behavioral techniques generally have reported excellent outcomes, with controlled studies reporting a reduction in headache frequency for both tension headache and migraines on the order of 40 to 90 percent (Kroger, 1977; Jessup, 1979). Nonhypnotic muscle relaxation has been shown to be effective in decreasing the amount of muscle tension both in the resting state and during headaches (Andreychuk, 1975; Adams, 1980). Biofeedback, utilizing either hand temperature or cranial pulses, has also been shown to be effective (Elmore, 1981). Multimodal approaches have generally produced significantly better results (Adler, 1976; Stambaugh, 1977; Hutchings, 1976).

Cancer Pain. Spiegel and Bloom (1983b) reported that a study of women with metastatic breast cancer showed that patients who received group therapy with training in self-hypnosis over a one-year period were able to reduce their pain experience by 50 percent when compared with a control group. In addition, at ten-year follow-up the treatment group had a mean survival rate of 36.6 months compared to 18.9 months for the controls, suggesting that the intervention may have important quantitative as well as qualitative effects (Spiegel, 1989a).

Other Pain. Hypnosis has been shown to be effective in reducing the pain and discomfort associated with repeated unpleasant medical interventions in children with cancer (Hilgard, 1982). Kuttner (1988) found that a hypnotic approach emphasizing storytelling and imagery was significantly more effective than behavioral techniques or standard medical practice in alleviating distress during bone marrow aspirations in young children with leukemia.

There is evidence that patients with chronic facial pain show a greater responsiveness to suggestion as measured by the Carleton University Responsiveness to Suggestion Scale (CURSS) than do normal controls (Stam, 1986). These patients had higher susceptibility scores than did controls, so that a high susceptibility score may be a good predictor of response to treatment among such patients.

In a study of nineteen patients with a variety of musculoskeletal disorders, Domangue (1985) reported significant reductions of pain and dysphoria following hypnosis. The reductions were associated with significant increases in plasma beta endorphin.

Barabasz and Barabasz (1989) evaluated the technique known as restricted environmental stimulation therapy (REST) in a sample of twenty patients with a variety of chronic pain syndromes. All the patients were initially rated as having low hypnotic susceptibility on the SHSS. Following exposure to the training technique, the subjects demonstrated significant increases in both SHSS scores and in pain reduction when compared to controls.

MODIFICATION OF CARDIOVASCULAR FUNCTION

Engel (1986) has suggested that the cardiovascular system can be seen as a behavioral system, formed by a series of interacting conditioned responses that function within a context. In other words, the system learns to respond to environmental cues and is influenced by other bodily conditioned responses. Learning, mediated by limbic-hypothalamic regulatory systems, shapes the nature of vascular dynamics.

Certainly the system demonstrates many learned responses. Sensitive measures of myocardial profusion indicate that significant transient changes in myocardial blood flow occur in response to stressful mental tasks (Deanfield, 1984). Psychological stress induces cardiovascular changes that are consistent with increased sympathetic nervous activity (Light, 1983).

Coronary-prone individuals exhibit distinctive patterns of cardiovascular and neuroendocrine responses for both the sensory intake and the processing components of cognitive function when compared with controls (Williams, 1982). Some individuals can show recurrent life-threatening cardiac arrhythmias in response to specific psychological stress, which may precipitate sudden cardiac arrest (Lown, 1982; Freeman, 1986).

Cardiac complications of hypertension appear to be more related to blood pressure responses to stressful situations than to baseline blood pressure measures (Devereux, 1983). Specific patterns of emotional expression coupled with a significant degree of baseline autonomic arousal may, in combination, be a reliable predictor of the risk for hypertension (Boutelle, 1987). Everyday conversations usually increase blood pressure significantly, and patients with hypertension have more marked increases than do controls (Lynch, 1981).

Although relatively little systematic work has been done on the use of hypnosis with cardiovascular disorders, what studies have been made suggest that alterations in peripheral and central vascular function may underlie a number of hypnotic effects (Banks, 1985; Barber, 1984). For example, a small pilot study showed that children trained in self-hypnosis could significantly alter their tissue levels of oxygen as measured by transcutaneous PO_2 measures (Olness, 1985). A careful single-case controlled study of a patient with Raynaud's disease showed a rapid and dramatic vasodilatation in response to hypnotic suggestion (Conn, 1984). Subjects who used a high degree of mental imagery seemed to be more susceptible to cardiovascular conditioning than subjects with poorer mental imagery ability (Arabian, 1983).

Hypertensive patients appeared to be significantly more effective at controlling cardiovascular responses to stressors in hypnosis than they were in the normal waking state; this was particularly true for subjects with more marked hypnotic ability (Bernardi, 1982). Normotensive subjects could either raise or decrease their blood pressure significantly with hypnosis, but they could only lower it with relaxation therapy (Sletvold, 1986). Patients who were able to reduce their blood pressure significantly using biofeedback techniques also showed a progressive increase in their ability to become internally absorbed and to withdraw from external stimuli (J. Cohen, 1983).

Hypertensive subjects also had characteristic patterns of increased cerebral blood flow that were most marked in the left hemisphere. During hypnosis, they could reduce cerebral blood flow more dramatically than could normotensive controls (Galeazzi, 1982). These changes were associated with decreases in vascular resistance and diastolic blood pressure in the rest of the body.

The role of exercise in regulating cardiovascular function may be related to hypnotic ability. Subjects with hypnotic ability could improve their aerobic performance significantly in response to posthypnotic suggestion (Jackson, 1979). Subjects with high hypnotic susceptibility significantly improved their performance in physical exercise using posthypnotic suggestion. But low susceptibility subjects could do virtually as well if they were given suggestions during the waking state. As in the case of pain control, these findings suggest that a variety of cognitive strategies can be effective but that no single approach is useful for all subjects. Similarly, subjects of varying hypnotic abilities improved their performance with similar instructions given in the waking state (Spanos, 1986b).

Friedman and Taub (1977, 1978) reported the results of a trial comparing hypnosis with biofeedback or a combination of both in essential hypertension. At the end of four weeks of treatment, all groups showed a significant reduction in blood pressure. But at six-month follow-up only the patients receiving hypnosis had maintained the reduction.

MODIFICATION OF RESPIRATORY FUNCTION

The respiratory system is another example of the combination of voluntary and involuntary mechanisms within a complex regulatory system. Breathing patterns, for example, vary with changes in emotional state. Bereaved individuals show characteristic abnormalities in respiratory control that are similar to those found in patients with major depression (Jellinek, 1985). Respiratory patterns are at the interface between emotional states and physiologic function.

Asthma

Asthma involves both allergic and conditioned responses to stimuli. There is some evidence that the two types of stimuli act in different ways and that hypnosis is specifically useful in modifying the conditioned aspects of asthma (Thorne, 1978). Highly susceptible subjects were more likely to be able to undergo an asthmalike attack in response to suggestion during hypnosis than were low susceptibles. This was true regardless of the subjects' history of asthma (Thorne, 1978).

The distinction between conditioned and allergic forms of asthma, however, is complicated by the fact that immune responses themselves can be conditioned. Animal studies show that histamine release, a major component of the allergic reaction, can be produced by classical conditioning procedures (Russell, 1984). Thus asthmatic attacks can be influenced by a combination of factors. Patients with asthma show a complex situation with specific sensitivity to allergens, increased generalized sensitivity of the autonomic nervous system, and conditioned responses to learned emotional or situational stimuli all playing a role in the disorder.

Current theories of the nature of asthma emphasize the interaction between immunologic and autonomic triggers of attacks (Barnes, 1987). Although modern treatments have greatly improved the management of many asthmatic patients, there is cause for concern owing to evidence of an increased mortality rate for asthma over the past few years (Burney, 1986). Overreliance on medication may have deemphasized the need for an awareness of emotional factors in the genesis of asthma as well as a relative neglect of the need to increase individual sensitivity to potential stressors and to provide appropriate training in effective breathing techniques (Wilkinson, 1988b).

Certainly, there is evidence that hyperventilation (which may cause bronchial constriction in those with hyperactive airways) can be produced in chronic asthmatic patients by their experiencing strong emotion. In one study using hypnosis, suggestions to recall feelings of anger or fear as well as suggestions to recall an asthmatic attack produced a substantial increase in the mean minute volume of respiration (Clarke, 1980), effectively reproducing the breathing pattern that occurs in the initial stages of an asthmatic attack. There is other substantial evidence for the role of emotions in precipitating these attacks (Bengtsson, 1984; Tunsater, 1984).

Hypnosis has been shown to alleviate the subjective distress of patients with asthma as measured by the number of attacks or the amount of medication that is needed (Maher-Loughnan, 1962, 1970), when compared to supportive therapy. In a study that randomly assigned asthmatics to either hypnosis or relaxation therapy, both were of benefit to the patients but the improvement in the hypnotherapy group was significantly greater (Maher-Loughnan, 1970). Moreover, only the hypnotic subjects showed improvement in physiologic measures of respiration (forced expiratory volume). Collison (1975) found that hypnotic susceptibility correlates positively with symptomatic improvement in asthma, but subjective improvement in asthmatic patients treated with hypnosis may not correlate with objective measures of air flow (Morrison, 1988).

Ewer and Stewart (1986) have reported a randomized control trial of hypnosis in patients with moderate asthma. Patients with a high hypnotic susceptibility showed a 74.9 percent improvement in bronchial hyperresponsiveness (to methacholine challenge), a 5.5 percent increase in peak expiratory flow rate, a 26.2 percent decrease in the use of bronchodilators, and a 41 percent improvement in daily ratings outside of the clinic. Twelve patients with a high hypnotic susceptibility score showed a 75 percent improvement, whereas a control group of seventeen patients and ten patients with a low level of hypnotic susceptibility showed no change in either objective or subjective measures.

More patients may be helped by a prolonged course of hypnotherapy than indicated by the Ewer study, underlining the care with which measures of hypnotic susceptibility must be interpreted. The patients treated by Maher-Loughnan showed a peak of improvement between the seventh and twelfth week of treatment, whereas the patients in the Ewer study were tested only at the end of six weeks, pointing up the need for adequate length of follow-up (Maher-Loughnan, 1984).

Hyperventilation

This responsivity of the respiratory system to suggestion is not limited to asthmatic individuals. Subjects who are told they are inhaling a substance that will cause breathing difficulty have significantly increased total respiratory resistance when compared with controls (Kotses, 1987). Ventilatory responses to CO_2 can be blunted in response to suggestion in the waking state and, to a greater degree, with hypnosis (Sato, 1986).

Changes in ventilatory pattern are also one of the mechanisms by which changes in emotional state can affect cardiovascular and other physiologic functions (Grossman, 1983). Hyperventilation is most common in patients with undiagnosed breathlessness, and chest pain with normal coronary arteries is associated with significant psychological distress (Bass, 1983). Between 10 and 45 percent of patients who have angiography for the investigation of chest pain and breathlessness will have normal angiograms (Bass, 1983; Kane, 1988). Approximately half of them may meet diagnostic criteria for an anxiety disorder, with or without panic attacks (Kane, 1988). Between two-thirds and three-quarters of the patients will also report symptoms of breathlessness or other features of hyperventilation (Bass, 1983; Roy-Byrne, 1989; Kane, 1988).

Hyperventilation, a learned system of dysfunctional breathing, can result in a host of physical and psychological symptoms (Lum, 1983). Patients with breathing abnormalities related to anxiety symptoms appear to have altered sensitivity to carbon dioxide (Bass, 1983; Gorman, 1988), but their hypersensitivity appears to be a disorder of conditioning rather than a biochemical alteration (Woods, 1988). It has been proposed that disturbances in CO_2 sensitivity and pCO_2 resting levels complete the circuit by predisposing the brain to increased sympathetic nervous system activity (Gorman, 1984). There appears to be increased peripheral nervous system activation in the actual attack but without evidence of sustained hyperactivity at other times (Shear, 1986).

Hyperventilation can be mimicked by forced breathing in some but not all patients (Cluff, 1984; Conway, 1988). Those who do not respond to the forced breathing with hyperventilation will respond to hypnotic suggestions of provoking situations (Conway, 1988). In other words, the breathing pattern itself was not sufficient to produce an attack unless the psychological and contextual cues were present. This differential pattern of response can also be distinguished by both personality measures (Conway, 1988) and blood gas response patterns (Salkovskis, 1986).

GASTROINTESTINAL DISORDERS

Irritable bowel syndrome (IBS) is one of the most common of gastrointestinal disorders (*Lancet,* 1984). Such patients have changes in bowel motility and abdominal pain associated with diffuse disorders of gastrointestinal motility that affect every part of the G.I. system. These patients typically are very poor at identifying visceral feedback correctly (Ritchie, 1973; Latimer, 1983; Whitehead, 1982). Generally, IBS responds relatively poorly to conventional drug therapies, and results of clinical trials aimed at affecting dietary measures, largely by increasing fiber ingestion, have been equivocal (Collins, 1988). A substantial number of IBS patients go on to a chronic course of greater or lesser severity.

Colonic motor activity in IBS patients shows a greater number of abnormalities both in the resting state and in response to stress (Kumar, 1985; Snape, 1986; Taylor, 1978; Whitehead, 1985). They have significantly higher motor activity in the colon in the resting state than do controls (Welgan, 1985). Both IBS patients and controls show significant increases in gut motor activity in response to stress, but only the IBS patients show a characteristic increase in 2–4 cycle per minute slow-wave activity.

The exact relationship between severity of psychological distress and severity of physical symptoms in IBS is not clear (Welgan, 1985; Latimer, 1983). Patients are more likely to have a psychiatric diagnosis than are patients with other gastrointestinal disorders (Young, 1976; Latimer, 1983). Some workers have reported a lack of a direct relationship between psychopathology and either colonic motility or severity of symptoms in IBS patients (Whitehead, 1980). Such patients do appear to manifest more emotional lability and a greater variety of symptoms than do other gastroenterology patients (Rosenthal, 1987). At present, we can conclude only that IBS patients are a heterogeneous group and that a multimodal approach to treatment that takes into account psychological, social, dietary, and physiologic factors is the only one that is justified by the evidence to date (Sammons, 1987).

Whorwell (1984) has reported successful treatment of IBS using hypnosis in a controlled study of a group of patients who had a severe chronic form of the disorder and had not responded to conventional therapies. Patients were randomly allocated to either psychotherapy or hypnotherapy groups. The psychotherapy patients did show a significant improvement in measures of pain, distension, and general well-being despite a lack of change in bowel habit. In contrast, the hypnotherapy patients showed a dramatic improvement in all measures, which persisted at two-year follow-up (Whorwell, 1987). Hypnotherapy, including suggestions for improved gastrointestinal function and pain reduction, was significantly better than hypnosis for simple deep muscle relaxation. Response to hypnotherapy did not correlate with measures of hypnotic susceptibility. The success rate was much higher in patients with more typical cases of IBS and those who were under the age of fifty. Harvey and his coworkers (1989) have reported a similar improvement following hypnotherapy in twenty of thirty-three patients with refractory IBS at three-month follow-up.

Another gastrointestinal disorder that has been investigated is duodenal ulcer disease. Colgan (1988) has reported a randomized trial of thirty patients with frequently relapsing duodenal ulcer disease. The subjects were treated for ten weeks with either hypnotherapy and ranitidine or the drug alone. At a twelve-month follow-up, all of the drug-only patients, but only half of the drug-plus-hypnotherapy patients, had relapsed. This is in keeping with the notion that hypnotic suggestion can reduce both baseline gastric acid and gastric acid response to stimulation (Klein, 1989; Stacher, 1975).

Also shown to be responsive to psychological intervention is the unpleasant and disabling anticipatory nausea and vomiting that is associated with chemotherapy for cancer (Carey, 1988). Both adolescent and adult cancer patients undergoing chemotherapy have been reported to have fewer symptoms of anticipatory nausea and vomiting following hypnotic interventions (Cotanch, 1985; Zeltzer, 1984). Hypnotic susceptibility scores have not been shown to correlate with treatment outcome (Zeltzer, 1984). Similar procedures, labeled relaxation with guided imagery rather than hypnosis, appear to be comparably effective (Lyles, 1982).

OTHER MEDICAL USES

Hypnotic intervention has been helpful for patients suffering from several other, unrelated disorders. Hemophiliacs composed one such group. Studies in subjects with normal bleeding time demonstrated that hypnotic training is not effective in reducing bleeding time in a laboratory situation (Hopkins, 1988). But over an eighteen-week follow-up, a group of hemophiliac patients who were taught self-hypnosis significantly reduced both their level of self-reported distress and the amount of the factor concentrate they required to control bleeding when compared with a control group of patients who did not undergo hypnosis (Swirsky-Saccetti, 1986). A thirty-month follow-up with hemophiliac patients demonstrated the effectiveness of group procedures for self-hypnosis in reducing distress and the amount of blood products required when compared to control groups in patients ranging from five to forty-eight years of age (LaBaw, 1975).

Hypnotherapy has also been used to prolong pregnancy and prevent premature delivery (Schwartz, 1963). In a prospective study, Omer found that frequency of physical complaints and the general level of anxiety were correlated with premature labor and premature contractions. A brief technique emphasizing the use of self-hypnosis was employed as an adjunct to pharmacological treatment. The prolongation of pregnancy was significantly higher for this group than for the medication-alone control group, and infant weight was also significantly greater (Omer, 1986a, 1986b, 1987a). On the other hand, a similar study designed to shorten postterm pregnancy reported no advantage in using hypnotic intervention (Omer, 1987b).

And, finally, a pair of randomized, carefully designed studies were conducted with a group of people who had warts. Subjects who were given hypnotic or nonhypnotic suggestions were significantly more likely to achieve wart regression than placebo or no-treatment groups

(Spanos, 1988). Pretreatment hypnotic susceptibility scores did not predict outcome.

CONCLUSIONS, PROBLEMS, AND POSSIBILITIES

The research on medical uses of hypnosis, though generally positive, leaves many major issues untouched. For our purposes, the domain of hypnosis can be divided into three broad areas. The first of these is hypnotizability or hypnotic susceptibility: the distribution of hypnotic ability in the patient population and, by implication, the way in which hypnotic susceptibility scales might be used to predict response not only to hypnosis but to other forms of cognitive and behavioral therapies.

Hypnotic Ability

There is a healthy theoretical controversy regarding the nature of hypnotic ability (for example, Spanos, 1986a), and clinical studies will be important in defining the nature of the debate in practical terms. Of particular significance is the nature of hypnotic ability and the means by which it may be measured. The prognostic role of hypnotic susceptibility scales is controversial (Bowers, 1986), although there is no question as to the potential importance of standardized measures of hypnotic ability. There continues to be an overall lack of correlation between hypnotizability and clinical outcome (Mott, 1979; Wadden, 1982). The debate between state and social cognitive theorists largely revolves around the weight that inherent hypnotic ability should be given versus response to expectations and contextual cues (Nadon, 1987). In the majority of cases, the benefits achieved appear to be due not only to the effects of the hypnotic state but also to the expectations of the patient and the quality of the relationship between patient and therapist (Brown, 1987; Spanos, 1986b; Stam, 1987). Brown and Fromm have defined hypnotic ability, taking these features into account:

Hypnotizability can be viewed as a quasi-stable trait, which some people have more of than do other people. Like any personality trait, hypnotizability is a relatively enduring characteristic that presumably exists independently of whether one has been hypnotized before. However, as with many traits, the degree to which this enduring characteristic is manifest varies with the situation. Expectation, motivation, attitude, anxiety, mood, and rapport with the hypnotist—all influence the degree of manifestation of this trait. (1987, p. 36)

There is a danger of simply equating hypnosis with a particular scale and not taking into account such factors as motivation, expectations, rapport, and context as part of the hypnotherapeutic field. Nevertheless, considerable progress has been made in modifying scales to the clinical setting (Bowers, 1986; Edmonston, 1986). Sensitively applied, hypnotizability scales play an important role in well-designed, randomized trials. The development of these scales clearly constitutes one of the more significant advances in the scientific study of hypnosis in medical conditions (Frankel, 1987). Despite their limitations, they will continue to be central to further research. The arguments against them do not constitute a dismissal of their value but, rather, the need to pursue their progressive improvement and modification for clinical purposes.

The Hypnotic Experience

The second area for consideration involves hypnosis as trance: the nature of the hypnotic experience. Some workers define trance as an altered state of consciousness or dissociation (Hilgard, 1977); others (Spanos, 1986a) have argued for a social-psychological approach that minimizes the putative differences between hypnotic state and everyday consciousness. Certainly, though there are changes in brain function during hypnosis, they are not unique to hypnosis nor are they uniform across all subjects. As previously noted (see chapter 5), the changes in brain function that occur in hypnosis are similar to the normal ultradian variations in activity and do not appear to differ from changes found in other types of absorbed concentration. This observation brings up the question of the uniqueness of hypnosis and the degree of overlap with other approaches such as relaxation, biofeedback, or nonhypnotic cognitive strategies and response-based imagery.

Although substantial and consistent psychophysiologic changes occur during hypnosis, there is no evidence for any changes that are specific to formal hypnosis (Sarbin, 1979). Physiologically, the effects of hypnosis seem to be mediated primarily by changes in blood flow (Barber, 1984), autonomic activity (Brown, 1986), and respiratory pattern (Wilkinson, 1988a). The evidence strongly suggests that social and psychological factors can influence physiologic processes, not through some magical legerdemain but through the usual everyday channels that connect body and brain.

One of the problems in establishing the role of hypnosis is our lack of understanding of how it works. A plausible mechanism of action is an important preliminary step in the general acceptance of any therapeutic modality. Workers have suggested that at least part of the hypnotic effect involves the reduction of anxiety, autonomic hypersensitivity, and conditioned responses (Davis, 1973; Horton, 1977; Brown, 1987).

There is evidence that changes in autonomic nervous system activity may affect the nature of sensory input. There appears to be an ongoing link between somatosensory input and sympathetic activity as measured by galvanic skin response (Hallin, 1983). Certainly, most hallucinogens and other drugs that affect the central nervous system (such as those that are used in healing ceremonies in other cultures) produce a modulation of autonomic nervous system activity (Joralemon, 1984). Drugs that influence the nervous system affect conditioned autonomic responses (Eikelboom, 1982). There is an inextricable link between perceptual state and sympathetic tone in subjective experience. Modification of that subjective experience through hypnosis may result in both perceptual changes and a resetting of the level of autonomic arousal.

The autonomic nervous system appears to be susceptible to psychophysiologic modification. Increases in arousal level may enhance sensitivity to autonomic feedback (Katkin, 1985). Similarly, certain cognitive skills are more available at specific arousal levels and may thus be more effective at learning to control particular physiologic measures such as heart rate (Levenson, 1981). This further underscores the important role that bodily cues and autonomic activity have in defining emotional states.

Those states appear to be mediated by a host of "information substances." The explosion of knowledge in the neurosciences has led to the development of a new perspective on how mind and body interact (Rossi, 1988). The traditional model of the nervous system consists of a complex wiring diagram of specific connections made up of pathways assembled from a synaptic arrangement of cells that communicate with each other through specific chemical transmitters and only at specific receptors, one cell to another in a particular order. The revolution in the neurosciences over the past decade has entailed the recognition of a far wider form of communication, which Schmitt (1984) has described as "parasynaptic." In this model, the classic neurotransmitters are augmented by a widening array of information substances, all of which function to convey information diffusely and at a distance. The distinction between the synaptic and parasynaptic systems is a difference in both spatial and temporal organization (Bloom, 1986). This diffuse system appears to work alongside and modulate the effects of the "more hard-wired" nervous system. Cell-to-cell synaptic transmission is analogous to telephone communication that occurs between one cell and another. In contrast, the revised model suggests that the process is more like that of radio or television being sent out diffusely in all directions and received by any system with the correct receptors.

A major conceptual shift in neuroscience has been wrought by the realization that brain function is modulated by numerous chemicals in addition to classical neurotransmitters. Many of these informational substances are neuropeptides, originally studied in other contexts as hormones, "gut peptides," or growth factors. Their number presently exceeds 50 and most, if not all, alter behavior and mood states. . . . We now realize that their signal specificity resides in receptors (distinct classes of recognition molecules), rather than the close juxtaposition occurring at classical synapses. Rather precise brain distribution patterns for many neuropeptide receptors have been determined. A number of brain loci, many within emotion-mediating brain areas, are enriched with many types of neuropeptide receptors suggesting a convergence of information at these "nodes." Additionally, neuropeptide receptors occur on mobile cells of the immune system; monocytes can chemotax to numerous neuropeptides via processes shown by structure-activity analysis to be mediated by distinct receptors indistinguishable from those found in the brain. Neuropeptides and their receptors thus join the brain, glands, and immune system in a network of communication between brain and body, probably representing the biochemical substrate of emotion. (Pert, 1985, p. 820s)

Significantly, it appears that these substances, particularly the neuropeptides, are most densely located in those structures specifically localized so that they may be involved in the modulation of emotion and perception (Pert, 1985). The neuropeptides function in the cerebral cortex in the sensory association processing areas and appear to have a critical role in the filtering of sensory input and selective attention (Lewis, 1981). Neuropeptides are also found in the brain stem and spinal cord where they appear to function as a type of modulating or gating system that affects the perception and expectation of pain (Pert, 1987). The limbic, hypothalamic, and pituitary systems have the highest concentrations in the brain of opiate receptors and these patterns correspond to areas responsible for emotional and motivational functions— the amygdala—and centers of physiologic homeostasis—hypothalamus-pituitary (Lewis, 1981; Pert, 1987).

Not only has a wide variety of new information substances been identified; the last decade has also seen a dramatic change in our understanding of traditional neurotransmitter-receptor interaction, which "requires that receptors not be considered in isolation but as components of complex neuronal circuits and, in particular, as the component that recognizes and transduces neurotransmitter signals into intracellular effects" (Hyman, 1988b, p. 262). Receptors, the specialized structures that serve to transduce the chemical message of the transmitter into intracellular information, can be modified by experience (Hyman, 1988a). Receptor sensitivities can be dramatically modified over time, so that though the signal of a neurotransmitter may be a relatively quick one, the results can be long-lasting.

It turns out that the brain may not be like a computer at all, unless it is one in which the hardware itself is undergoing constant modification. In addition to conduction along a hard-wired network, transmitters can change the set of channels available for information processing and thereby facilitate some pathways and inhibit others. These modifications may be long-lasting and may subserve important functions, such as selective gating of sensory inputs, short-term memory, and, speculatively, perhaps the effective coloration of experience. (Hyman, 1988a, p. 165)

Therapeutic Benefits of Hypnosis

The third area for our discussion is hypnosis as hypnotherapy: hypnosis as it is used in the clinical context as a modality that can be integrated with other therapeutic approaches. If hypnotic skills are restricted to a relatively small population, these findings are of limited clinical interest. For a substantial number of other patients, however, there may be a significant advantage to a form of rehearsal and training in the hypnotic technique. There is significant recent support for the hypothesis that hypnotic skill can be thought of as a set of social and cognitive skills potentially modifiable by training and the context in which they are used (Spanos, 1986a). Subjects who receive cognitive training in hypnotic skills can significantly improve their hypnotic susceptibility scores (Gfeller, 1987; Gorassini, 1986; Spanos, 1986a, 1986b) and also improve their clinical response (Stam, 1987). A high degree of rapport and interpersonal contact with the trainer significantly improves this response (Lynn, 1987b). Similarly, successful treatment response with biofeedback appears to depend on personality characteristics and interpersonal style (Ford, 1985), suggesting a common therapeutic thread shared by different modalities.

Spinhoven (1987) has suggested that hypnosis can be defined as either an antecedent variable (that is, the difference between hypnosis and other states of consciousness) or as a subject variable (that is, the inherent hypnotic talent of an individual subject). Examining hypnosis as an antecedent variable is complicated by the degree of heterogeneity of individual responses and the lack of any external validating measure that reliably discriminates between the hypnotic and nonhypnotic contexts (Spanos, 1986a). There are characteristic differences between excellent hypnotic subjects in hypnosis and simulating subjects, but there is substantial overlap for many subjects of low or moderate hypnotic ability between times at which they are hypnotized and times at which they are not (Spanos, 1987a, 1987b). In the absence of reliable external validating criteria, the problem is a significant one. It becomes even more complex in a clinical setting when hypnosis is being compared with some other treatment modality, such as behavior therapy or biofeedback, which also involves instructions for relaxing, letting go, following a sequence of suggested steps, and using imaginative processes extensively (Spinhoven, 1987). Frequently, the only difference between a hypnotic induction and an imagination-based behavioral therapy will be how they are labeled.

The question also arises as to whether one treatment is inherently more effective than the other, or whether there are particular patients who benefit from one but not the other. Good hypnotic subjects may spontaneously use their hypnotic abilities in the absence of hypnotic induction (Barber, 1984). Because of these difficulties, most of the research has focused on hypnosis as a subject variable through the use of hypnotic susceptibility scales. Broadly speaking, the research done to date has not been able to elucidate a clear predictor of outcome (Holroyd, 1982; Miller, 1985; Neff, 1983; Spanos, 1985a). The results indicate that tests of hypnotic susceptibility do not predict which patients will respond preferentially to hypnotic or nonhypnotic treatment, nor does combining biofeedback and hypnosis show an advantage over either technique alone (Sigman, 1988). As Sigman suggests, our preoccupation with differences in technique may obscure the differences in personal ability and context that are the determining factors (Marino, 1989). Further development of susceptibility scales, perhaps linked with psychophysiologic markers, may enhance their clinical value (Hilgard, 1982).

The cognitive and affective aspects of hypnosis are nonspecific. It appears that relaxation, the development of positive imagery and the interruption of negative cognitions (catastrophizing), an increased sensitivity to physical cues, and an enhancement of self-esteem appear to be the common factors involved in therapeutic effectiveness. In addition, the perceived quality of the therapeutic relationship seems to be a critical variable (Lynn, 1987b). The diversity of approaches suggests that "hypnosis does not in itself imply a specific therapy, but rather a special context within which a variety of therapeutic approaches can be applied" (Hart, 1988, p. 201). Certainly, hypnosis is best viewed not as a panacea but simply as a useful adjunct to other forms of therapy.

Perhaps the greatest clinical challenge remains the need to suit the treatment to the patient and not the other way round (Dance, 1988). Milton Erickson frequently warned against the inherent limitations of a monochromatic treatment approach, or what he termed the "procrustean bed of psychotherapy" (Erickson and Rossi, 1979, p. 233). In their thoughtful review of the subject, Daniel Brown and Erica Fromm (1986) advocate a multimodal approach to the control of psychobiologic function in a number of different disorders. They combine hypnosis with cognitive and behavioral measures, biofeedback, and psychodynamically oriented psychotherapies. The goal is to provide a treatment program open to critical evaluation that may ultimately help determine which elements are particularly effective given the individual needs of the patient. Recognizing that illness is a multifactorial biologic, psychological, and social process, the worker will adopt a multimodal approach in which treatment will be weighted toward those factors that will be most useful in each clinical situation.

There is growing evidence that treatments that integrate cognitive features with increased sensitivity to bodily cues may be considerably more effective than either treatment alone. For example, though cognitive treatment and biofeedback both were found to be effective for decreasing blood pressure in hypertensives, those receiving the first treatment achieved better results in emotional expression and those receiving the second had greater decreases in blood pressure levels (Achmon, 1989). Such therapy is more likely to be effective for long periods of time if relaxation techniques are integrated with cognitive strategies (Patel, 1988). The marked variability that most patients have shown in their response to one aspect of therapy also supports the notion of a multimodal approach (Achmon, 1989).

A closer integration of hypnotherapy and other behavioral approaches, then, is essential. In order to achieve this, four broad issues must be addressed successfully. The first is ascertaining the role of hypnotic ability in responses to both hypnotic and nonhypnotic therapies, and the consequent prognostic power of hypnotic susceptibility scales. The second is establishing the degree of overlap between hypnosis and other forms of therapy. To this end, trials comparing hypnosis with other forms of therapy need to be undertaken to identify the common critical variables. Third, more studies are needed of cognitive training to enhance hypnotic ability, which would, it is hoped, increase its therapeutic efficacy. And finally, we must conduct many more carefully designed clinical trials to further establish the effectiveness of hypnotherapy in a number of medical disorders.

8 VERSIONS OF SELF: MULTIPLE PERSONALITY DISORDER

I saw that of the two natures that contended in the field of my consciousness, even if I could be rightly said to be either, it was only because I was radically both.

R. L. Stevenson,
The Strange Case of Dr. Jekyll and Mr. Hyde

One of the most controversial topics in clinical hypnosis is the spontaneous generation of alternate versions of self: multiple personality disorder. Certainly no other psychiatric disorder engenders so much controversy: some investigators insist that it usually goes undetected, whereas others question its existence. The evidence, though incomplete, suggests that multiple personality does occur as an attempt to integrate the consequences of traumatic experiences in individuals with high hypnotic ability. The evidence also suggests, however, that the form of the disorder is a result of contextual cues, expectations, and cultural values. The self, in all of its manifestations, is a social product.

MISS BEAUCHAMP

In the spring of 1898 a twenty-three-year-old student, whom the world came to know as "Miss Beauchamp," consulted a prominent Boston psychiatrist, Morton Prince. Miss Beauchamp was anxious and unhappy. She complained of a host of physical pains and a lack of energy. She had few friends, and her life was one of lonely isolation. She read voraciously and was particularly addicted to the popular romantic novels of the time. Prince describes a picture of "a neurotic, sensitive, visionary child, brought up in an unsympathetic atmosphere. . . . She never gave expression to the ordinary feelings of everyday child life; never spoke to say she was tired, hungry, or sleepy. She lived within herself and dreamed" (Prince, 1906, 1920, quoted in Kenny, 1986, p. 139).

Miss Beauchamp was the pseudonym of Clara Fowler. Using Prince's account as a source book, medical historians have uncovered a great deal of Fowler's story. Her father was an explosive and abusive man. When she was thirteen, her mother, with whom she had not been close, died. After three unhappy years Clara ran away from home. Prior to consulting Prince, she had been involved in a prolonged unhappy relationship (which Prince vaguely refers to as "traumatic") with a man many years older than herself.

Prince felt that he was treating a conventional, if extreme, case of neurasthenia, a popular diagnosis of the time, which purportedly was the result of the taxing demands of excessive intellectual work on the frail female constitution. Having little success with conventional treatments, Prince decided to resort to hypnosis. It was shortly thereafter that during hypnosis a remarkable thing happened:

> I was startled to hear her . . . speak of herself in her waking state as "She." . . .
> "Are you 'she,'" I said.
> "No, I am not."
> "I say you are."
> Again a denial. (Prince, 1906, quoted in Kenny, 1986, p. 142)

Over Prince's objections a new personality, calling herself "Sally," began to emerge. At first Sally spoke only during hypnosis, but gradually she began to appear spontaneously with greater and greater frequency. The character of Sally as she emerged was everything that Clara Fowler was not. Clara was serious, withdrawn, and unexpressive; Sally was witty, lively, and flirtatious. In short, all the things that Clara Fowler was not, Sally became. The notion that the new personality would somehow be a compensation for the original one was quite obvious. Within the framework of the hypnotic relationship with Prince, a new version of her personality emerged.

"Hypnosis—being an 'altered' state—granted Miss Beauchamp the poetic license to experiment with the content of her selfhood" (Kenny,

1986, p. 145). Kenny has pointed out that Sally, in fact, was also remarkably similar to Dr. Prince: witty, extroverted, and very much a social animal. Sally and Dr. Prince clearly had a great deal in common. Using the Sally personality as an adviser and collaborator, Prince recounts the gradual integration of the various aspects of Clara Fowler's personality. At the end of therapy, Clara Fowler no longer had a trace of a discrete Sally personality. She was confident, happy, and, above all, definitely one person. This self she described as an integration of her original personality with a later version. She married a psychiatric colleague of Prince's and led an active family and social life as a prominent Boston hostess.

"In the symbolically transformed shape of medical disorder Prince [had] encountered one of the representative problems of his age and became the inadvertent director of a play with a peculiarly creative cast of characters; the climax, as in the novel, took the form of self-realization, a partial resolution of existential and objective contradiction" (Kenny, 1986, p. 130).

Kenny proposes that multiple personality is "an idiom of distress" that has arisen as a result of social definitions of the self and the ways in which that self can be disordered. "Every society poses questions of identity and value that can lead to instability in the content of selfhood" (Kenny, 1986, p. 9).

In his fascinating social and historical account of some of the most famous cases of multiple personality disorder, Kenny (1986) paints a vivid picture of nineteenth-century America as a society intoxicated with a heady brew of Puritan guilt, utopianism, rapid cycles of economic boom and decline, and changes in the social roles of women. Kenny also shows the origins of a possible model for multiple personality in the nineteenth century's obsession with possession both in the fundamentalist Christian sense and in the attempts to reach another "spirit world" through the agency of mediumship.

Late-nineteenth-century psychology contained a hidden agenda that emanated from issues of wider public concern, most particularly the position of women in the new urban industrial world. The contemporary study of multiple personality also has a hidden agenda that can be detected in the complex of issues to which the problem is connected. As in the nineteenth century, psychic dissociation leading to multiplicity is frequently attributed to trauma; however, now the focal point is childhood sexual abuse. The changes set afoot in the nineteenth century in the structure of the family and patterns of work are still running their course toward an uncertain future. (Kenny, 1986, p. 15)

THE PHENOMENOLOGIC MODEL OF MULTIPLE
PERSONALITY DISORDER

After decades of virtual obscurity, multiple personality disorder (MPD) has become the object of a dramatic resurgence of interest in North America. During the middle part of the century, use of the diagnostic label was rare. Even clinicians who were associated with the disorder in the public's mind rarely came across a case (Thigpen, 1984). The concept is one that reliably engenders a lively controversy. A debate rages about how common MPD actually is. Some clinicians (for example, Bliss, 1985) insist that the disorder is usually misdiagnosed and goes unsuspected by the majority of doctors. For example, Bliss reports an incidence of about 10 percent or more in a sample of 150 consecutive psychiatric patients (1985). In contrast, Thigpen and Cleckley (1984) say that of literally thousands of patients referred to them over a twenty-five-year period because of their well-known interest in the disorder only one could be diagnosed as having MPD after their initial report on Eve Black. On the other hand, critics (see Kenny, 1986; Spanos, 1985b) believe that the resurgence of interest is a social and cultural phenomenon that results from patients' behavior being shaped by societal pressures and credulous clinicians.

For MPD, DSM-III-R, the current psychiatric diagnostic system, lists the following criteria:

(a) The existence within the individual of two or most distinct personalities or personality states (each with its own relatively enduring pattern of perceiving, related to, and thinking about the environment and self).
(b) At least two of these personalities or personality states recurrently take full control of the individual's behavior. (American Psychiatric Association, 1987)

Kluft (1987) suggests that direct questioning of the patient is typically met with denial. Although some evidence suggests that the diagnosis is increasing in frequency, there is also substantial clinical evidence that patients may actively conceal features of the disorder because they are embarrassing, frightening, or otherwise unacceptable (Kluft, 1987; Bliss, 1986; Braun, 1986a).

Associated features that, though less specific, can alert the clinician to the possibility of the diagnosis include repeated changes in diagnosis, complex mixtures of physical and emotional symptoms, rapid shifts in the level of function, and failure of conventional treatments (Putnam, 1984). Histories of childhood physical and sexual abuse should also suggest the diagnosis (Beahrs, 1988). In addition, when compared with other psychiatric patients, those with the MPD diagnosis have been reported to have a significantly higher frequency of complaints of amnesia, auditory hallucinations, headaches, undiagnosed physical symptoms, sexual dysfunctions, and histories of rape and childhood physical and sexual abuse (Coons, 1986; C. A. Ross, 1989a). Patients with MPD are more commonly female at a rate of 4–9:1 (Kluft, 1987; Bliss, 1986).

These patients have significantly more unexplained physical symptoms than do other patient groups (C. A. Ross, 1989a, 1989b). The variety of nonspecific somatic symptoms common in MPD may be associated with childhood histories of sexual abuse (Goodwin, 1989; C. A. Ross, 1989a, 1989b). This is of particular interest given the significant number of MPD patients who meet criteria for the diagnosis of somatization disorder (C. A Ross, 1989a). Patients with somatization disorders show a dysfunction in the focus of attention when compared with controls (James, 1987). Furthermore, those with conversion symptoms show a marked impairment in sympathetic tone as reflected by their galvanic skin responses when compared with controls or with patients with anxiety disorders (Horvath, 1980). In combination these two studies suggest possible focal right hemisphere EEG involvement in dysfunctions of attention and sympathetic tone (both of which are mediated by neural circuits involving the right hemisphere).

The personalities emerge with distinctive styles of expressing themselves and usually possess separate names, gender, age, family histories, and life-styles. They may have entirely different occupations, sets of friendships, and social networks. Differences in I.Q., handedness, handwriting style, and other features have been reported (Kluft, 1987). Although early writers described cases in which the personalities appeared to be complementary to one another, recent authors report that the single most common form of MPD presentation is that of an alter personality who functions as a "persecutor" (Beahrs, 1982), intent on punishing or injuring the original personality for some real or imagined transgression. The manner of presentation is typically distinct from the "host" personality. "Their voices, vocabularies, speech patterns, accents, pitch, rhythm, and even preferred languages may vary. The movement characteristics of each alter may be sufficiently distinct as to constitute a virtual 'action signature.' Their facial expressions, both when 'neutral' and when affectively engaged, may be different on a dramatic and consistent basis" (Kluft, 1987, pp. 211–212).

Kluft reports (1985) that in about 40 percent of patients the disorder runs a chronic course; for the remainder the appearance of symptoms may be episodic. In his series of patients, only 20 percent originally presented with clear-cut symptoms, 40 percent fit Putnam's group of patients who had unusual psychiatric histories, and another 40 percent were discovered only by his using highly specialized diagnostic protocols (Kluft, 1987). They had been seen by the clinician for an average of 6.8 years between their initial mental health contact and the diagnosis of MPD.

These patients are more likely than others to report spontaneous alterations in cognition, affect, memory, or behavior in their daily lives (Carlson, 1989). Loewenstein (1987) has demonstrated that experiential sampling, a method of subjective report over time, can distinguish significant variations in the patterns of a single MPD patient. The patient's variety of responses over time were the most varied within a single subject ever recorded.

The physiologic differences between the various MPD personalities can be surprising. For example, a careful study of ten MPD patients showed significantly more variability in visual function across alter personalities than did control subjects who were asked to impersonate MPD patients (Miller, 1989). On average, the MPD subjects had 4.5 times the number of changes in optical function between alter personalities than did the controls.

The episodic nature of MPD is seen by some clinicians as similar to the course of seizure disorders (Tucker, 1986). Patients with temporal lobe epilepsy also frequently report dissociative symptoms with transient episodes of disorientation, amnesia, and dramatic behavioral and emotional changes (Schenk, 1981; Mesulam, 1981). Ross (1987) has reported a positive correlation between reports of temporal lobe symptoms and hypnotic induction profiles. The more likely the subjects were to report temporal lobe experiences, the more likely they were to show a high degree of hypnotic susceptibility. Schenk (1981) found that one-third of a sample of patients with temporal lobe epilepsy exhibited some form of dissociative phenomena (ranging from isolated symptoms to a full-blown MPD picture). Experiences of multiple personality and of demonic possession were often found in individuals with periodic abnormalities of the EEG in the region of the temporal lobe (Mesulam, 1981).

There is some further evidence of altered brain function in MPD. Regional cerebral blood flow measures identify reliable individual characteristics, such as response to arousal (Mathew, 1984). In a study of regional cerebral blood flow in a patient with MPD, Mathew and his coworkers (1984) found changes in brain activity limited to the right temporal area. This finding is significant in that MPD has been found in patients with temporal lobe epilepsy who show a similar blood flow pattern (Schenk, 1981). This region is also part of the temporal parietal circuit in the right hemisphere, which is responsible for the sense of personal involvement in awareness (Kissin, 1986). This finding is consistent with the notion that MPD patients do not in fact have gross cerebral impairment but a relatively subtle change in affective and memory processes. But as this is a report of a single case study, it must be interpreted cautiously.

On the other hand, EEG studies of two multiple personalities showed that the differences between the alters was no greater than those for a control subject who was simulating (in this case, the control was the investigator himself, who mimicked the personalities he had observed with one of the patients). The changes seen in the EEG record are typical of any altered mental state with associated changes in concentration, mood, and muscle tension. One would expect to observe the same sort of differences between a professional actor's EEG record while he was performing a role onstage and when he was in the normal waking state (Coons, 1982).

Putnam studied the cerebral evoked potential responses to visual stimuli in ten patients compared to simulating controls. In contrast to Coons, Putnam found that there were differences between the MPD patients and the controls with respect to both amplitude of the measures and latency of the responses, suggesting a more durable and innate difference than Coon's study (Herbert, 1983). Therapeutic integration in MPD may be associated with specific change in the pattern of evoked potentials. Braun (1983) has presented evidence in two MPD patients of a change of visual evoked potential patterns as a result of hypnotherapy.

Mutations of the Self: The Structure of Dissociation

Multiple personality and other forms of dissociation form a central part of William James's classic *Principles of Psychology*. Like his friend Morton Prince, James was fascinated by the implications of these disorders for the understanding of the relationship between memory and personal identity. Under the heading of "alternating" personality, James examined the histories of a number of famous cases of nineteenth-century individuals with multiple personality disorder. In his discussion of these remarkable cases, James emphasizes two particular "mutations of self" seen in MPD patients: alterations of memory and alterations in perceptual and motor function (James, [1890] 1983, p. 352).

James notes that these two mutations interacted, resulting in a situation in which the various states of consciousness were distinguishable by various memory contents and by the way in which they processed information. In discussing a case of French psychiatrist Pierre Janet's, James compares Léonie 1 and 2, the first two character states, with Léonie 3— the more fully integrated state that Janet achieved under further hypnosis: "Léonie 1 knows only of herself; Léonie 2, of herself and of Léonie 1; Léonie 3 knows of herself and of both the others. Léonie 1 has a visual consciousness; Léonie 2 has one both visual and auditory; in Léonie 3 it is at once visual, auditory, and tactile" (p. 367).

In their theorizing, James and his contemporaries used the term "subliminal consciousness" to refer to a wide range of thought from which our normal consciousness is only a "selection" (Taylor, 1983, p. 41). In James's view, consciousness can be divided among a number of separate but potentially equal partners. In this formulation the arrangement of dissociations is not on the basis of any particular predetermined unconscious hierarchy but can fit any heuristic pattern of behavioral or psychological needs. The only constraints are the inherent limitations of overall neurologic capacity, on one hand, and the existing range of possibilities for individual learning and social role, on the other.

James describes the mind as "a confederation of psychic entities." The various members of this mental confederacy have access to sensory input or cognitive processes that are not directly available to "the ordinary waking self" but might be contacted during hypnosis (Taylor, 1983, p. 42). Thus, they saw hypnosis as a potentially useful therapeutic tool in integrating the abilities of the confederates by allowing them to communicate more easily between themselves. This view was highly popular in the prevailing utopian ethos at the end of the nineteenth century. The idea of vast untapped human potentials residing within the mind fit very well with the liberal belief in the perfectability of humanity.

James cites numerous famous instances of multiple personality including Janet's case of Léonie:

This woman, whose life sounds more like an improbable romance than a genuine history, has had attacks of natural somnambulism since the age of three years. She has been hypnotized constantly by all sorts of persons from the age of sixteen upwards, and she is now forty-five. Whilst her normal life developed in one way in the midst of her poor country surroundings, her second life was passed in drawing-rooms and doctors' offices, and naturally took an entirely different direction. Today, when in her normal state, this poor peasant woman is a serious and rather sad person, calm and slow, very mild with everyone, and extremely timid: to look at her one would never suspect a personage which she contains. But hardly is she put to sleep hypnotically when a metamorphosis occurs. Her face is no longer the same. She keeps her eyes closed, it is true, but the acuteness of her other senses supplies their place. She is gay, noisy, restless, sometimes insupportably so. (Janet, quoted in James, [1890] 1983, p. 366).

Apparently the hypnotic Léonie (Léonie 2) also developed quite a sharp wit and delighted in scathing impersonations of the notables who came to witness her "demonstrations":

She refuses the name of Léonie and takes that of Léontine (Léonie 2) to which her first magnetizers had accustomed her. "That good woman is not myself," she says, "she is too stupid!" To herself, Léontine or Léonie 2, she attributes all the sensations and all the actions, in a word all the conscious experiences, which she has undergone in somnambulism, and knits them together to make the history of her already long life. To Léonie 1, . . . on the other hand, she exclusively ascribes the events lived through in waking hours. I was at first struck by an important exception to the rule, and was disposed to think that there might be something arbitrary in this partition of her recollections. In the normal state Léonie has a husband and children; but Léonie 2, the somnambulist, whilst acknowledging the children as her own, attributes the husband to "the other." This choice was perhaps explicable, but it followed no rule. It was not till later that I learned that her magnetizers in early days, as audacious as certain hypnotizers of recent date, had somnambulized her for her first accouchements, and that she had lapsed into that state spontaneously in the later ones. Léonie 2 was thus quite right in ascribing to herself the children—it was she who had had them, and the rule that her first trance-state forms a different personality was not broken. (pp. 366–367)

Memory. For both James and Janet, the cohesion of the loose confederacy of the self depends on memory. Memory is the matrix of personal identity. The sense of self is carried by memory through time. Alterations in memory (as seen in MPD) can lead to discontinuity in personal experience and in the sense of identity. Much of the original interest in MPD stemmed from the fact that patients were often amnesic for large chunks of their behavior. This led to the conclusion that a "disassociation" had occurred, that executive control had in fact been "taken over" by another personality. Recent evidence, however, suggests that the amnesia produced is much more flexible than was once supposed.

Silberman and his coworkers (1985) studied memory function in MPD using an interference paradigm (the degree to which recall of information is influenced by prior and subsequent learning). The patients were able to compartmentalize information significantly more easily than controls, and this was true both for the dissociated and the nondissociated state. But the MPD patients' overall ability to memorize information was no different from controls. Further, the information learned in one alter was, to some degree, available to the individual in other personality states.

Thus, the amnesia produced by the dissociative "barrier" appears to be flexible. Personal salience influences recall in hypnosis in a nonlinear way. It would appear that the barrier may be significantly strengthened when the information to be kept out of conscious awareness is either irrelevant (does not have a personal meaning) or at odds with significant conscious attitudes (Sheehan, 1982). Both episodic and procedural memory seem to be influenced by different mechanisms in hypnosis, reflecting the importance of personal context (Sheehan, 1982). Information that is more significant to the individual is more greatly influenced by hypnosis (Shields, 1986). In or out of hypnosis, both amnesia and recollection are more effective when the individual is motivated to forget or remember (Thorne, 1974).

Subjects with instructions for posthypnotic amnesia can still guess at significantly better than chance levels about the content of the amnesia (Bartis, 1986). Hypnotic amnesia can be breached and events recalled if the contextual variables are altered. Task demands that prevent using strategies that maintain amnesia significantly increase recall (Radtke, 1987). Amnesia in hypnosis may be due to disruption of particular retrieval processes, but the information may still be available if another strategy is used (Wilson, 1986).

A similar case obtains for hypermnesia—the ability to remember in far greater detail. Hypermnesia may occur even though the mind is consciously occupied with other tasks (Gardiner, 1989). Conscious thought suppression may actually improve retention (Wegner, 1987). A significant number of highly hypnotizable subjects will integrate suggested material with existing memories (Laurence, 1986b). Laurence and his coworkers suggest that this occurs most frequently in highly hypnotizable subjects with a propensity for dual cognitive functioning of dissociation—that is, individuals who are more likely to show the "hidden observer effect" or to report duality in hypnotic age regression. Although hypnosis can be used to improve recall of a particular event, it appears to be the nature of the instructions, not the hypnosis per se, that functions as a memory aid (Yuille, 1987). Certainly, eyewitness recall may be significantly improved or worsened by hypnosis (Register, 1987). The use of hypnosis cannot only alter memories but in some cases manufacture them entirely (Dywan, 1983; Laurence, 1983).

Hypnosis per se, without specific suggestions, does not function as a particularly powerful retrieval cue for items learned in hypnosis (Kihlstrom, 1985). Memory improvement during hypnosis may reflect the fact that individuals who are susceptible to hypnosis tend to use more flexible cognitive strategies than do people who are less susceptible (Crawford, 1983a). Subjects who are taught different cognitive strategies for memory can make substantial improvements in their performance on related tests (Ericsson, 1982). Emotional arousal per se does not necessarily affect memory one way or the other (Baker, 1987). The emotional arousal associated with memory must be specific to the information and its significance. The critical feature seems to be the ability to reproduce the original cognitive strategy or emotional state that was experienced at the time of learning (Rossi, 1986a).

"Memory" is not a faculty—a psychic tool at the disposal of ego—but an immanent aspect of all goal-directed activity that binds the task together in relation to its end. Precisely because of this immanent quality we are normally not aware of "remembering," and are only caught short when we cannot remember something. Memory is generally in relation to an activity, and hence to how an occasion is defined; for this reason memory is as much a social as a psychological fact. (Kenny, 1986, pp. 17–18)

Hypnotic alterations of this construction are similar to those that occur in the normal waking state (Pettinati, 1988). This construction is vulnerable to a complex variety of cognitive and emotional influences (Bowers, 1988). In fact, it is these very influences that, while making memory unreliable, also make it personally significant (Frankel, 1988). The sense of personal identity is constructed from the ongoing interaction of memory and experience. It is not simply a biological given but an active social and personal achievement.

Sensory and Motor Function. Janet had noted that, like the amnesias, the various paralyses and anesthesias of hysteric patients could be reversed by hypnosis (James, [1890]1983, p. 362). He proposed that as with memory these other functions were not "lost" but were only temporarily unavailable, being related to another, dissociated, state of mind. Janet believed that the disturbances of sensation were related to traumatic amnesias for the same class of sensation. In effect, he postulated a sensory loss in memory with one particular sense and its associated (state-dependent) memories markedly diminished. Similarly, symptoms such as automatic behavior or hallucinations could be seen as a partial interruption of the dissociation. The full restoration of the sensory information therapeutically through hypnosis resulted in a filling out and completion of the existing personality: "When you restore her inhibited sensibilities and memories by plunging her into the hypnotic trance—in other words, when you rescue them from their 'dissociated' and split-off condition, and make them rejoin the other sensibilities and memories—she is a different person" (James, [1890] 1983, p. 363).

James recognized parallels between the various sensory deficits found in hysterical patients and the "negative hallucinations" artificially produced in hypnosis. In both cases, a specific type of sensory input was restricted from conscious awareness. At the same time, both hysterical patient and hypnotic subject would demonstrate by concurrent behavior that they had in fact registered the information at another level. For example, subjects who were told that they were no longer able to see a chair directly in front of them would report that they could not do so, yet they would avoid the obstacle successfully while moving about the room. This is in direct contrast to subjects simulating hypnotic behavior who inevitably will "accidentally" stumble into the chair (Bowers, 1976). Thus, in the trance state, perception that is excluded from awareness continues to influence behavior.

Messrs. Pierre Janet and A. Binet have shown that during the times of anaesthesia, and coexisting with it, sensibility to the anaesthetic parts is also there, in the form of a secondary consciousness entirely cut off from the primary or normal one, but susceptible of being tapped and made to testify to its existence in various odd ways. . . .

The apparently anaesthetic hand of these subjects, for one thing, will often adapt itself discriminatingly to whatever objects may be put into it. . . . M. Binet found a very curious sort of connection between the apparently anaesthetic skin and the mind in some Salpêtrière-subjects. Things placed in the hand were not felt, but thought of (apparently in visual terms) and in no wise referred by the subject to their starting point in the hand's sensation. . . .

These individuals, namely, saw the impression received by the hand, but could not feel it; and the thing seen appeared by no means associated with the hand, but more like an independent vision, which usually interested and surprised the patient. . . .

Messrs. Bernheim and Pitres have also proved, by observations too complicated to be given in this spot, that the hysterical blindness is no real blindness at all. . . . M. Binet has found the hand of his patients unconsciously writing down words which their eyes were vainly endeavoring to "see," i.e., to bring to the upper consciousness. Their submerged consciousness was of course seeing them, or the hand could not have written as it did. . . .

It must be admitted, therefore, that in certain persons, at least, the total possible consciousness may be split into parts which coexist but mutually ignore each other, and share the objects of knowledge between them. More remarkable still, they are complementary. Give an object to one of the consciousnesses, and by that fact you remove it from the other or others. (James, [1890] 1983, pp. 201–204)

James notes the change in the "ratio of the senses" as it occurred in one of Janet's subjects, Lucie. There was a marked contrast between Lucie 1, the preexisting state, and Lucie 3, the state noted in hypnosis.

Her sensibility became perfect, and instead of being an extreme example of the "visual" type, she was transformed into what in Prof. Charcot's terminology is known as a motor. That is to say, that whereas when awake she had thought in visual terms exclusively, and could imagine things only by remembering how they looked, now in this deeper trance her thoughts and memories seemed to M. Janet to be largely composed of images of movement and of touch (p. 364)

In addition, while in hypnosis, Lucie related these changes to childhood memories of shock and illness. In essence, Janet concluded that Lucie had not been frightened out of her wits; rather, she had been frightened out of her feelings. Lucie had reacted to the trauma by a restriction of conscious awareness that eliminated bodily awareness.

Patients with somatization disorders also show a dysfunction in the process of attention when compared with normal controls (James, 1987). Studies of brain function (in the form of cerebral blood flow) showed a substantially different pattern of the organization of attention in response to stimuli in fourteen patients with somatization disorder when compared with a similar number of matched controls. This would suggest that the normal attentional processes are restricted in such patients when they are experiencing their symptoms. These differences held true both for evoked potentials and regional cerebral blood flow. Furthermore, patients with conversion symptoms showed a marked impairment in their galvanic skin responses when compared with controls or with patients with anxiety disorders (Horvath, 1980). Thus there is evidence of focal right hemisphere EEG abnormalities and dysfunctions in attention and sympathetic tone (both of which are mediated by neural circuits involving the right hemisphere). Given the involvement of the right hemisphere areas in the initiation of trance states (see chapter 5), there is at least suggestive evidence for the involvement of spontaneous hypnotic states in the development of hypnotic states.

These patients also show inconsistent and contradictory motor performance results that are not at all like the responses seen in patients with lesions of the peripheral or central nervous system (Knutsson, 1985). In this respect, their symptoms are similar to the differences between hypnotic phenomena such as amnesia, hallucination, or other forms of "trance logic" when compared with the situations they mimic (Spanos, 1986a).

Hallucinations, whether during hypnosis or out of it, are highly responsive to contextual cues (Young, 1987; Hilgard, 1977). Intense absorption does appear to be associated with the experience of visual hallucinations (Sheehan, 1982). Alterations in level of physiologic arousal and expectation appear to be particularly important factors (Asaad, 1986). Hallucinations are more frequent in highly emotional circumstances such as life-threatening situations or the loss of a spouse (Siegel, 1984; Mueser, 1987; Greeley, 1987). These hallucinations differ from those found in major psychiatric disorders both qualitatively and quantitatively (Andrade, 1986).

Hypnotized subjects and simulating subjects show different responses to suggestions of perceptual restriction such as hypnotically induced deafness, and both groups show striking differences from controls (Nash, 1987). Although hypnotized subjects show differences in perceptual processes when compared with subjects in the waking state, the differences are not similar to those found in subliminal perception or dichotic listening studies (Nash, 1987; Kihlstrom, 1987). This suggests that unconscious processes are not wholly amorphous but have a discrete structure.

In a detailed study of the subjective experiences of subjects in trance, Sheehan (1982) has demonstrated that hypnotic subjects' responses do differ from simulators or from controls in the waking state, but they also differ significantly from the actual experience of the suggested event. In experimental conditions, subjects perceive the experimental situation as a problem that is to be solved. This is not to say that the experiences are any more or less literally true, but rather, that the personal need for meaning and the intensity of the emotional state may combine to make the problem solving more personally relevant and useful.

A Four-Factor Theory

Richard Kluft (1984) has proposed a four-factor theory for MPD that accounts for many of the clinical features. The first factor is a marked talent for dissociation. Patients with MPD usually have high scores on tests of hypnotizability (Bliss, 1985; Lipman, 1985). These patients also report more spontaneous dissociative experiences including "extrasensory and supernatural" experiences, sleepwalking, and childhood imaginary playmates than do patients with other psychiatric disorders (C. A. Ross, 1989a). There is also a correlation between scores on formalized testing of hypnotic ability and subjective reports of spontaneous experiences (Carlson, 1989). Thus, MPD patients display a greater degree of hypnotic ability in response to standardized testing and report more dissociative experiences in their daily lives than do other groups.

If dissociation is defined as the "lack of the normal integration of thoughts, feelings, and experiences into the stream of consciousness and memory" (Bernstein, 1986, p. 727), then another measure of dissociation is the degree to which subjects are able to attend to two separate tasks at the same time. Zamansky and Clark (1986) found that subjects of low hypnotizability scores were much more sensitive to the effects of interruptions and distractions than those with medium or high scores. Using a paradigm that involved simultaneously listening to a story and identifying a series of tones, Zamansky and Bartis (1985) found that 40 percent of the highly hypnotizable subjects but none of the moderately hypnotizable subjects were able to perform the task. These findings suggest that although there appears to be a strong correlation between dissociation and hypnotic ability they are not identical.

The second factor is exposure to a severe and emotionally overwhelming physical or mental trauma during childhood. Spiegel (1986) has reviewed the evidence suggesting traumatic origins for MPD. There is substantial evidence of a positive relationship between hypnotic ability and childhood physical or sexual abuse (Hilgard, 1979; Nash, 1984; Sexton, 1988). For example, individuals who have been abused as children are significantly more hypnotizable than either controls or individuals who have had a family disruption by divorce or death (Nash, 1986).

There is parallel evidence that supports a positive correlation between a history of childhood abuse and the later development of dissociative disorders in the clinical literature (Putnam, 1986; Carlson, 1989). Severe physical or mental abuse during childhood is found in the history of virtually all MPD patients in a number of studies (Bliss, 1986; Braun, 1986b; Putnam, 1986). Patients with MPD are more likely to report histories of physical and sexual abuse during childhood than other patient populations (Kluft, 1985; Spiegel, 1986; C. A. Ross, 1989a). In a study of ninety-eight female psychiatric inpatients, Chu and Dill (1990) reported that 63 percent of the subjects said they had been the victims of physical and/or sexual abuse, and that 83 percent of abused subjects had significantly elevated dissociative symptom scores. In a large sample of college students, Josephine Hilgard (1979) found a positive association between childhood physical trauma and hypnotic ability in another study. College students who reported severe physical or psychological abuse during childhood were also more likely to report. frequent spontaneous dissociative experiences (Sanders, 1989).

The nature of the interaction between hypnotizability and exposure to traumatic experience remains an open question. Josephine Hilgard (1979) proposed that there were two developmental pathways for hypnotic ability: either severe childhood physical or psychological abuse or a capacity for intense experiential absorption reflected in what Hilgard termed "imaginative involvement," which developed from early childhood. Whether this indicates MPD patients develop hypnotic ability in the response to trauma during a critical period of childhood or represents an inherently greater biologic hypnotic ability remains unresolved.

In reanalyzing Josephine Hilgard's data, Frischholz (1985) found that the combination of reports of high imaginative involvement and childhood punishment yielded a substantially higher correlation with hypnotic ability than either variable alone. Similarly, in the Zamansky and Bartis (1984) study, 60 percent of the highly hypnotizable subjects were unable to perform the dissociation task efficiently. Furthermore, one-quarter of the subjects in Perry's sample who reported few spontaneous dissociative experiences scored in the medium or high range of hypnotic ability (Carlson, 1989). Thus, it seems reasonable to conclude that although most individuals who report a large number of spontaneous dissociative experiences will demonstrate significant hypnotic ability, there are others who do not report such experiences but remain good hypnotic subjects (Carlson, 1989).

The third factor proposed by Kluft is the existence of personal, family, and social influences that encourage the use and development of dissociative skills. Dissociative experiences are certainly highly responsive to context (Spanos, 1985b, 1986d) and are far more frequent in cultures that value and encourage such experiences than in cultures that do not (Winkelman, 1986). Both the frequency and the specific features of dissociative experiences are influenced by contextual demands (Dobkin de Rios, 1989). There is also evidence that clinical interactions can provide sufficiently strong contextual cues to encourage the development of the MPD syndrome. Within the experimental situation, some role-playing college students may develop features of MPD that result in consistent differences in response to testing (Spanos, 1985b, 1986d).

The fourth factor in Kluft's theory is an absence of restorative or integrative experiences. The evidence suggests that contexts that encourage integration and personal development minimize the psychological disturbance that results from exposure to traumatic experiences, whereas an environment that permits further trauma by denying or devaluing the individual's experience increases psychological morbidity (Spiegel, 1986; Dobkin de Rios, 1989).

In summary, the dissociations seen in MPD appear to be a fundamental psychobiologic mechanism that most individuals may display to a varying degree but that is also sensitive to contextual cues. The evidence suggests that dissociative phenomena arise in a context, and that context is a particular social setting and the way in which it frames potential responses. Psychological and physiologic studies of various hypnotic phenomena support this interpretation. For example, studies of hypnotic age regression show that the induced state is not a true return to childhood but, rather, a more widespread and nonspecific use of alternative social, cognitive, and psychophysiologic strategies of information processing (Spanos, 1986d; Aravindakshan, 1988; Nash, 1987). The process of dissociation in MPD appears to be one of protection and repair (Spiegel, 1986). In that sense it is a function, a work-in-progress. The manifestations of alternate states of consciousness can be seen as versions of reality, a recursive process combining both stability and change. It is this process that is central in dealing with emotional trauma.

A PSYCHOBIOLOGIC MODEL: POST-TRAUMATIC STRESS DISORDER

Posttraumatic stress disorder (PTSD), as defined by DSM-III-R (American Psychiatric Association, 1987), is the result of exposure to an overwhelmingly stressful situation. The origins typically involve either natural disasters or extreme human violence. Such exposure produces a reaction in even the healthiest of individuals. In this way, the reaction is considered "normal," much like grief experienced at the death of a loved one (Andreasen, 1985).

Horowitz suggests that there is a predictable course of events that involves a period of emotional distress followed by alternating phases of denial (when the individual attempts to carry on as usual) and intrusion (in which memories, feelings, and thoughts related to the experience flood back into awareness). How the individual finally integrates the experience depends not only on the nature of the stress but also on the experiences both prior to the event and after the stress. (This includes the long-lasting effects of the stressor.) The PTSD syndrome involves both exposure to a horrible experience and a challenge to the person's self-image and his or her expectations of the world and of other people (Brown, 1986). Thus the symptoms represent a reaction to the stress and an attempt to accept and integrate the experience (Horowitz, 1986). The symptoms themselves can produce a vicious cycle by impairing other areas of the person's life (Green, 1985), thus blocking attempts at resolution.

Spiegel (1989b) has suggested that MPD can be conceptualized as an extreme form of chronic post-traumatic stress disorder. In his studies, patients with PTSD and patients with MPD showed significantly higher scores of hypnotic ability than did patients with other psychiatric disorders. Stutman (1985) also found significantly higher hypnotizability scores and mental visual imagery scores in PTSD patients than in controls. There are other suggestive parallels as well.

In addition to increased scores on tests of hypnotic ability, dissociative symptoms including decreased concentration and level of function, episodes of amnesia or confusion, and flashbacks, or brief, vivid, visual hallucinations of the traumatic situation commonly occur (Horowitz, 1986). These types of visual hallucinations are more common in patients who score highly on vividness of mental imagery and on impact of the event emotionally on scales measuring their response to the stressful event (Burstein, 1986). Patients with the disorder also frequently have unexplained chronic physical pain (Benedikt, 1986), sleep disturbances related to frightening dreams (Kramer, 1986), and increased physiologic responses to verbal accounts of events similar to the trauma (Pitman, 1987).

Spiegel (1989b) has drawn an analogy between the major symptom clusters of PTSD and the absorption, dissociation, and heightened sensitivity to context that are three major components of hypnosis. The intrusiveness and power of traumatic imagery are similar to the focused attention of hypnosis. Similarly, dissociation may blunt the emotional power of a trauma at the cost of making it inaccessible to the main state of consciousness. The increased physiologic sensitivity to traumatic cues is similar to the heightened sensitivity to suggestion found in trance.

The recurrent vivid imagery associated with strong emotion may be the central mediating mechanism in PTSD (Brett, 1985). The imagery is the brain's enactment of a search for meaning and completion (Horowitz, 1986). The evidence suggests that the recurrence of flashbacks or other stressful associations with traumatic experience are not simply passive replays of the event but attempts by the brain to make sense of and eventually overcome the trauma experience (Horowitz, 1986). This is also true of the nightmares and other sleep disturbances experienced (Wilmer, 1982).

Emotional blunting, amnesia, avoidance, and dissociation are seen as attempts to modulate the consequences of both the trauma and the subsequent reexperiencing of it. Similarly, intrusion by the intense imagery and affect related to the trauma can also be interpreted either as a further assault on the individual or as evidence of a gradual reintegration of the experience. Dissociation, typically with attendant amnesia and alteration of perception, cognitive style, and behavior, may thus be conceptualized as an intermediate or transitional step between these two alternatives (Horowitz, 1986). Achieving a more permanent balance appears to involve alterations in the quality of the imagery as well as in the intensity of the emotional responses (Spiegel, 1988c; Friedman, 1988). This appears to involve a reappraisal of the significance of the symptoms and of the meaning of the trauma as well as a greater sense of control over the symptom (Kingsbury, 1988; Spiegel, 1988c).

Kolb (1987) has suggested that PTSD is the result of a sensitizing conditioning response that dampens habituation or the ability to adapt to new stimuli. Patients can show a combination of reduced sensitivity to some cues and heightened responses to others. They have a higher threshold to startle response but an increased response to cues that are over that threshold (Kramer, 1989). This is consistent with the notion that these patients have generally blunted response to most cues but respond dramatically to stronger or more specific stimuli. Disturbances in orienting responses are paralleled by difficulties in maintaining the level of sleep (R. J. Ross, 1989). Patients also have longer REM periods, a greater REM density, and a greater variance in the REM latency—the time between falling asleep and the onset of the first REM episode (Ross, 1990).

Lactate infusions (which will produce panic attacks in patients with a panic disorder) will also produce flashbacks in PTSD symptoms in patients who have episodes of panic within the disorder (Rainey, 1987). The production of flashbacks in subjects with PTSD (the flashbacks were associated in most cases with the development of a full-blown panic state) suggests that the level of arousal is critical in the return of the intrusive imagery as well as the emotional and cognitive state (Rainey, 1987). Taken together, these features strongly suggest changes in arousal mechanisms resulting in a very dramatic physiologic reexperiencing of a traumatic situation in response to subsequent cues. In this sense, the PTSD syndrome is not only psychological but neurophysiologic as well, altering the brain's processing of future events by resetting physiologic mechanisms (Kolb, 1988).

The neurophysiologic changes found in PTSD support the notion of a central disturbance in attentional processes. The features of the syndrome can be conceptualized as a phasic alternation between the hyperarousal that occurs in response to acute trauma and typically accompanies reexperiencing of elements of the trauma and the compensatory restriction of arousal and avoidance of stimulation that accompanies the numbing response (Wilson, 1989). Underlying the psychological changes appears to be a biologic dynamic instability in which autonomic nervous system activity alternates between sympathetic stimulation with high levels of the biogenic amines being released and the numbing phase in which amine and opioid depletion are accompanied by parasympathetic dominance (van der Kolk, 1985).

Research into the psychobiology of PTSD has focused on two areas. The first is the evidence for alterations in release of the catecholamines epinephrine and norepinephrine. These substances are released in response to stress as part of the "fight or flight" mechanism both within the brain itself and, via the peripheral nervous system, throughout the rest of the body. These changes can be studied by measuring physiologic indexes to arousal such as heart rate or blood pressure increases and circulating levels of the hormones or of their metabolites or by measuring changes in receptor sensitivity. (Because of the difficulty in determining receptor activity within the central nervous system, receptor studies are usually done on circulating white blood cells or platelets and are thus indirect. Newer brain imaging techniques that can demonstrate metabolic activity within the brain itself may give us a more direct way of studying receptors within the living brain.) Increased catecholamine release may be related to a number of PTSD symptoms including increased startle responses, mood disturbances, troubled sleep, recurrent nightmares, and vivid flashbacks.

These patients excrete high levels of the urinary metabolites of the neurotransmitters norepinephrine and epinephrine (Giller, 1989). They also have significantly lower levels of the platelet enzyme MAO and lower CAMP signal transduction (Lerer, 1987). The increase in sympathetic arousal results in increases in EEG rhythm, heart rate, blood pressure, respiratory rate, muscle tension, and the release of stress hormones and other information substances (van der Kolk, 1985; Kolb, 1987). The cortisol excretion rate, however, which is also typically increased during stress, is relatively reduced (Mason, 1986). As reduced cortisol levels are typically seen in many subjects trying to cope with a severe chronic stress, Giller and his coworkers (1989) have suggested that the norepinephrine/cortisol ratio might be used to discriminate individuals with PTSD from those with other diagnoses.

The level of norepinephrine release is monitored by specific alpha-2 receptors that function to provide negative feedback and slow down norepinephrine release. Yohimbine is a drug that specifically blocks the alpha-2 receptor. Whereas administration of yohimbine has a mild stimulant effect on normal controls, administration to PTSD patients leads to increased anxiety including panic attacks and dissociative experiences including flashbacks (Krystal, 1990). Patients may have a 40 percent decrease in their platelet alpha-2 receptors when compared with controls (Perry, 1989). This "down regulation," or decrease in the number of binding sites, is in sharp contrast to the picture seen in major depression where a substantial number of patients demonstrate an "up regulated" picture in which there is increased binding activity. In addition to the alterations in receptor activity, transduction of the signal across the cell membrane by the adenylate cyclase system in platelets and lymphocytes is found in PTSD in contrast to controls (Lerer, 1990).

The long-term changes in response to stress that occur in PTSD are typically highly specific for exposure to stimuli which resemble the original stressor. Viewing a combat film evoked significant increases in blood pressure, heart rate, and emotional lability as well as peripheral blood levels of epinephrine in these patients (Murburg, 1990). Responses of plasmic catecholamine and their metabolites in response to exercise are also different when compared to controls (Hamner, 1990b). Patients may have higher resting heart rates and slightly higher resting levels of plasma catecholamines (McFall, 1990; Hamner, 1990a). These changes may be related to abnormally high twenty-four-hour urinary levels of catecholamines and their metabolites as well as low twenty-four-hour cortisol levels and increased cortisol receptors on circulating lymphocytes in PTSD patients (Southwick, 1990).

The second system that has been implicated in PTSD is that of the endogenous opiate system in the brain. Endogenous opiates are released in response to extreme stress in both animals and humans. The release of the opiates as a response to stress seems to be related to a blunting of painful stimuli. Stress-induced analgesia appears to be mediated by opiate mechanisms and can be blocked by the administration of the opiate antagonist naloxone (Lewis, 1980). In humans, this analgesic response is associated with a perception that the stress is uncontrollable (Bandura, 1988). Noting these factors and observing that lack of control over the imagery distinguishes PTSD patients from controls, Pitman and his coworkers (1990) studied the analgesic response in Vietnam veterans with PTSD to a film of violent combat. They found that when compared with controls, the PTSD patients reported a 30 percent decrease in pain intensity immediately following the videotape. This decrease in pain ratings did not occur when the patients were concurrently given naloxone. Persistent and prolonged opiate release may be related to the experiences of emotional numbing and decreased response to pain that is seen in PTSD patients. The alternation of periods of arousal and increased sensitivity to specific stimuli alternating with emotional numbing might be associated with a persistent imbalance between the systems that regulate catecholamines and the endogenous opiates.

These patients appear to have abnormalities in endorphin regulation. In one study, approximately 30 percent of patients reported a decrease in pain responses that could be blocked by the opiate antagonist naloxone (van der Kolk, 1989). Patients are also reported to display significantly higher serum levels of the beta endorphin in response to an exercise test when compared with matched controls (Hamner, 1989). Van der Kolk (1985) has suggested that this analgesic response, apparently mediated by endogenous opiates, may be partly accountable for reinforcing the sustained arousal level of PTSD patients.

The imbalance between endogenous opiate release and noradrenergic activity may thus be related to the phasic reexperiencing of trauma-related imagery and emotion and may be involved in the dissociative states that develop in these patients (Spiegel, 1988c; Burges Watson, 1988). It has been suggested that the physiologic evidence of hyperarousal in PTSD patients is related to heightened activity in the noradrenergic systems that modulate activity in the hippocampus and amygdala, and that such increased activity is reinforced by the surges in endogenous opiates that occur in reexposure to traumatic situations (Friedman, 1988; van der Kolk, 1989). This hypothesis is in keeping with the findings of increased hypnotic susceptibility in these patients (Spiegel, 1988c).

In a study of six subjects with PTSD, Brende reported that hypnotically induced imagery was associated with increased right hemisphere activity, hypervigilance with increased left hemisphere activity, and numbing with decreased right hemisphere activity (1982). These findings support the notion that the overintrusion and numbing phases represent separate and complementary approaches to processing traumatic experiences. In addition, they support Spiegel's hypothesis that dissociative mechanisms mediated by the right hemisphere are responsible for post-traumatic flashbacks.

Rossi has proposed that state-dependent learning and memory phenomena are central both in traumatic dissociation and in therapeutic hypnosis (Rossi, 1986a; Rossi and Cheek, 1988). He has pointed out evidence that suggests the enhancement and potentiation of learning and memory that occurs in states of high arousal. This would account both for the vividness of intrusive imagery and affect as well as the way in which such material, because of its state-bound nature, can spontaneously emerge in subsequent similar states of arousal. Thus, intrusive material can be conceptualized as state-bound patterns of information released whenever arousal reaches a certain critical level. This model parsimoniously accounts for the frequency of both affective disturbance and somatic symptoms (either as the direct consequence of autonomic nervous system disturbance or as a physical reexperiencing of the intrusion of traumatic memories) and the decreased threshold for further dissociation (Braun, 1984; Spiegel, 1989b).

The features of PTSD and MPD are both symptom and cure. They represent an intermediate step in the movement toward coming to terms with the traumatic event (Horowitz, 1986; Auerhahn, 1984). In this sense, they are analogous to Rothenberg's (1988) creative processing in which events with at least two strong and competing emotional valences are held for the same events and represent an unstable intermediate step in the journey toward resolution. Many people do make good adjustments after a traumatic experience (Hendin, 1984). Patients with PTSD may be able to make an adjustment but remain vulnerable to reactivation of their experiences and onset of the disorder after a significant delay similar to the manner in which a subject may demonstrate a posthypnotic response (Solomon, 1987).

Wilson (1989) points out that effective cultural rituals universally include not only cognitive restructuring and emotional support but highly patterned means for altering the level of arousal. On a physiologic level, this would allow for the deconditioning of the traumatic responses and a resynchronization that may help reestablish a physiologic equilibrium. The treatment process, whether for combat veteran or incest victim, extends beyond the clinical setting to involve the attitude of the society toward the patient.

THE TRANSCULTURAL MODEL: POSSESSION STATES

Trance serves a pervasive function of deepening and enriching personal involvement in many cultures. It can be a fluid and creative way of maintaining and altering the web of relationships. In a cross-cultural survey of 488 societies, Bourguignon reported that "ninety percent have one or more institutionalized, culturally patterned forms of altered states of consciousness" (1973). The goal of trance is integration, both at the personal level by bringing forward unconscious processes and at the interpersonal level by establishing a common vehicle for the expression of important social themes that is available to all members of the group.

In literate cultures institutionalized trance is relatively uncommon outside the contexts of hypnosis, spiritual ceremonies, or dissociative disorders. The use of trance in oral cultures is far more varied and typically involves a wide number of medical, religious, social, and psychological forms. In oral societies trance is frequently a central part of the social role of women. Particularly, it provides a forum in which women's interests and values can be expressed and their key role in the maintenance of culture confirmed. Through all these uses trance is seen as a significant and valued part of the community life and is usually organized in a highly systematic collective way.

A Case Study: The Mayotte

Michael Lambek has provided us with a remarkable depiction of a society in which trance plays such a critical role in his studies of the Mayotte, the inhabitants of the Comoro archipelago off the coast of Madagascar (1981). In this relatively isolated culture, there is a highly structured and elaborate system of social communication that has evolved from the widespread use of trance. Possession states involve as many as one-third of the female population and perhaps 10 percent of the males (Lambek, 1981, p. 56). Among the Mayotte, possession is a common occurrence with an explicit time course, including well-defined onset, process, and resolution, and an implicit cultural function.

As the population of the islands is a heterogeneous mix composed of peoples from southern Africa, the Middle East, and the islands of the

Indian Ocean, there is much need for a constantly active system of social and personal integration. As a result,

what we perceive today is merely a moment in a long process of cultural fusion, fission, and refusion along new lines. Furthermore, the ethnic and linguistic labels have relatively little immediate sociological significance. Intermarriage and bilingualism are common, and group membership in Mayotte is defined according to principles of residence, ownership, and participation in ceremonial exchange networks rather than more abstract ascriptive criteria. Mayotte is an open society: despite the great cultural heterogeneity there is a vigorously affirmed social unity, based on Islam and a common loyalty to the island as an indivisible whole. (Lambek, 1981, p. 2)

The result is a society with a delicate balance that must be constantly stabilized and adjusted. While recognizing the need for such adjustments, the Mayottes attribute them to the needs of the "spirit world." But far from being a heavenly phenomenon, the world of the spirits is closely linked to daily human life. These spirits are decidedly humanlike and must be related to rather than worshiped.

The spirits come into direct contact with the Mayottes through the process of a ritualized form of possession. The afflicted individual (the Mayotte consider possession to be a form of disease) is "taken over" by a spirit who behaves differently, speaks with a different voice, and uses different characteristic gestures. The behavior of the spirits is usually quite outrageous within the highly formalized Mayotte terms of reference.

It is not so much that a weak person, helped by a spirit, can become suddenly powerful, but that the spirits, by their very natures, throw into question the whole moral basis of power. Spirits are potent yet parasitic, educated yet extortionist, self-seeking and self-motivated, vain, ungenerous, untrustworthy, querulous, and irresponsible. Treating with the spirits requires knowing when to be tactful and patient and when to put your foot down and be self-assertive in turn. (p. 33)

In a tightly regulated society, the spirits express the less socially desirable characteristics of the individual. Moreover, they appear in individuals, typically women, who are in some way socially disadvantaged. Thus they are the antithesis of the ideal Mayotte: self-centered rather than generous, flamboyant rather than polite, and disrespectful rather than exhibiting the highly developed sense of social responsibility that is typical.

The spirit possessions challenge and subtly balance the existing social order. During possession the individuals are allowed a latitude of behavior that would be unthinkable at other times. Although most of the possessed are female, the possessing spirits are typically male. Their behavior, in its very self-indulgence and eccentricity, both confirms that the possession state is different from a normal waking state for the whole community and provides a forum in which such behavior is socially acceptable. Whatever happens during trance is the responsibility of the spirit. In fact, the "host" is almost always amnesic for what has happened.

The drama of possession, diagnosis, and cure follows a carefully structured scenario. Although the circumstances of each case are highly individual, the general stages are quite fixed. Patient, family members, and healer all have a role to play in the development of the individual, the family, and the culture.

Whenever possession occurs, a local healer, adept in the ways of the spirit (and the human) world, is summoned for a formal ceremony. The ceremony involves the whole community, but there is no audience in our sense of the word. Each person becomes actively involved in some form or other. As with any other communal task, there are specialists for particular roles, but everyone participates. In an oral culture, each relationship is grounded in a larger web of active participation.

In possession, "therapy" involves the development of a relationship among the patient, the healer, the patient's family, and the spirit. The first step is the spirit's announcement of a name. The name declares a symbolic personality, social role, and kinship pattern, and thus helps define what type of negotiations are likely to take place. Also, by allowing the use of a name, the spirit indicates its willingness to enter into negotiations and abide by the rules of the ritual.

The spirits themselves also have a highly developed kinship pattern. Spirits will announce themselves to be friend, husband, child, or parent of other spirits in the community. These kinship patterns emphasize the communal aspect of the trance experience, despite its intensely personal nature. These declared affinities of the spirits have a profound impact on social relationships regardless of the relative social relationships of the human hosts. Thus, these relationships serve also to alter subtly the overt social structure and to remind all involved of their obligations.

Possession allows for the voicing of the unspeakable. Trance functions as a creative forum in which personal and social conflicts can be expressed and worked through. Spirit possession is a form of psychotherapy in which every member of the community may participate.

The second step involves a process of negotiation whereby, in return for meeting the spirit's demands (usually for special foods or other luxuries), the illness is resolved. It is important to note that this means not that the spirit disappears but that the symptoms of discord cease. The process of therapy largely involves the working out of a clearly defined relationship with the spirit. During this process, the negotiations lead to a more clearly defined personality manifestation of the spirit, who gradually agrees to take on a more responsible attitude toward his host. Patient and spirit coexist from that point onward in a synergistic manner.

In the third stage this relationship flourishes, with the spirit, in return for the occasional bribe, resolving disputes when conflicts arise between humans. In this final stage, the actual trance episodes are usually infrequent. Patient and spirit have agreed on the rules of the game and both typically abide by their end of the bargain.

It is clear that, for the Mayotte, possession trance provides what Kenny (1986) has called "an idiom of distress." Using this idiom, a wide variety of physical, emotional, and interpersonal difficulties are given a coherent structure, meaning, and format for resolution. Although the spirits initially appear to be boorish houseguests, they in fact provide an important personal and social mechanism for balancing the needs of the individual with those of a complex society. The possession metaphor reframes the difficulties of an individual in a manner that is both coherent and culturally acceptable.

Coming as it does frequently at the time of marriage, possession can editorialize on the nature of the relationship and provide badly needed information that might be intolerable to the fragile male ego if approached directly. Possession implicitly reminds the more socially dominant male of the responsibilities and obligations as well as the privileges of his position and demonstrates that the relationship is a fluid one, subject to ongoing negotiations. The trance state models a creative tension, a working relationship.

Thus, it serves also as a crucible of shared learning. Relationships can be worked out (even if this working-out is mostly implicit and covert) by the people directly involved and with the active participation of the community and the experienced healer; moreover, the unconscious processes are cultivated. The individuals are encouraged to deal with the situation using the widest possible range of creative resources available to them. The unconscious processes that are utilized become more and more active with the development of a full-fledged, distinct personality on the part of the spirit. They are not limited to the strict playing out of what are relatively inflexible social roles and obligations overtly offered them by the Islamic marriage laws and the need to maintain a reliable system of land claim agreements.

Thus, the possession state serves both an individual psychological function and a wider social and cultural one. This serves to underline the notion that the various forms of trance serve to align the needs of the individual with the needs of the larger community. In situations that are delicately balanced or changing rapidly, both the individual and the society depend heavily on custom and continuous negotiation. Trance serves in this world both as a repository for the precedents for a variety of conflicts and as a means for conflict resolution.

Possession is an autonomous, culturally constituted system. It is not the product of a few deviant individuals, nor necessarily the symptom of a deeply divided society. Virtually every member of Mayotte society comes into contact regularly with spirits, either by direct possession or by interaction with the spirits when they possess friends, neighbors, curers, or kin. The relationships formed by an individual in trance have a social reality; they mesh with the ties of kinship, alliance, and locality to form a single whole. From this perspective, men also participate in possession, but simply in different roles from the women. Possession is thus a basic aspect of the social structure, not a by-product of it. (Lambek, 1981, p. 69)

Personal and Social Synchrony

It has been suggested that the endogenous opiates may provide the connection between the social context of trance and the physiologic manifestations (Frecska, 1989). Changes in the levels of endogenous opiates accompany physical or psychological stress and appear to be involved in the brain's attempt to modulate the effects of stress (Maier, 1986; Margules, 1979). Endogenous opiates also seem to be involved in the establishment and maintenance of the infant-mother bond (Panksepp, 1980, 1985). These mechanisms may continue to be important for maintaining the intensity and synchrony of relationships throughout life. Many of the induction techniques used in a variety of cultures appear to stimulate the release of endogenous opiates (Prince, 1982a, 1982b; Winkelman, 1986). Frecska and Kulcsar (1989) propose that trance induction procedures result in the release of endogenous opiates, which promote personal well-being and strengthen social bonds. Their psychobiologic model also suggests that the intense relationship and synchrony found in healing rituals creates a state of expectation, a context that enhances opiate release.

Social relationships are an important way in which biological rhythms are synchronized (Hofer, 1981, 1984). The maintenance of relationships can be thought of as the mutual synchronizing of these rhythms when they are disrupted by trauma (Field, 1985). Most healing rituals appear to share an aspect of traumatic physical or psychological events in that they, too, influence levels of endogenous opiates in the brain (Frecska, 1989; Winkelman, 1986). The healing ceremony can be conceptualized as a revivification of the stressful event that provides a socially supported context for healing and integration.

TRANCE AND SELF

In a recent summary of work on multiple personality disorder, Beahrs (1988) has made a number of useful points: (1) MPD is a distinct pathological condition with a complex and multivariate etiology; (2) massive childhood trauma (particularly physical and sexual abuse) is found in the overwhelming number of patients; (3) the phenomena of MPD closely resemble those found in the hypnotic state; (4) the initial presentation of the MPD patient may vary and seems to be associated with the life stages and experiences of the individual at the time; (5) MPD is treatable (hypnosis may be useful in identifying and integrating aspects of the personality, but treatment must also involve a comprehensive approach); (6) the current diagnostic criteria do not distinguish adequately between the full-blown dissociations seen in MPD and the "roles" and "ego states" that are universal; and (7) the presentation of MPD is highly responsive to the psychosocial context, an aspect that is not adequately dealt with by most writers on the subject.

With acceptance by the scientific community a major goal of the burgeoning MPD movement, it is easy to understand that those aspects of dissociative disorder that make it appear loose, fuzzy, or quasi-mystical would be avoided like the plague. The contextual perspective is often viewed as an attack on the reality of MPD, while it is feared that the continuity of dissociation and everyday living could work against broad professional acceptance by diffusing the defining boundaries of the construct. These concerns are unfortunate. MPD is "real," by clear operational criteria as reliable as most in psychiatry, and the data and consensus increasingly impressive. If MPD is not quite what it seems, this does not minimize its existence, validity, or importance, but may point the way toward new understanding and approaches to treatment intervention. (Beahrs, 1988, pp. 229–230)

The degree to which a society sanctions the use of trance appears to influence the prevalence of possession states or MPD. Such states are mòre frequent in societies in which dissociative states are accepted or actively encouraged and are much less frequent when this is not the case (Bourguignon, 1989). The actual prevalence of the disorder in any one culture may well reflect an interaction between social acceptance and the severity of the trauma experienced and the individual degree of hypnotic ability of the patient. A society in which these experiences are not accepted may well demonstrate a higher overall threshold for the expression of the disorder involving a more intense exposure to individual trauma or a greater relative degree of hypnotic ability.

Lewis (1989) has suggested that possession is a form of hypothesis-making or problem-solving activity. Whenever existing social structures are being challenged, either because they are too rigid or too chaotic, possession cults and other forms of dissociation flourish. Dissociation can be seen as the first step in a process of individual and social healing. Just as dissociation provides each individual with a form to express and work out their own concerns, it also provides a mechanism by which these concerns can be used to shape the social community. Dissociation is a method by which personal identity, responsibility, and privileges can be negotiated. Regardless of the particular cultural framework, the stage is set for a means by which an individual, working through personal trauma, influences both the microcosm and the macrocosm.

A related issue in both PTSD and dissociation is the question of vulnerability to the disorder. Attempts to explain why all who are exposed to trauma are not at equal risk have focused on the interaction between the nature of the experience of the stress or on a vulnerability, possibly related to previous stressors, in the individuals who developed the disorder. In animals, the response to exposure to stress has been found to be influenced by previous exposure to stress as well as whether the stress is escapable or inescapable (Charney, 1990). This would suggest that both a history of previous exposure to stress and the degree to which the stress is perceived as being controllable are critical for the development of the disorder. In humans, children and adolescents who have been abused physically or sexually demonstrated higher baseline heart rates and blood pressures and down regulated alpha-2 receptors (Perry, 1990). Furthermore, women with a history of childhood sexual abuse have significantly blunted responses of the hormones cortisol and prolactin in response to intravenous clomipramine challenge (Corrigan, 1990), suggesting that the biologic effects of trauma may persist for decades. Similarly, in a survey of fourteen hundred women, 13 percent reported exposure to significant traumatic events (Resnick, 1990).

The MPD diagnosis is not just a clinical matter dealing with phenomenologic or biologic issues but has profound social implications as well (Beahrs, 1982). Close to the heart of the concept is the changing role of women (Rivera, 1989). The overwhelming majority of patients with MPD are women, and it can be seen that there is a widespread use, in a variety of cultures, of dissociative processes by women to underline and negotiate both personal distress and wider social needs (Lewis, 1989). Second, the growing evidence for a strong link between childhood violence and sexual abuse and the later development of MPD parallels a growing awareness in society of the extent and impact of this pervasive social problem. In this light, MPD can be conceptualized both as a personal reaction to trauma and as part of a larger social agenda which links the psychological and social dimensions (Rivera, 1989).

The critics of the MPD concept have always emphasized the possibility that the syndrome is frequently a creation of the therapeutic collaboration (Kenny, 1986). Under the influence of therapeutic suggestion and the sanction given by the clinical situation, the patient begins to organize various behaviors and experiences into a coherent alternate personality. Spanos (1985b, 1986d) gives experimental evidence to support the notion of multiple personality as a social role enactment shaped by what goes on between patient and therapist as well as by the expectations and impressions the patient arrives with. This would not minimize the seriousness or the significance of the clinical observations but would emphasize the important part that contextual cues have in the hypnotic process. Experimental subjects who are encouraged to develop another personality (either with or without hypnosis) adopt many of the features of the MPD patients. Spanos concludes that, for an able subject, the creation of an alter under hypnotic conditions is a relatively easy task. But context is again critical, as hypnosis without specific suggestion does not appear to influence the features of the disorder (C. A. Ross, 1989c).

With the increased popularity of the diagnosis and growing public awareness, some MPD patients have had their cast of characters proliferate. It is hard not to see this population boom (going from two or three personalities to, in some cases, over two dozen) as being a response to their uniqueness being challenged (Kenny, 1986). Given the current social focus on the diagnosis and the natural desire of individuals to respond to social expectations and to secure a sense of meaning and understanding of their predicament in a clinical setting, it seems unlikely that a substantial number of MPD patients and the proliferation of alters in some of them are not functions of their interactions with therapists. Whether this constitutes an iatrogenic illness or a creative therapeutic intervention is open to interpretation. Reification of the MPD concept may or may not turn out to be a useful clinical event. It is important, however, to recognize the great sensitivity of these patients to their context and their ability to creatively elaborate symptoms expected of them.

A central problem the diagnosis of MPD raises relates to our definition of personality. Implicit in the traditional concept is the description of the personality as an entity (a thing located in space rather than a process followed through time). As Bennett Braun observes: "The concept of MPD is easier to comprehend when the personalities are perceived as thought processes" (1986a, p. xii). Rather than distinct entities, dissociated "personalities" can thus be understood as procedures or roles adopted and developed in response to particular social contexts. Such contexts appear to include severe physical or psychological trauma, family or societal injunctions that prevent open dissent, and particular contexts (whether in the clinician's office or the spiritualist's seance) that encourage refinement of the role.

The elaboration of disparate psychological events into a coherent personality with a large measure of autonomy is a universal human experience. It is one of which we all have personal experience from our childhood, and it is intrinsic to our cognitive representations, or metaphors, of personal and social experience. James speculated that "split off" experiences would also tend to the form of personality particularly if encouraged by social structures ([1890] 1983, p. 222). Moreover, the process is one that tends to propagate itself. "Once baptized, the subconscious personage . . . grows more definitely outlined and displays better her psychological characters. In particular she shows us that she is conscious of the feelings excluded from the consciousness of the primary or normal personage" (Janet, quoted in James, [1890] 1983, pp. 222–223).

Within this context, the therapist or experimenter can be an influential guide and mentor. Patient and therapist can often be seen as participating in a creative collaboration and alternating in the roles of author, director, and performers of the drama. The ways in which we organize experience are determined by the metaphors we use. The metaphors of personal experience and of dramatic structure are universal (though not exclusive) descriptions of the process. They not only describe but by generating expectations actually define the form these experiences will take.

The ritual use of trance, possession states, and MPD share some common characteristics in their presentation. Typically, each evolves gradually over time, and the full manifestation requires an initiation procedure and progressive rehearsal of the role (Ervin, 1988). The role becomes both more elaborate and more coherent with repeated practice. This implies a learning process in which feedback from the society helps shape further manifestations. In MPD, this elaboration can take the form of either a richer unified personality or the proliferation of alters.

I perceive the more important and subtle issue to be that of the relations between "mind" and society, between concept and self-experience—those processes that result in the parceling up of an apparently unitary flow of consciousness (James's "stream of thought") into sensibly discontinuous experience in accord with culture, role, and the individual vicissitudes of fate. I therefore also perceive that multiple personality is in one sense genuine, but in another spurious. (Kenny, 1986, p. 183)

THE HYPNOTIC SELF

Social acceptance of possession encourages individual cultivation and expression of dissociative abilities. Various transcultural studies suggest that these phenomena are important mechanisms for both personal and social equilibrium (Lewis, 1989). Trance may permit the socially disadvantaged (particularly women) to participate in social and political processes from which they would otherwise be barred (Lewis, 1989). There is clear evidence, from a variety of cultures, that the content of spirit possession and other related systems reflect the ongoing concerns of the greater community.

Our sense of self and of others is fluid and constantly being modified by the contextual frame. Social roles must be constantly renegotiated. This may be particularly true in response to severe trauma. Trauma appears to promote dissociation or the spontaneous use of hypnotic skills in an effort to repair or reestablish models of self and others. There appears to be a dynamic interaction in this process between individual hypnotic ability, the severity of the trauma, and accepted social manifestations of trance behavior. In a real sense, we are constantly creating versions of ourself and these versions depend upon circumstances. What remains the same is a core of individual abilities and experiences. How they are expressed is always a matter of negotiation.

9 A HYPNOTIC SUGGESTION

Hypnotism and hypnosis are the terms applied to a unique,
complex form of unusual but normal behavior which can probably
be induced in every normal person under suitable conditions. . . .
but again, some of them are difficult subjects.

Milton Erickson, 1980a

The work of Milton Erickson clearly illustrates two
significant aspects of the hypnotherapeutic interaction.
The first is the role of suggestion in absorbing attention,
establishing rapport, and effecting therapeutic change.
The second is the nature of ideodynamic response, the
ability of the brain to create meaning from contextual
cues. Erickson's clinical work involved careful observation,
flexible communication, and emphasis on the creative use
of unconscious resources. Drawing attention to practice
rather than theory, this work underlines the collaborative
process that is central to hypnotherapy. The notion that
the patient-therapist interaction is the source of therapeutic growth is the most potent hypnotic suggestion of
all.

SUGGESTION AND IDEODYNAMIC RESPONSES

In the spring of 1882, Hippolyte Bernheim, professor of
medicine at the University of Nancy and one of the leading experts on

hypnosis in nineteenth-century France, received a surprise visit in his consulting room. A patient, whom Bernheim had treated for an extremely painful and disabling sciatica unsuccessfully for over six months, reappeared to announce that he was cured. The incurable disability was gone. During the physical examination, the patient cheerfully went through a variety of contortions to demonstrate his newfound flexibility and freedom from pain. Equally astonishing, and perhaps for the great professor somewhat mortifying, was the origin of this dramatic cure. The patient's symptoms had been relieved during a single visit to a humble general practitioner by the name of Ambroise Liébeault, practicing in the sleepy village of Pont Saint Vincent.

To Bernheim's credit, he did not dismiss the case as an isolated incident but decided to pay Liébeault a visit. Bernheim discovered a busy, rather nondescript general practitioner's office (Liébeault often saw more than fifty patients in a single morning) and a decided absence of scientific rigor. Liébeault employed hypnosis extensively but in a highly original fashion. Abandoning the elaborate mesmeric passes and incantations fashionable at the time, Liébeault had opted for a very informal and conversational style of hypnotic induction. The scene was described by J. M. Bramwell, a later English visitor to Liébeault's office:

Two little girls, about six or seven years of age, no doubt brought in the first instance by friends, walked in and sat down on the sofa behind the doctor. He, stopping for a moment in his work made a pass in the direction of one of them, and said: "Sleep, my little kitten," repeated the same for the other, and in an instant they were both asleep. He rapidly gave them their dose of suggestion and then evidently forgot all about them. (Bramwell, 1903, p. 32)

Bernheim was impressed, if not by the setting, at least by the results. He and Liébeault became friends and colleagues in what came to be known as the "Nancy school" of hypnosis. Their theories came into conflict with those of Charcot and his Parisian colleagues. The result was a lively controversy that persists among theorists to this day.

Jean-Martin Charcot at the Salpêtrière Hospital in Paris was the individual most responsible for providing hypnosis with a degree of scientific respectability (Ellenberger, 1970). He did this not by his research on the subject, which was negligible, nor by his theories on the matter, which were simplistic and incorrect, but simply by the fact that as a distinguished neurologist and charismatic speaker he lent the aura of his reputation to the field. Charcot equated hypnosis with hysteria and believed that in his demonstration he was revealing a form of nervous system pathology.

In a famous painting by Pierre Brouillet, Charcot is shown conducting rounds at the Salpêtrière demonstrating a patient in a hysterical fit induced by hypnosis before a group of his colleagues (Ellenberger, 1970). The painting is a veritable who's who of the history of neurology. Assisting Charcot is Joseph Babinski; the others watching attentively include Gilles de la Tourette, Pierre Marie, Paul Richer, and Charles Féré. The unidentified patient is demonstrating the third stage of Charcot's model of hysteria with unfailing exactitude. What the painting also reveals is that on a back wall of the lecture room hangs a large poster in plain view to the patient, displaying exactly the posture she is flawlessly demonstrating. It is ironic, as Edmonston (1986) has pointed out, that though Bernheim and the Nancy school appear to have won the theoretical war with Charcot and his Parisian followers, Charcot's name is much better known and Brouillet's painting (largely because of its frequent reproduction in introductory psychology texts) is the only part of the controversy that is known to most of us today.

A commentary on the dispute between the two schools was written by a young Viennese neurologist who had been a student of Charcot's, Sigmund Freud. He translated Bernheim's book on suggestion into German, and in the summer of 1889 visited him in Nancy. In his introduction, Freud wrote:

Dr. Bernheim . . . maintains that all the phenomena of hypnotism have the same origin: they arise, that is, from a suggestion, a conscious idea, which has been introduced into the brain of the hypnotized person by an external influence and has been accepted by him as though it had arisen spontaneously. On this view, all hypnotic manifestations would be mental phenomena, effects of suggestions.

. . . If the supporters of the suggestion theory are right, all the observations made at the Salpêtrière are worthless: indeed, they become errors in observation. The hypnosis of hysterics would have no characteristics of its own; but every physician would be free to produce any symptomatology. . . .

It is worth while considering what it is which we can legitimately call a "suggestion." No doubt some kind of mental influence is implied by the term; and I should like to put forward the view that what distinguishes a suggestion from other kinds of mental influence, such as a command or the giving of a piece of information or instruction, is that in the case of a suggestion an idea is aroused in another person's brain which is not examined in regard to its origin but is accepted just as though it had arisen spontaneously in that brain. . . . In other words, it is a question in these cases not so much of suggestions as of stimulation to *autosuggestions*. (Freud, [1888] 1959, pp. 14–21)

Charcot and his followers emphasized the pathological and stereo-typed model of hypnosis. In contrast, the Nancy school emphasized the continuity between hypnosis and normal consciousness and underlined the central role that rapport and suggestion had in hypnosis. Above all, they emphasized the role of verbal suggestion by the therapist in stimulating "ideodynamic" responses on the part of the patient (Rossi, 1986a).

Bernheim viewed the way in which the brain responds to suggestion as the key to the hypnotic experience. He theorized that in hypnosis the mind functions by

transforming the idea received into an act. . . . In the normal condition, every formulated idea is questioned by the mind. . . . In the hypnotized subject, on the contrary, the transformation of thought into action, sensation, movement, or vision is so quickly and so actively accomplished, that the intellectual inhibition has not time to act. When the mind interposes, it is already an accomplished fact, which is often registered with surprise, and which is confirmed by the fact that it proves to be real. . . . There is, then, exaltation of the ideo-motor reflex excitability, which effects the unconscious transformation of the thought into movement, unknown to the will.

. . . There is also, then, exaltation of the ideo-sensorial reflex excitability, which effects the unconscious transformation of the thought into sensation, or into a sensory image. . . .

The mechanism of suggestion in general, may then be summed up in the following formula: increase of the reflex ideo-motor, ideo-sensitive, and ideo-excitability. (Bernheim, [1886] 1957, quoted in Rossi and Cheek, 1988, p. 5)

The ideomotor concept derives from the sensorimotor reflex described by the nineteenth-century neurologists. Bernheim envisioned a process in which the sensory arms of the loop are replaced by a suggestion that takes on the force of direct sensory input. Thus, thinking about a movement tends to produce the movement. Bernheim's contribution was to postulate that in hypnosis the therapist's suggestions, as interpreted by the patient, can affect the ideodynamic responses without conscious mediation.

The one hundred years of the history of hypnosis since Bernheim can be seen as a gradual elaboration of his ideas, marking a transition from a view of hypnosis as a weakened mental state induced by the "magnetism" of the hypnotist to the contemporary view that hypnotherapy involves a complex collaborative process in which both individuals are creatively and cooperatively involved (Gilligan, 1987; Rossi, 1988). Indeed, Rossi has suggested that various forms of psychodynamic psychotherapy, including Freud's development of the free association method in psychoanalysis, or Carl Jung's development of the active imagination techniques, can be seen as the attempt by these innovative minds to break away from the limitations of the narrow models of hypnosis and of mental function and to develop more subjectively permissive techniques of therapy. In the modern era, clinicians such as Cheek and Erickson have extended the use of ideodynamic phenomena for similar purposes. The clinical techniques of Milton Erickson illustrate the wide potential value of these approaches.

As Bernheim pointed out, ideomotor activity is only one variety of ideodynamic responses. It captures our attention simply because it is an external, visible manifestation. Ideodynamic phenomena are central to our understanding of the nature of hypnosis. They are also central to the understanding of the nature of hypnotic suggestion: the manner in which the words of the therapist can induce motor, emotional, sensory, or cognitive changes in the subject in the absence of apparent conscious volition.

The notion of ideomotor responses is central to most of the current experimental approaches to hypnosis, the hypnotic susceptibility scales that are routinely used, and the way in which the data are interpreted (Sheehan, 1982). Sheehan's careful studies of subjective experiential responses to hypnotic suggestions show that there is a wide degree of difference among subjects' reactions to ideomotor suggestion. The individual subject may use a variety of cognitive strategies that depend on different attentional and imagery processes. But above all, the degree of rapport between subject and investigator appears to be the critical variable. A high degree of mutual involvement can often stimulate subjects to more creative responses as well as induce them to attempt tasks that are unpleasant and normally aversive. This ability for mutual synchronization to deal with painful or frightening tasks is clearly a cornerstone of hypnotherapy.

Ideomotor phenomena provide a way to conceptualize how the brain organizes communication. As we have seen (in chapters 2 and 3), there is a wide variety of subtle motor and sensory activities that change subsequently in the service of maintaining a communication rhythm. There may be an optimal synchronization between mental events and physical responses occurring at the level of the microdynamics of the interaction. Stimuli that are synchronized with the phases of the cardiovascular pulse pressure produce more prominent potentials in the brain, particularly in the right hemisphere (Sandman, 1984). Alterations in the respiratory pattern can reduce measures of physiologic and psychological arousal significantly (Cappo, 1984). Ideodynamic responses represent the internal synchrony of brain processes with the rhythm of interaction. That activity, usually below the level of conscious awareness, is concerned with maintaining the interaction by interpreting and expressing a frame for the context. Far from being peripheral to human understanding, we have also seen that that frame can be developed in a highly sophisticated way for a variety of social purposes.

Similarly, the synchronization of physiologic responses appears to be important in hypnotic induction. The physiologic manifestations of the development of trance (or of the related phase of the ultradian rhythm) can be used as part of an ideodynamic feedback loop to enhance this synchronization. A study that measured physiologic change in both therapist and patient showed that synchronization of respiration, cardiovascular responses, muscle responses, galvanic skin response, and EEG was strongly correlated with successful hypnotic induction, and lack of synchronization resulted in a failure to create a trance state (Bányai, 1985). Rapport, the sense of shared experience, appears to be the meaning in the rhythm.

IDEODYNAMIC RESPONSES AND THE HYPNOTIC EXPERIENCE

In discussing altered states of consciousness, Charles Tart (1983) suggested that there are specific emotional, cognitive, perceptual, attentional, and social factors that, taken together, serve to stabilize a particular state. Hypnosis is one technique for altering the state of consciousness in which some aspects of human awareness and abilities can be emphasized. For this to happen, hypnosis must of necessity do two things. First, it must disrupt the normal state of consciousness, and second, it must provide a patterning for a new and altered state. As with the use of other tools, the results of hypnosis will depend on both the experience and technique of the users and the task to which the tool is directed.

In a similar vein, Erickson and Rossi (1976, 1979) have emphasized the need to depotentiate habitual modes of awareness and to access and utilize unconscious processes in hypnosis. They describe a five-stage model of hypnotherapy that involves (1) absorption of attention; (2) the depotentiation of conscious processes; (3) the enhancement and gaining of access to unconscious processes (which involve ideomotor responses, a state of arousal via the activation of the sympathetic nervous system, and an ultradian repatterning); (4) a synthesis (or reframing); and (5) a ratification of the trance experience.

These steps result in the effective mobilization and sequencing of cerebral resources. The cognitive resources available for information processing are discrete and measurable (Wickens, 1983; Poppel, 1988). Absorption in a particular task—the ability of the brain to limit the amount of attention paid to distracting stimuli—produces a corresponding increase in the strength of information processing (Wickens, 1983). In this sense, "depotentiation" of conscious processes enhances hypnotic responding by freeing up greater information-processing resources for the task at hand. Electrophysiologic studies suggest that different aspects of information processing require reliably consistent different lengths of time. The greater the amount of information-processing resources that are available to the task enhances the electrophysiologic responses to decision-making processes (Woods, 1980). These measures of cognitive processing are also related to clear psychophysiological correlates that reliably mark out both the intensity and the stage of the processing (Cohen, 1985).

The ability to involve oneself in everyday imaginative activities does seem to be related to hypnotic abilities (Tellegen, 1974; Rhue, 1989). Hypnotizable individuals tend to report more intense differences in subjective experience during altered states of consciousness. Moreover, the intensity is augmented by the formal hypnotic induction (Kumar, 1988). Josephine Hilgard (1979) suggested that a composite ability she called imaginative involvement is predictive of hypnotic ability. Individuals possessing this quality tend to be avid readers of fiction, enjoy watching and performing in the arts, have deep religious personal commitments, and are mentally active in a number of imaginative ways. Hilgard noted several characteristics including enjoyment of the moment, a time-limited escape from the world of reality (with a tendency toward a strong reality orientation at other times), and active involvement (unlike the stereotyped picture of the hypnotic subject as passive and dependent).

The ability for imaginative involvement and absorption is a significant predictor of hypnotic ability (Nadon, 1987). Moreover, these predictors are strongly associated with the person's experiencing similar styles of thinking in the waking state and during dreaming (Nadon, 1987). Absorption appears to relate to differential response in hypnosis, meditation, biofeedback, and marijuana intoxication. In hypnosis, absorption correlates with increased and more vivid imagery, inward and absorbed attention, positive affect, decreased self-awareness, and increased alterations in other aspects of subjective experience (Pekala, 1985).

Internal absorption and hypnotizability is related to the vividness of mental imagery (Wallace, 1990). Although hypnosis per se does not necessarily enhance imagery after a formal induction, there is some evidence that it and other cognitive training methods can enhance the use of imagery significantly (Spanos, 1986b). Hypnotic subjects, however, are more likely to accept the changes as genuine (Spanos, 1968). This also appears to be true for other forms of hypnotic experience (Hilgard, 1977).

In a systematic study of the use of imagery and enhancing hypnotic response, Kirsch (1987) found that parallel imagery (imagery that supported the hypnotic suggestions) enhanced or decreased response according to the expectations of the subjects. If they had been told that such imagery would enhance the response, their responses were greater; if they had been told that it would inhibit response, the responses were diminished. In contrast, counterimagery (imagery incompatible with the suggestions) inhibited responses in subjects when they were told that it would but had no effect when the subjects were told that it would enhance their responses. This suggests that the nature of the suggestions and the nature of the imagery play a significant part, but the subject's expectation is also an important variable.

Normal subjects who score highly on spontaneous visual and auditory imagery scales are more likely to have visual or auditory hallucinations in response to hypnotic suggestion (Young, 1987). Similarly, psychiatric patients who are hallucinating are more likely to respond to hypnotic suggestions for auditory (but not visual) hallucinations than are nonhallucinating psychiatric patients (Young, 1987).

It has been suggested that the use of imagery and relaxation techniques in the hypnotic induction, though not affecting traditional behavioral measures of hypnosis, significantly changes subjective reports of the experience (Mitchell, 1986). Strategies that use imagery followed by cognitive procedures are more effective for altering unpleasant moods than cognition followed by imagery (Means, 1986–1987).

Retention of information learned in hypnosis is not related to hypnotic susceptibility but is related to the degree of absorption and vividness of the imagery associated with the items (Sweeney, 1986). Similarly, although subjects with both high and low hypnotic susceptibility scores use similar memory strategies in dealing with visual imagery, during the hypnotic state subjects with high hypnotic susceptibility scores have access to different strategies, particularly those that emphasize distinctions or "object difference"—arranging information in an antithetical structure (Crawford, 1982b). This is illustrated by the differences between cooperative hypnosis (sometimes called heterohypnosis) and self-hypnosis. Both involve absorption and internal focus, but self-hypnosis stimulates a more expansive, free-floating attention with the development of much richer imagery, and traditional heterohypnosis involves focused concentration and sensitivity to the stimuli coming from the hypnotist (Fromm, 1981; Johnson, 1981).

THE CONSCIOUS-UNCONSCIOUS DISTINCTION

Franklin has suggested a relationship between emotional involvement and attention or absorption in the information being received (Franklin, 1988). The level of arousal and degree of absorption is the result of an interaction between the cortex, the limbic system, and the reticular formation of the brain stem, integrating cognitive, emotional, and physiologic information. According to this model, emotional evaluation and physiologic patterning determine which way information is processed. Franklin suggests that this is an interplay of conscious and automatic processes, and involves an active balance between the two.

While helping to redefine the nature of clinical interactions, ideodynamic phenomena also help clarify what we mean by the terms *conscious* and *unconscious*. Traditional models of human cognition that emphasize narrow problem-solving processes are inadequate. Creativity, even the quirky form that makes each of us unique, is more complex (Csikszentmihalyi, 1988). Human brain activity involves the constant interaction of conscious and unconscious processes. In this sense, consciousness can be conceptualized as an additional level of flexibility in self-regulation (Bateson, 1987).

Baars (1988) has described consciousness in terms of a "global workspace" through which the distributed specialized functions of the brain can be integrated. Conscious brain activity can be thought of as a blackboard available to all the various subsystems of the brain. The activity of each subsystem may or may not be available to the others. Thus conscious activity provides a meeting place in which these subsystems can produce an integrated society.

In his description of the workspace, Baars includes both conscious and unconscious processes. In contrasting the two, he points out the

relative inefficiency of conscious activity but indicates that these processes also

have great range, relational capacity and context sensitivity. Furthermore, conscious events have apparent internal consistency, seriality, and limited capacity.
In contrast to all these aspects of conscious functioning, unconscious processors
are highly efficient in their specialized tasks, have relatively limited domains, are
relatively isolated and autonomous, highly diverse, and capable of contradicting
each other; they can operate in parallel, and, taken together, unconscious processors have very great capacity.

There is a remarkable match between these contrasts and a system architecture used in some artificial intelligence applications, called a global workspace
in a distributed system of specialized processors. This organization can be compared to a very large committee of experts, each speaking his or her specialized
jargon, who can communicate with each other through some global broadcast-
ing device, a large blackboard in front of the committee of experts, for example.
(Baars, 1988, p. 117)

The fundamental unity of conscious and unconscious processes can
be observed clearly in problem-solving activity. Baars characterizes the
common pattern of problem solving as a triad involving (1) a conscious
stage in which the problem is identified, (2) an unconscious stage in
which cognitive resources are allocated according to unconscious goal
context, and (3) a conscious identification of the solution. Any sharp
distinction between voluntary and involuntary processes simply ignores
the important part that automatic activity plays in all behavior. Adapting the ideomotor theory to modern cognitive models, Baars points out
the important role that unconscious goals (schemata) and context (or
frames) have in shaping voluntary activity. Our current models deem-
phasize the traditional sharp distinction between conscious and unconscious processes and instead focus on the way in which the two streams
constantly interact in achieving any goal.

The cognitive schema is a complex representational state that provides a goal or intention that is constantly being compared with the
ongoing frame. Such a schema may or may not be conscious. Baars
describes ideomotor control of thought and action as a process in which
"conscious goal images without effective competition serve to organize
and trigger automatically controlled actions, which then run off without
further conscious involvement" (1988, p. 247).

In a real sense the action that results from this complex set of momentary
conscious and unconscious constraints is a solution posed by problems triggered by the conscious goal, and bounded by numerous physical, kinetic, social,

and other contextual considerations. It makes sense therefore to treat voluntary control as a kind of problem solving. (p. 258)

It has been suggested that the role of conscious activity and voluntary action can be conceptualized in terms not of what we can do but of what it prevents. Far from being a rare or isolated activity, ideomotor behavior can be seen as the primary way in which the brain operates. The vast majority of our activities, even those we assume to be most voluntary (such as speech), are initiated and maintained by unconscious processes. Libet (1985) has suggested that the role of the conscious will is not to initiate an act but rather to select and control the outcome. The role of conscious activity is a permissive one in this view, either inhibiting or permitting implementation of the activity that emerges unconsciously.

As we have seen, this fits with the evidence of brain activity in hypnosis, which suggests that hypnotic ability depends largely upon "letting go" or responding without inhibition to the contextual cues (see chapter 5). On the other hand, a major component of lack of hypnotic ability may be an interference by conscious processes that actively inhibit hypnotic responsiveness. In order to achieve this role, the level of conscious activity must be closely related to the level of arousal and attentional processes. As we have seen, the links between cortical and subcortical activity provide a basis by which the full brain can be involved.

Baars points out the importance of contextual feedback in both altering and stabilizing this system. He defines context as

unconscious systems that evoke and shape conscious experience. . . . In a sense, contexts can be thought of as information that the nervous system has already adapted to; it is the ground against which new events are defined. Consciousness always seems to favor novel and informative messages. But recognizing novelty requires an implicit comparison to the *status quo,* the old knowledge that is represented contextually. (1988, p. 135)

Ideomotor activity demonstrates the importance of the nonverbal frame in initiating and maintaining the hypnotic state. But ideodynamic theory may also provide a connecting link with the maintenance of cognitive schema. Ideomotor theory suggests that responses occur whenever ideas or suggestions take on the characteristics of vividness and sensory input. Baars (1988) suggests that the ability of perceptual and imaginal activity to influence cognitive schemata is related to the brain's ability to integrate cognitive schemata. Suggestions that fit within the interactional frame and that do not violate cognitive sche-

mata are likely to produce ideomotor activity unless they are deliberately inhibited.

Learning can be interpreted "as a change in context, one that alters
the way the learned material is experienced" (Baars, 1988, p. 135).
Context has a pervasive influence in initiating, maintaining, and shaping conscious experience. In this sense, the major role of attentional
processes is to determine the appropriate context and the way in which
information will be processed. "Thus we are compelled to view even a
single conscious experience as part of a dynamic, developmental process of learning and adaptation. Increasingly it seems that the system
underlying conscious experience is our primary organ of adaptation"
(Baars, 1988, p. 221).

In a real sense, then, metaphor can be seen as a form of ideomotor
control over abstractions. "In general, an imageable metaphor seems to
serve the function of evoking and recruiting conceptual processes that
are more abstract and often more accurate than the image itself. These
abstract entities may be impossible to experience qualitatively. Hence
the need for visual figures, audible words, and concrete metaphors"
(Baars, 1988, p. 285).

Baars defines hypnosis as "a state in which ideomotor control operates without effective competition" (p. 287). This sort of focusing resources can be achieved only by absorption in a context that is so vivid it
effectively or selectively inhibits all other possible competition.

Thus we can enter an absorbed state either if consciousness is dominated by a
very strong context, or if there is a drop in competition from alternative contexts. In fact, most actual absorbed states have both of these features. In watching a fascinating movie our experience is being structured by the story line,
which continually generates new expectations about future events that need to
be tested. At the same time we may relax, postpone some pressing concerns, and
thus lower the urgency of competing topics.

One implication is that we are always in the absorbed state relative to our own
dominant context. (p. 288)

Baars links hypnosis with this type of absorption in "a new, imaginative context that dominates experience for some time to the exclusion of
other events" (p. 289). Hypnosis can thus be seen as a state in which
there is a strong link between a cognitive schema and the interactional
frame. Baars suggests that suggestibility or sensitivity to cues can then
be seen merely as the consequence of ideomotor control in an absorbed
state in which there is minimal competition of other concerns.

In sum, hypnosis may simply be ideomotor control in a state of absorption. But absorbed states are quite normal and, in a general sense, we are all absorbed in our own top-level contexts. The major difference seems to be that highly hypnotizable subjects are quite flexible in the topics of their absorption, while most people are not. Perhaps we should turn the usual question around. Instead of asking what is different about hypnosis, we might ask: Why is flexible absorption so difficult for three-quarters of the population? What is it that is added to a "ground state" of absorption, which we all share, that resists flexible ideomotor control? (p. 292)

In an absorbed state, conscious experience is unusually resistant to distraction. Baars's ideomotor theory, derived from the earlier theorists, suggests "the notion that conscious goals are inherently impulsive, and tend to be carried out by default unless they are inhibited by other conscious thoughts or intentions" (p. 379).

In this view, all the phenomena that are associated with the hypnotic state can be seen as forms of ideodynamic communication. This includes the full range of trance behavior, which may range from simple finger signals indicating yes or no to specific questions to the development of various types of complex emotional, cognitive, or sensory experiences. The occurrence of these phenomena indicate that the therapist and patient are in a close rapport and collaborative relationship.

At first glance, the ideomotor model may suggest that hypnosis is a state very different from normal waking consciousness. But though ideomotor behavior appears to violate our perception of consciously and deliberately controlled behavior, this may be more a reflection of the limitations of our model of conscious and deliberate control than a statement about hypnosis as a special state. In a careful review, Lynn (1990) has demonstrated that the automatic behavior shown by hypnotic subjects is highly sensitive to contextual cues and typically follows the same social and psychological parameters as do our other, ostensibly deliberate, behavior. Just as we have shown with unconscious learning, ideomotor behavior is a normal and, indeed, essential part of everyday cognition and behavior. It is only when our attention is drawn to such behavior in hypnosis that it seems in some way remarkable. Whether we describe it as cognitive flexibility (Crawford, 1983a) or increased internal sensitivity (Rossi, 1990), hypnosis appears to be encouraging less restricted styles of thinking, feeling, and behaving. Erickson's (1976) homey definition of hypnosis as "helping the patient to get out of his own way" aptly describes the basis of the naturalistic approach.

ERICKSON'S NATURALISTIC APPROACHES

The work of Milton Erickson has been critical in the development of the cooperative approach. Erickson has been the single most influential clinician in the development of hypnotherapy in the past quarter century (Baker, 1988; Zeig, 1988). His perception and enhancement of individual responses in the development of hypnotic behavior paralleled his creative use of metaphor and highly patterned verbal structures (Kirmayer, 1988). The result was a flexible approach that permitted a variety of possible responses. Erickson emphasized that hypnotic techniques were not important in themselves but, rather, served to stimulate internal absorption and involvement of ideomotor and ideosensory processes:

These techniques are of particular value with patients who want hypnosis, who could benefit from it, but who resist any formal or overt effort at trance induction and who need to have their obstructive resistances bypassed. The essential consideration in the use of ideomotor techniques lies not in their elaborateness or novelty but simply in the initiation of motor activity, either real or hallucinated, as a means of fixating and focussing the subjects' attention upon inner experiential learnings and capabilities. (Erickson, 1980a, 1:138)

Erickson later used his observations to develop nonverbal, or "pantomime," techniques of hypnotic induction (1:331–339) as well as to augment his elaborate verbal inductions (1:340–359, 366–377). In these works, Erickson emphasized the importance of the process of communication, which is often obscured by our bias toward the content of communication. He communicated with gesture, facial expression, gaze, tone of voice, and respiratory pattern. He also observed the same nonverbal features in his patient to monitor the ongoing hypnotic state. As a result he achieved a high level of rapport in the form of a synchronization of nonverbal communication.

The following example demonstrates Erickson's recognition of a subject's ideodynamic response that was outside of the putative hypnotic task. Erickson then utilized this idiosyncratic response to develop further trance phenomena. He describes it this way:

During his [Erickson's] first demonstration of the hand-levitation technique of trance induction to that 1923–1924 seminar group, a special finding was made by the writer of the spontaneous manifestation in a volunteer subject of hallucinated ideomotor activity. She had volunteered to act as a subject for a demonstration of what the writer meant by a "hand-levitation trance induction." While she and the group intently watched her hands as they rested on her lap, the

writer offered repeated, insistent, appropriate suggestions for right hand levitation, all without avail. Silent study of the subject in an effort to appraise the
failure of response disclosed her gaze to be directed into midair at shoulder
level, and her facial expression and apparent complete detachment from her
surroundings indicated that a deep trance state had developed. She was told to
elevate her left hand voluntarily to the level of her right hand. Without any
alteration of the direction of her gaze, she brought her left hand up to shoulder
level. She was told to replace her left hand in her lap and then to watch her right
hand 'slowly descend' to her lap. When it reached her lap, she was to give
immediately a full verbal report upon her experience. There resulted a slow
downward shifting of her gaze, and as it reached her lap, she looked up at the
group and delightedly gave an extensive description of the 'sensations' of her
hallucinatory experience, with no realization that she had actually developed
her first known trance state, but with an amnesia for the reality of the trance
experience as such, though not for the content.

   She asked to be allowed to repeat her experience and promptly did so. This
time the group watched her eye and facial behavior. Again there was no hand
movement, but all agreed that she developed a somnambulistic trance immediately upon beginning to shift her gaze upward. This conclusion was put to test
at once by demonstrating with her the phenomena of deep hypnosis. (1:137)

   Erickson's model emphasizes the effects achieved rather than the
techniques used. He advocated what he called a *naturalistic approach* to
hypnotic induction. This concept is based on the idea that the hypnotic
experience is an extension of normal human experience, "the common
everyday trance." Using careful observation of the individual, Erickson
attempted to develop trance naturally out of the immediate context,
paying minute attention to subtle behavioral cues. Although hypnotic
suggestions are not the equivalent of subliminal stimuli, it appears that
hypnosis does improve sensitivity for subliminally perceived facial car-
icatures (Kunzendorf, 1986–1987). This suggests that face-to-face
communication with its subtle changes in facial expression is enhanced
during the hypnotic state. Erickson used simple alterations of common
behavior as part of an absorbing hypnotic induction:

Erickson: And now I want you to shake your head No. [Erickson models head
shaking.] Your name isn't Ruth, is it? [Erickson shakes No.] [Ruth shakes No.]
And you aren't a women, are you? [Ruth shakes her head No.] And you aren't
sitting down, are you? [Ruth shakes her head No.] And you aren't in trance, are
you? [Ruth shakes her head No.] (Erickson, 1981, pp. 166–167)

   In a behavioral example, the "handshake induction," a normal handshake was changed imperceptibly by Erickson into a nonverbal suggestion of the development of arm catalepsy and, by extension, hyp-

notic trance by placing the induction within the context of an innocuous social situation (a handshake) suddenly altered and utilized (Erickson, 1980a, 1:331).

As Edmondston (1986) has observed, Erickson used an elaborate combination of contextual cues as hypnotic inductions. O'Hanlon (1987) lists a number of such cues including voice, breathing, and tonal synchronization, and mirroring of the patient's posture, gesture, or vocabulary. Similarly, these cues function as a form of conditioning in which hypnotic behaviors can be systematically reinforced. No individual element is particularly "hypnotic"; it is the combination of all these elements that produces the most effective therapeutic context. "The apparently bewildering array of innovations in Erickson's approaches to trance induction all share this one significant feature in common: They illustrate how indirect suggestions and minimal cues that evoke and utilize the subject's own associations are the real basis of the hypnotherapist's skill" (Erickson, 1980a, 1:134).

Erickson was tone-deaf and spoke with a highly characteristic rhythm. He habitually stressed syllables in his speech that produced a heightened form of the patient's own words. Similarly, he often spoke in rhythm with the patient's breathing. Students who worked with him have often acquired, either consciously or unconsciously, a similar rhythm that they slip into when using their "trance voice" (Gilligan, 1987). Edward Sapir, the father of modern linguistics, once observed that Milton Erickson's speaking rhythm was one that he had heard only in a recording of a Central African tribe (Erickson, 1980a, 1:134). A child of eight observed to Erickson: "Every night my mommy sings me to sleep, but you breathe me to sleep" (1:361).

When, as a boy, Erickson observed changes in people's breathing patterns that he could not fully understand, he began to experiment with deliberate alterations in breathing pattern as a form of unconscious communication. For example, he tried to learn how to alter his breathing in such a way that classmates would hum or yawn.

At church old Mrs. Snow (probably in her early 40's) was much in demand as a soloist for weddings, funerals, and weekly services. She also was a regular attendant at community sings. I could never understand why Mrs. Snow put extra syllables into words nor why she did such peculiar breathing, because when she began that kind of breathing, so did other people, even if they didn't sing. When I asked her about it, she gave me irrelevant answers about the thoracic, diaphragmatic, and abdominal breathing, but what I wanted to know was why people listening would tighten their throats and change their breathing. I often noticed that people would change their breathing and then begin to hum and then to sing. I also noticed that when people hummed, others would join in, even waving their hands or feet—for which I felt no urge. . . .

Everybody breathed; nobody paid any attention to their breathing unless ill; and yet breathing was on a par with humming, singing, and vocalization of any sort. Also, breathing was basic to vocalization of any sort. Breathing was basic to vocal behavior, but nobody seemed ever to recognize it as such.

[This] . . . served to convince me further that people communicated with each other at "breathing" levels of awareness unknown to them. I did not then have an adequate vocabulary nor a clarity of concepts to come to a good understanding, even for myself. But I did know that communication with another could be achieved in a nonverbal and actually unrecognized fashion, but that there had to be definitive stimuli to achieve this end, and that it was best accomplished without the awareness of the other person. (1980a, 1:363–364)

Written accounts and videotaped excerpts of Erickson's work all testify to the subtle and effective way in which he responded to and worked with the rhythm of the interaction. Erickson's observational capacities are legendary. Zeig (1980) describes him as a cat, focusing intently on the moment-to-moment changes in the interaction. This focus allowed him to make interventions with a rhythmic inevitability. His mastery of nonverbal forms of communication allowed him to shape the context so that it was in synchrony with personal rhythms. In this sense, his approach bridged the conceptual gap between interpersonal communication and subjective experience.

Erickson's ability not only to observe nonverbal cues but to use his voice, gestures, and facial expression are also central to his approach. He used what he referred to as the *"interspersal technique"*—using particular voice tones and volume or particular postures consistently in an alternating pattern as a way of encouraging a dissociative experience (Erickson, 1980c, 4:262). A hypnotist's using two different tones of voice—one when talking about the "conscious mind" while describing an external orientation and one when talking about the "unconscious mind" while focusing on an internally oriented description—can encourage an especially vivid state of focused absorption in which creative problem solving may occur.

It is this active aspect of unconscious learning that Erickson's language seems designed to reach. The work on unconscious learning provides indirect support for Erickson's contention that his goal in hypnotherapy was to bypass normal conscious awareness and communicate directly with the unconscious mind (Erickson, 1976b). He apparently intuitively understood the compelling nature of oral poetry, the use of intriguing and compelling language to effect change.

Erickson emphasized that the value of his varied and creative language was in the development and maintenance of the trance state (Erickson and Rossi, 1981, p. 188). Commenting on the response of one of his patients to an elaborate verbal pattern, Erickson said:

For this subject, as in other instances in which this type of technique has been employed, the utilization of the reality situation was of such character that she could formulate no subjectively adequate responses. This resulted in an increasing need to make some kind of a response. As this desire increased, an opportunity for response was presented to her in a form rendered inherently appropriate and effective by the total situation. Thus the very nature of the total situation was utilized in the technique of induction. (1980a, 1:204)

Erickson recognized the importance of the flow of language in achieving his hypnotherapeutic goals. In discussing the use of language to alter the emotional state of a patient traumatized by painful childhood experiences, he said:

From the hideous and negative beginning of the last section a markedly positive ending comes in this section. There is admixture of a happy childhood game, of the poetry of youth, the aim of adulthood, all combined by poetic nuances that could not be disputed. She could not find any single thing to dispute. She was caught in a flowing stream of ideas journeying a rough emotional passage but ending pleasantly. (Erickson and Rossi, 1979, p. 434)

Erickson's use of language was wordplay in the fullest sense of the term. Language for him was indeed play: a shared process that actively involved each person. His use of words was an active invitation for the listener to participate at both the conscious and the unconscious levels. It was a variation of the forms of play that are so important in childhood learning and development. Just as children's play is a very serious business, this form of wordplay can be used in the service of critical growth and learning in the adult.

It was the flexibility of Erickson's language that was at the heart of his creative clinical approach. At the same time, this flexibility has led to considerable ambiguity in characterizing his approach. He has been described, on the one hand, as a highly directive and authoritarian therapist who sculpted elaborate, detailed therapeutic dramas for his patients (for example, Hilgard, 1988) and, on the other, as the archetype of the nondirective and permissive figure using only the most indirect language (McCue, 1988). A third view of Erickson has combined features of these two positions, suggesting that he was a Svengali-like individual merely cloaking his highly directive approach in ostensibly indirect language (for example, Bander and Grinder, 1975). Moreover, critics of the Ericksonian approach have pointed out numerous variations in his different accounts of the same case history (Hilgard, 1988; McCue, 1988). It is but one of the many paradoxes of Milton Erickson that so many different views should exist of an individual who was perhaps the most closely scrutinized and observed therapist in history. This confusion is puzzling in a therapist who was so open in his clinical work and who left behind a considerable volume of audiotapes and visual recordings as well as an extensive body of writings.

Resolution of the paradox comes, in part, by placing Erickson's work in the clinical context. Clearly, he used both highly directive approaches and indirect suggestion according to the needs of the situation as they arose (Kirmayer, 1988). Erickson was guided by the perceived needs of the context and the ongoing feedback he received from his patient. In this, he was following the well-established technique of the oral poet, who makes dramatic changes in emphasis each time he tells a new version of an old story (Lord, 1960). Insisting on the "original" version is akin to expecting a jazz improvisation to conform to a musical score. This flexibility may make it difficult to characterize the Ericksonian approach in simple terms, but it underlines his contention that therapy must be guided by the individual needs of the particular patient (Erickson and Rossi, 1979).

One of the most important of all considerations in inducing hypnosis is meeting adequately the patients as personalities and their needs as individuals. Too often the effort is made to fit the patients to an accepted formal technique of suggestion, rather than adapting the technique to the patients in accord with their actual personality situations. In any such adaptation there is an imperative need to accept and to utilize those psychological states, understandings, and attitudes that each patient brings into the situation. To ignore those factors in favor of some ritual of procedure may and often does delay, impede, limit, or even prevent the desired results. The acceptance and utilization of those factors, on the other hand, promotes more rapid trance induction, the development of more profound trance states, the more ready acceptance of therapy, and greater ease for the handling of the total therapeutic situation. (Erickson, 1980a, 1:175–176)

UTILIZATION

As Hilgard has pointed out (1984), Erickson's most significant contribution was his flexible use of a variety of what have come to be known as strategic interventions in therapy with individuals, couples, or families. His influence extends beyond traditional hypnotherapy. Current strategic family therapy owes a great deal of its technical development to his influence on systems theorists in the 1950s and 1960s (Zeig, 1988).

In contrast to traditional psychodynamic methods, Erickson minimized the value of the process of interpretation by the therapist and acceptance of this interpretation by the patient's conscious mind. He emphasized the importance of techniques that discourage conscious analysis. By thus "depotentiating" the conscious mind, these therapies are more likely to facilitate unconscious processes. Erickson apparently used these techniques frequently when he felt that conscious limitations prevented the patient from full therapeutic involvement.

The past cannot be changed, only one's views and interpretations of it, and even these change with the passage of time. Hence, at best, views and interpretations of the past are of importance only when they stultify the person into a rigidity. Life is lived in the present for the morrow. Hence, psychotherapy is properly oriented about life today in preparation for tomorrow, next month, next year, the future, which in itself will compel many changes in the functioning of the person at all levels of his behavior. (Erickson, quoted in Beahrs, 1971, p. 74)

Erickson emphasized the notion of *utilization*—that is, the use of the patient's beliefs, behavior, or personality as the stuff of therapy (O'Hanlon, 1987). The rapid development of synchronization and rapport paved the way for an approach to therapy that was typically brief and goal-oriented. Rather than viewing overtly noncompliant behavior as potential resistance that had to be overcome, Erickson approached it as an important communication from the patient that could be accepted and then transformed (see Haley, 1973, p. 28).

In characterizing Erickson's general approach, Gilligan has emphasized the importance he placed on respecting and utilizing the unique personality and situation of each patient. Gilligan suggests that "the traditional concept of resistance is better viewed as behavioral feedback indicating a need for further pacing by the therapist" (1987, p. 97). As Erickson pointed out:

The reasons for these difficulties derive from the fact that hypnosis depends upon inter- and intrapersonal relationships. Such relationships are inconstant and alter in accord with personality reactions to each hypnotic development. Additionally, each individual personality is unique, and its patterns of spontaneous and responsive behavior necessarily vary in relation to time, situation, purposes served, and the personalities involved. (1980a, 1:139)

Erickson also noted the variability of trance induction in the clinical setting. Utilization requires not only acute observation but flexibility in order to be able to actually utilize whatever is presented. Erickson combined traditional hypnotherapeutic techniques with a variety of strategic, behavioral, and cognitive style interventions. O'Hanlon lists fifteen techniques Erickson utilized in altering behavioral patterns. For example, his approaches to symptom control frequently involved alterations in the behavioral sequence of the symptom or alteration of the circumstances in which the symptom occurred (O'Hanlon, 1987). Erickson's goal was to elicit abilities and skills and then to link them to the problem context. He viewed this as a form of both explicit and covert posthypnotic suggestion.

Subjects are systematically trained in different types of hypnotic behavior. In training subjects for hypnotic anaesthesia for obstetrical purposes, they may be taught automatic writing and negative visual hallucinations as a preliminary foundation. The former is taught as a foundation for local dissociation of a body part and the latter as a means of instruction in not responding to stimuli. Such training might seem irrelevant, but experience has disclosed that it can be a highly effective procedure in securing the full utilization of the subjects' capabilities. (1980a, 1:143–144)

CONFUSION TECHNIQUES AND INDIRECT SUGGESTION

Although a predictable rhythm is the basis for interactional synchrony, disruptions of the rhythm can also be used creatively. Disruptions of rhythm or violations of the rhythmic expectations increase arousal and these can lead to either increased or decreased credibility (Burgoon, 1988). Thus, surprise, ambiguity, and other forms of rhythmic or prosodic incongruity all lead to heightened arousal, which in turn increases the sensitivity to the communication. These features are seen as increasing the importance of the interaction with more intense positive or negative emotional evaluations (Burgoon, 1988). Thus, these types of violations, by heightening awareness, raise the stakes for the outcome of the interaction. If rapport and a collaborative context have been achieved, this can result in a greatly enhanced therapeutic expectation. Outside of that context, however, the results may be disastrous.

The combination of naturalistic inductions and elaborate storytelling results in communication with a high degree of ambiguity. Erickson used more verbally elaborate and complex *confusion techniques* to establish rapport with patients who could not easily accept the therapeutic situation. Rather than negating such behavior as "resistance," he regarded it as verbal ambiguity that could lead to a state of increased hypnotic sensitivity. For example, he might begin a session with the casual statement, "Please do not go into a trance until you have seated yourself comfortably in the chair" (Erickson, 1983, p. 185).

A number of forms of communication can be used to encourage people to make their own meanings. Erickson used the technique of describing a friend or previous patient who had a similar problem (the "my friend John" technique; see Erickson, 1980a, 1:340). In this way issues could be opened up that were too sensitive to deal with directly. O'Hanlon (1987) cites the ways in which Erickson would use jokes, riddles, puns, stories, and other forms of indirect communication to elicit these sorts of creative responses. He used these techniques to suggest new possibilities, to evoke latent abilities, and, through interspersal, to sow suggestions in a way that would not elicit conscious resistance.

The ambiguity of indirect suggestion appears to function at two levels, both absorbing conscious attention and facilitating unconscious responses (Erickson, 1976b). Ambiguity is the vehicle for expressing conflicting feelings simultaneously (Barton, 1984). Response to indirect approaches and confusion techniques are also strongly influenced by the level of rapport. Both verbal and nonverbal ambiguity produce confusion in states of poor rapport, but the same strategies increase comprehension in situations in which there are high degrees of rapport (Burgoon, 1988). The permissive suggestion thus allows for both greater individual response and greater cooperative participation. Tied to the immediate context, indirect suggestion creates a more pervasive response than direct suggestion, while the subjective experience serves to underline the "naturalness" of the response. This may serve to encourage some individuals to develop alternate cognitive strategies to bypass conscious limitations. Clinical studies of Ericksonian approaches, however, have only partially supported the use of indirect and facilitating language for some patients who are unable to utilize direct suggestion.

Indirect suggestion appears to play a greater role in altering the subjective, experiential component of hypnosis, and it may have less of an effect on the behavioral components (Lynn, 1987a). Some studies have found that indirect wording enhances response to suggestion (Alman, 1980; Stone, 1985; Spinhoven, 1988); others have found that direct and indirect suggestion produce equivalent responses (Lynn,

1987a; Matthews, 1985). Indirect suggestion may more dramatically alter the personal experiential components of hypnotic response (Matthews, 1985; Lynn, 1987a). Woolson (1986) also suggests that this relationship occurs despite the fact that exposure to indirect induction produces less of a subjective difference between the hypnotic and normal waking state. Stone and Lundy (1985) found that indirect suggestions that were combined with "neutral" and "irrelevant" comments on the immediate experience of the individual were more effective. Permissive techniques have been reported to be more effective in inducing hypnotic analgesia (Barber, 1977; Crowley, 1980; Gillett, 1984; Frichton, 1985), although a recent well-designed study found no difference between direct and indirect hypnotic suggestions for pain control (Van Gorp, 1985). Indirect suggestion may result in greater compliance in the hypnotic condition and may enhance response to posthypnotic suggestion (Alman, 1980); direct suggestion, on the other hand, results in greater compliance in the nonhypnotic condition (Alman, 1980; Stone, 1985; Woolson, 1986).

In summary, it appears that no particular technique is in itself more potent than any other. Direct and indirect suggestions and confusion techniques can all be effective inasmuch as they enhance the hypnotic ability of an individual within a particular context. Erickson used whatever approach the situation required (Hammond, 1988). Confusion techniques may be more relevant in the clinical situation when there is a conflict surrounding the goal of the hypnotherapy than during an experimental paradigm in which the goal has been set by the research design. Motivation, rapport, and degree of involvement are enhanced not by a specific technique but by flexibility on the part of the hypnotherapist. As Erickson's long-standing collaborator Ernest Rossi has observed:

While it was true that Erickson's early research papers were replete with ingenious ways of manipulating people, I never saw him do anything particularly outrageous. Quite the contrary, in the last decade of his life when I studied with him, he would usually facilitate therapeutic trance only after he had observed that the patient's physical and mental processes had "quieted down." (1990, p. 11)

A simple view of indirect suggestion seems to suggest two important factors. First, subjects are sensitive not only to suggestions but to the way in which they are delivered and the context in which they appear. Even slight manipulations of voice tone have a significant effect on the response to suggestions (Gehm, 1989). The degree of rapport as measured by the synchrony of the nonverbal cues and the degree of psycho-physiologic patterning constitutes an important reinforcement for the context of the hypnotic message (Bányai, 1985). Second, the context in which hypnosis is presented provides a frame around which hypnotic experiences are interpreted. In his use of indirect suggestion, Erickson emphasized the value of multiple repetitions, approaches from differ-ent directions, and, above all, a context of positive expectation as the keys to effective communication (Erickson and Rossi, 1976). In this sense, indirect approaches clearly constitute a potent enhancement of direct suggestion (Lachnit, 1989; Gudjonsson, 1989; Stewart, 1990). The question is not whether indirect suggestion is superior to direct approaches but, rather, emphasizes that nonverbal and contextual cues have a potent influence on the way even simple communications are interpreted.

THERAPEUTIC SUGGESTION

As hypnotic behavior arises from everyday behavior, Erickson believed that the therapeutic aspects of the interaction arise from enhancing the particular skills and orientation of the individual. Because trance is a natural skill or ability, psychological growth is an inherent capacity of each human being. The challenge to the therapist, then, becomes the need to establish a context in which change can be supported and encouraged. For all his creativity and linguistic skill, Erickson believed that the truly original work is done by the patient (1979).

Just as each patient is unique, so will each individual's approach to trance be unique. Hypnosis is not a unitary state, nor is there a single conceptual model that accounts for the variety of responses subjects will demonstrate (Balthazard, 1985). Cognitive, perceptual, emotional, and attentional processes can all be altered to a lesser or greater extent. The changes in each of these areas can operate along a continuum from negligible to extreme. For example, visual hallucinations occur in a proportion of subjects, being more common in those who are highly susceptible (Hilgard, 1976). But even when the hallucinations are ex-tremely vivid, the individual will still behave both as if the hallucination were there and as if it were not. For example, hypnotized subjects will not try to sit on a hallucinated chair, whereas subjects who are simulat-ing hypnosis will (Spanos, 1986a). The subject is able to maintain a formation of a hallucinatory experience as highly individualized

(Sheehan, 1982), perceiving that the experience is both genuine and not genuine at the same time.

The suggestions received influence the subjective experience, with a directive, compulsory style of suggestion leading to more involuntary responses, and permissive, indirect approaches tending to emphasize the naturalness of the experience. Each subject uses his own expectations in combination with the type of suggestions to develop a particular strategy (Sheehan, 1982).

Thus, there is a wide degree of individual variation in hypnotic response; it is an active interpretive process reflecting the way in which the individual understands the context (Sheehan, 1982). Hypnotic subjects show greater responsiveness to persuasive communication than do subjects with less ability in either the trance state or out of it (Malott, 1989), though that responsiveness is increased significantly in the hypnotic state. At any one time, hypnotic ability to respond to suggestion appears to be a combination of individual attributes and contextual cues (Malott, 1989). Subjects' attributions of their hypnotic responsiveness are closely tied to their reported rapport with the experimenter (Lynn, 1987b). Moreover, subjects who are rated as being highly susceptible report significantly greater positive rapport than do subjects with low susceptibility (Lynn, 1987b). Context and personality also interact. Extroverted subjects are more hypnotizable in a group situation and, conversely, introverted subjects are more hypnotizable in a one-to-one situation (Preston, 1982). Hypnotic response always appears to be an interaction between an individual aptitude and the way in which circumstances either enhance or detract from that ability.

Sheehan has thoughtfully criticized the way that standardized behavioral scales can limit our understanding of factors such as individual cognitive style, rapport, and degree of absorption with a particular task (1982). The most detailed psychometric analyses of the data from experimental hypnotic studies clearly suggest that there is no single underlying hypnotic dimension and that any hypnotic response is a complex interplay of several factors for each individual (Balthazard, 1985).

Particular situational variables (e.g., the nature of the hypnotic test task) may determine the actual behavior that emanates from a subject's use of a specific cognitive style, and mobility in their use emphasizes an important source of diversity. The data tell us that individuals who use a style as it suits the hypnotic situation at hand may well show considerable variation in their response. . . . The problem-solving nature of the hypnotic experience is indexed in part by the extent to which input from suggestions appears to be processed by the subject together with cognitions about reality features of his or her environment.

. . . It appears that susceptible subjects can skillfully extract meaning from what the hypnotist is suggesting and from features of their environment such as their personal identity, past history, and other events occurring outside the framework of suggestion established by the hypnotist. . . . The fact that attention seems more directed than we have acknowledged in the past does not at all suggest that viewpoints focusing on the automaticity of response or occurrence of dissociation are untenable. But the data do imply that such theories have underestimated the fluidity of barriers that exist between the different streams of awareness and the higher order nature of cognizing that occurs when input from unattended consciousness breaks into conscious awareness. (Sheehan, 1982, pp. 265–266)

Although subjects who have a positive attitude about hypnosis can score in the low, medium, or high range of hypnotic susceptibility, negative attitudes about hypnosis are strongly associated with low scores (Spanos, 1987a). Individuals who have negative beliefs about hypnosis or who fear what may happen to them during a trance state invariably have low scores of hypnotic susceptibility. In keeping with Gruzelier's (1985) electrophysiologic work, this suggests that negative emotional responses to the context of trance are associated with active neurophysiologic inhibition of hypnotic ability. Similarly, more subjects are likely to refuse the same intervention when it is labeled as "hypnosis" than when it is labeled as "relaxation" (Hendler, 1986).

Such observations have supported the clinical notion that, despite earlier reports of the relative stability of hypnotic susceptibility, hypnotic abilities can be modified by appropriate training (Diamond, 1982, 1987) via behavioral techniques, explanation, and practice, and by an enhanced rapport between patient and therapist (Kinney, 1974; Spanos, 1986a, 1986b; Gfeller, 1987). Training procedures can substantially increase hypnotic susceptibility scores for subjects in both medium and low susceptibility groups. This improvement in scores is particularly enhanced in the low susceptibility group if they are exposed to a high degree of involvement with the experimenter and are able to establish a strong degree of rapport (Gfeller, 1987). Hypnotic skill training can involve encouraging positive attitudes about hypnosis, practicing the use of imagery, and coming to see hypnotic behavior as an active response on the part of the individual (Spanos, 1986a). Each component appears to play a part; the combination of all three is significantly more effective in improving hypnotic ability scores than the use of only one.

Subjects who score poorly on tests of hypnotic susceptibility can, in fact, be taught similar cognitive strategies that will increase the amount of experience of amnesia, whereas subjects who initially experience significant amnesia can, in fact, be taught to retrieve pertinent information (Spanos, 1986b). Similarly, although hypnotic ability is related to the degree of hypnotic analgesia, subjects who score poorly on hypnotic susceptibility can be taught substantial pain control through the use of other cognitive techniques such as distraction. Spanos concludes that these studies "emphasize the active, goal-directed nature of subjects' responding, the importance of their motivations to adopt and maintain the 'good subject' role as this is defined to them, and the crucial influence of contextual cues in shaping the interpretations and self-presentations that constitute 'appropriate' responding" (Spanos, 1986b, p. 466).

The evidence suggests that measures of hypnotic susceptibility are important clinical and research tools but that what they measure is, as with other psychological variables, a matter that requires careful interpretation. Ernest Hilgard, one of the individuals primarily responsible for the development of useful standardized measures of hypnotic ability, has emphasized that care must be taken, particularly in the clinical setting, to choose the appropriate instrument (1982). Further identification of hypnotic phenomena will require convergent enquiry combining subjective responses, behavioral measures, and psychophysiologic validation (Orne, 1981).

It is easy to speak of "an altered state of consciousness" or of "dissociation" as if we know precisely what these terms mean. The evidence suggests that the trance state involves substantial changes in cognition, emotion, perception, and physiologic regulation. But these changes do not exist in a vacuum. Intermingled with them will be the surrounding context for the individual: their previous history, current concerns, and the quality of the interaction and degree of rapport they experience with the hypnotherapist. Hypnotic states can be reliably identified as producing both qualitative and quantitative changes over time, but there are substantial differences in the ways that different individuals respond (Sheehan, 1982).

Rossi suggests that we use the term *sensitivity*, not *suggestibility*, to describe a patient's responses in hypnotherapy (1988). In this view, suggestion is a two-way process, part of an interpersonal field. Both patient and therapist are actively, not passively, involved, and creation occurs on both sides. Rossi suggests that the therapist, in effect, completes a biofeedback loop for the patient, acting as a transducer for the patient's communication and returning it as a new source of input for the recursive process. In this view, trance is a repetitive iterative process that is fundamental to neurologic organization and to cognition (Hofstadter, 1979).

Recursive functions are built into our nervous system; it is found, for example, that the output of a nerve cell often feeds back to the same cell to modulate its further activity. This recursive function is found to be a fundamental feature of virtually all of our sensory and motor processes at the cellular and molecular levels. . . . the essential operation that allows for the generation of ever new forms of complexity. . . . [It is] the essence of all processes of self-reflexivity, self-awareness, and self-reflection. Ultimately, the recursive function leads to the creation of meaning and identity for society as a whole, as well as for individuals. (Rossi, 1988, pp. 33–34)

ORAL POETRY

Hilgard (1984) notes that whereas traditional psychodynamic theories emphasize communication with the conscious mind, Erickson presupposed an ability to talk directly to unconscious processes. In this way, interspersal and confusion techniques could be effective in eliciting unconscious cooperation and promoting experiential learning even in the face of conscious skepticism or resistance. Hilgard also notes Erickson's technique whereby he would offer an opportunity for experiential learning that was ostensibly different but in fact structurally related to the presenting clinical problem. This learning would occur either within the relationship in therapy with Erickson or as a homework assignment. Similarly, stories and metaphors could be used to induce hypnotherapeutic trance or to provide a metaphorical structure that paralleled the patient's current difficulties. The trance induction itself could serve as a metaphor for therapy. For example, he used the technique of teaching arm levitation in hypnotic trance as a metaphor for a patient who was suffering from sexual impotence (O'Hanlon, 1987).

As Hilgard (1984, 1988) points out, anyone looking through Erickson's voluminous writings for an explicit statement of his theoretical underpinnings will be disappointed. Instead, one will find a wealth of highly individual, creative clinical techniques, case examples, and varied approaches. Above all, one will perceive a sensitive, imaginative mind constantly trying to produce a greater flexibility and variety, suiting the words and actions of the therapy situation to the individual needs and requirements of each patient.

Richard Van Dyck has suggested that though Erickson did not explicitly contribute to the theory of psychotherapy, his work may be considered an endowment for a "treasure of examples on how to adapt unique circumstances and effect a change" (in Zeig, 1980, p. xiii). These examples are similar only in the sense that Sherlock Holmes's cases are similar: a problem is laid out and then resolved in what initially appears to be a flash of intuition or magic. But Erickson's description reveals his systematic use of painstaking observation and attention to the factors that make each therapeutic intervention and each patient unique.

Erickson's originality was reflected in his use of language. O'Hanlon (1987) quotes Zeig's observation that Erickson frequently used antithetical concepts and verbal structures to provide a forward rhythm to the hypnotic induction. The prosodic rhythm gives forward drive to the narrative; it brings people along through its abilities to pattern and synchronize. The most moving poetry can involve highly intricate patterns of words or a simple line of monosyllables ("To be or not to be"). Which will work best depends simply on the dramatic needs and context. There is no magical incantation. The magic resides in the brain's hypnotic ability to respond to an appropriate suggestion at the proper time. In this sense, Ezra Pound was quite correct: the meaning *is* in the rhythm.

Erickson exhibited a further hallmark of the oral poet in that no two versions of the same story were ever identical. Erickson used contextual cues and ongoing feedback from his listener to improvise and develop his stories in a way that seemed most meaningful in the current context. Again, as with the oral poet, the distinction between performer and audience blurs. Erickson viewed trance as a period of creative reorganization (Rossi, 1987). In a very real way, the patient actively guided Erickson's therapeutic approaches.

The nature of hypnotherapy involves the linking of hypnotic phenomena with therapeutic goals. It is the therapeutic context that makes the connection compelling ("When your eyes close you will go deeply into a trance"; "When you awaken tomorrow morning you will have a new understanding about this problem"). Hypnotherapy, like all forms of psychotherapy, involves the extension of existing clusters of metaphor, the creation of new meaning. This aspect is often termed "reframing": the alteration not of memory or experience but of the evaluation we make of it.

Reframing is the creation of new meaning. To reframe "means to change the conceptual and/or emotional setting or viewpoint in relation to which a situation is experienced and to place it in another frame which fits the 'facts' of the same concrete situation equally well or even better, and thereby changes its entire meaning" (Watzlawick, 1974, p. 95). Reframing is a means for altering the frame of reference into which a particular event has been categorized. As we have seen, metaphor is an ongoing mechanism for doing this. Erickson's particular contribution to this approach was to unite the proposed change with existing motivations, needs, and abilities of the individual. By doing so, he encouraged change in a direction that emphasized the individuals' or couples' strengths rather than their psychological weaknesses.

The induction and maintenance of a trance serve to provide a special psychological state in which patients can reassociate and reorganize their inner psychological complexities and utilize their own capacities in a manner in accord with their own experiential life. . . .

Therapy results from an inner resynthesis of the patient's behavior achieved by the patient himself. It is true that direct suggestion can effect an alteration in the patient's behavior and result in a symptomatic cure, at least temporarily. However, such a "cure" is simply a response to the suggestion and does not entail that reassociation and reorganization of ideas, understandings, and memories so essential for actual cure. It is this experience of reassociating and reorganizing his own experiential life that eventuates in a cure, not the manifestation of responsive behavior which can, at best, satisfy only the observer. (Erickson, 1980c, 4:38)

Erickson's assumption was that individuals have abilities in other areas that they are not using in the problem situation. Hence, metaphor, with its ability to extend knowledge, was an ideal vehicle for this sort of transfer (Haskell, 1987). Erickson used stories and situations that paralleled the nature of the problem confronting the patient. Although occasionally the isomorphism was related to a story, it could also be related to a particular task assignment or style of interaction or hypnotic phenomenon. The use of hypnosis or the intervention or the homework prescription could all be metaphorical in their structure.

Stories can be used to achieve rapport, give advice, increase self-awareness, stimulate motivation, reframe or redefine a problem, or, via the interspersal technique, serve as an induction to traditional hypnosis. Stories, which are particularly effective in bypassing habitual conscious mental sets, make the information presented more memorable by virtue both of the associated imagery and the narrative sequence. Above all, the metaphorical approach encourages the patient's own individual responses and creativity rather than prescribing some externally imposed solution (Zeig, 1980). Metaphor is, in effect, a transduction process (information changes level in both directions) between our perceptual experience and our cognitive and emotional evaluation of that experience.

Erickson's use of stories in combination to achieve a cumulative effect was similar in approach to the work of the playwright or film director who builds toward an effect by a combination of scenes. Erickson's work was a therapeutic version of Sergei Eisenstein's theory of montage, in which the juxtaposition of two images can result in the creation of a third association that results from the gestalt properties of the whole. The human response is naturally to try to make a connection between the various elements. That connection builds inevitably from the connections already made.

To excerpt a single story from Erickson's work is rather like presenting a single scene from Shakespeare. One gets an idea of the way in which language is used and perhaps the flavor of the approach, but it cannot do justice to the way in which the whole structure works upon the participants. In Erickson's work, one story flowed seemingly naturally from another, so that a series of gradually elaborating themes and motifs formed an overall coherent structure. Each element of his work built upon the previous elements, with prosody, language, and storytelling working upon one another (see Zeig, 1980).

Erickson's stories were constructed so that they fit within the patient's frame of reference. In this way, they constituted what Rossi has referred to as a "growing edge" for the personality (1988). Beginning with a base in the person's current understanding, they showed a natural way of extending beyond those limitations. This process extended beyond solving the immediate problem and included formulating a new attitude toward problem solving in general. Thus, it became a springboard for a new form of change, a generative change that saw development and transformation as an inevitable extension of everyday human abilities.

Now there is another case: In October, 1956, I was invited to address a national meeting of psychiatrists on the subject of hypnosis at Boston State Hospital in Boston.

Dr. L. Alex was on the staff and he was the chairman of the program committee. When I arrived, he asked me if I would not only lecture on hypnosis, but would I demonstrate.

I asked him whom I should use for a subject and he said, "Members of the audience." I said, "That won't be entirely satisfactory." He said, "Well, why don't you walk around the wards and find a subject that you think would be satisfactory."

I went around the wards until I saw a couple of nurses talking. I watched one of the couple and noted all of her behavior. After they finished talking, I went to the one nurse, introduced myself, and told her I was lecturing before the meeting on hypnosis and would she be willing to be my hypnotic subject. She said she didn't know anything about hypnosis, had never read about it, had never seen it. I told her that was fine, it would make her an even better subject. She said, "If you think I could do it, I will be very happy to do it." I thanked her and said, "That's an agreed upon promise." She said, "Certainly."

Then I went and told Dr. Alex about the nurse named Betty who was going to be my subject. And he reacted very violently. He said, "You can't use that nurse. She has been in psychoanalytic therapy for two years. She is a compensated depression." ("Compensated depression" means a patient who is very seriously depressed, but who has resolved to continue. No matter how bad they feel, how unhappy they feel, they are going to do their work.)

Dr. Alex added, "And she is suicidal. She has already given away her personal jewelry. She is an orphan. She has no siblings, and her friends are the other nurses at the hospital. She has given away her personal property, and a lot of her clothes. She has already sent in her letter of resignation." (I don't remember the date of her resignation. I think it was October 20th and this was October 6th.) "After she resigns on the 20th, she is going to commit suicide. You can't use her."

The analyst, Dr. Alex, all the staff and the nurses pleaded with me not to use Betty. I said, "Unfortunately, I accepted Betty's promise, giving her mine in return. Now if I go back on my promise and don't use her, being depressed, she may consider that the final rejection and commit suicide this evening and not wait until the 20th." I held my ground and they yielded.

I told Betty where to sit in the audience in the auditorium. I gave my lecture. I called on various members of the audience to demonstrate a little something about hypnosis here and there—various phenomena. And then I said, "Betty, please stand up. Now walk slowly up to the stage. Continue on directly in front of me. Now don't walk too fast or too slowly but go a little bit deeper into a trance with each step you take."

When Betty finally arrived on the stage in front of me, she was already in a very, very deep hypnotic trance. I asked her, "Where are you, Betty?" She said, "Here." I said, "Where is here?" She said, "With you." I said, "Where are we?" She said, "Here." I said, "What's there?" (Erickson points out to an imaginary audience.) She said, "Nothing." I said "What's there?" (Erickson gestures behind him.) She said, "Nothing." In other words, she had a total negative hallucination for all of her surroundings. I was the only visible thing to her. So I demonstrated catalepsy and glove anesthesia. (Erickson pinches his hand.)

Then I said to Betty, "I think it would be nice if we went out to the Boston Arboretum and made a visit there. We can do it very easily." I explained all about time distortion—how you could shorten time or expand time. So, I said, "Time has expanded and each second is a day long."

So, she hallucinated being in the arboretum with me. I pointed out that the annuals were dying now since it was October. The perennials were dying since it was October. I pointed out that the change of colors of the leaves was taking place, since the leaves turn color in October in Massachusetts. I pointed out the shrubs, bushes and the vines of various trees, and pointed out how each bush, each shrub, each tree had a differently shaped leaf. I spoke about the perennials coming back to life next spring. The annuals being planted next spring. I talked about the trees and their blossoms. The kind of fruit on the trees. The kind of seed and how the birds would eat the fruit and distribute the seed which might sprout under favorable conditions and grow to be another tree. I discussed the arboretum thoroughly.

Then I suggested we might like to go to the Boston Zoo. I explained I knew there was a baby kangaroo there and that we could hope it would be out of its mother's pouch so that we could *see* the baby kangaroo. I explained to her that baby kangaroos are called "joeys." They are about an inch long when born. They climb into the mother's pouch and attach themselves to the nipple. Then a physical change occurs in the mouth of the inch-long baby kangaroo and it can't let loose of the nipple again. And so it nurses and nurses and nurses and grows. I think it spends about three months in the mother's pouch before it looks out. We looked at the kangaroos. We saw the baby kangaroo was looking out of the pouch. We looked at the tigers and their cubs, the lions and their cubs, the bears, the monkeys, the wolves, all of the animals.

Then we went to the aviary and looked at all the birds there. I spoke about the migration of birds—how the Arctic tern spends a short summer in the arctic zone and then flies to the southernmost tip of South America—a trip of 10,000 miles. The bird spends the winter, which is summer in South America, and does it by a guidance system no man can understand. The Arctic tern and various birds instinctively knew how to migrate thousands of miles without a compass— a thing men couldn't do.

Then we went back to the State Hospital and I had her see the audience and talk to Dr. Alex. I didn't awaken her. I had her in the trance state. I had her discuss the feeling of heaviness that Christine mentioned and others mentioned feeling. And she answered questions for them. Then I suggested that we really ought to walk down the street to the Boston Beach.

I spoke about the Boston Beach being there long before the Puritans settled Massachusetts. How the Indians had enjoyed it. How the early colonials had enjoyed the beach. How it was a place of pleasure today and had been in the past for countless generations—how it would be a place of pleasure and happiness far into the future.

I had her look at the ocean and see the ocean very quiet, and then there were storm waves on it, then huge storm waves on it, and then I had her watch the ocean quiet down. I had her watch the tide come in and go out. Then I suggested we go back to the Boston State Hospital.

I demonstrated a few more things about hypnosis and then I thanked her very profoundly in the trance for having helped me so much—having taught the audience so much. I awakened her and did my thank you all over again, and sent her back to the ward.

The next day Betty did not show up at the hospital. Her friends were alarmed. They went to her apartment. There was no note, no sign of Betty, no uniform there . . . just ordinary clothes. Finally, the police were called in, and Betty's body could not be found anywhere. She had completely disappeared and Dr. Alex and I were blamed for Betty's suicide.

The next year I lectured in Boston. I still got a lot of blame for Betty's suicide. So did Dr. Alex.

Five years later almost everybody had forgotten about Betty except Dr. Alex and me. Ten years later, never a word about Betty. Sixteen years later in July, 1972, I got a long distance call from Florida. A woman's voice said, "You probably won't remember me, but I am Betty, the nurse you used to demonstrate hypnosis at the Boston State Hospital in 1956. I just happened to think today that you might like to know what happened to me." I said, "I certainly would." (Group laughter.)

She said, "After I left the hospital that night, I went down to the Naval Recruiting Station and I demanded immediate induction into the Nursing Corps of the Navy. I served two enlistments. I was discharged in Florida. I got a job in a hospital. I met a retired Air Force officer and we were married. I now have five children and I'm working in the hospital. And the thought came to me today that you might like to know what happened to me." So I asked if I could tell Dr. Alex. She said, "If you wish. It makes no difference to me." We have carried on an active correspondence ever since.

Now then I went to the arboretum and had her hallucinate the arboretum, what was I talking about? Patterns of life: life today; life in the future; blossoms; fruit; seeds; the different pattern of each leaf for each plant. We went to the zoo and I was again discussing life with her—youthful life, mature life, the wonders of life—migration patterns. And then we went to the seashore where countless generations in the past had found pleasure, where countless generations in the future would find pleasure, and where the current generation was finding pleasure. And the mysteries of the ocean: the migration of whales; sea turtles, like the migration of birds, something that man can't understand, but fascinating.

I named all the things worthwhile living for. And nobody knew I was doing psychotherapy except me. They heard all the things I said, but they just thought I was demonstrating time distortion, hallucinations—visual and auditory. They thought I was demonstrating hypnotic phenomena. They never realized I was intentionally doing psychotherapy. (Zeig, 1980, pp. 148–153)

Part of the allure of hypnosis is that it deals with functions and capacities that appear to be beyond most normal abilities. We have seen, in fact, that most of these extensions derive from the normal abilities and functions of the brain. Even the more "dramatic" aspects of hypnotic suggestion such as analgesia or amnesia have been shown to be highly goal-directed cognitive responses to the social and psychological demands of the test situation (Spanos, 1986a). Hypnosis is thus a tool that is composed of normal human capacities. It is inherently neither good nor bad, and the results depend on the circumstances in which it is used (Gilligan, 1987). There is a correlation between overall hypnotic responsiveness and relative mental health, on one hand (Zlotogorski, 1987), and the ability to utilize hypnotic suggestions for the development of a positive self-concept, on the other (Koe, 1987).

The concepts of hypnotizability and dissociation, once considered to be interchangeable, are both undergoing redefinition (Laurence, 1986a; Frankel, 1990). There does seem to be a discontinuity between the more universal hypnotic phenomena that are related to the common everyday trance and the profound dissociative states that occur in response to overwhelming trauma (Weitzenhoffer, 1989). Whether referring to such extreme symptoms (Spanos, 1986d) or with more "normal" hypnotic responses (Council, 1986), contextual cues, in particular those provided by the therapeutic relationship, will have a critical effect on their expression.

Cognition, affect, and behavior in hypnosis are more sensitive to contextual cues and the processes of social psychology than was first recognized. Brain function in hypnosis appears more and more not as a special state but as an ongoing process that, according to how the situation is defined, focuses existing resources in order to deal with pertinent tasks. Again, hypnosis in this context appears magical not because of any inherent "special" state but because of our rather narrow definition of what we are capable of. If the contextual cues permit, then hypnotic subjects can simply bypass typical conscious limitations. For example, contextual cues appear to play an important role in success in pain reduction. In a quantitative EEG study of brain function during hypnosis or acupuncture used to relieve experimental pain, Saletu (1987) has demonstrated that the EEG changes during hypnosis were highly dependent on the wording of the hypnotic suggestions. Direct verbal suggestion and encouragement prior to hypnosis significantly increase reported hypnotic analgesia (Stewart, 1990). Ultimately, the importance of hypnosis is greatest as a demonstration not of some sort of supernatural powers but of an expansion of our understanding of what normal human consciousness involves and how it is influenced by communication.

Hypnosis encourages us to look at all human communication in two specific ways—first, to pay close attention to the actual structure and rhythm of the interaction as it develops over time. We are often biased toward the content or meaning of an interaction (as it is interpreted in the light of our theoretic preconceptions), and hypnosis reminds us that these interpretations must constantly be informed by the ongoing flow of words, tone, gesture, and facial expression. Second, hypnosis helps us recognize the importance of experiential factors in human learning. The more involving and absorbing a procedure is, the greater the resulting impact is on the individual (Acosta, 1990). Profound changes in attentional processes, cognitive strategies, and emotional responses all occur most readily when an individual is absorbed in a process that appears to be personally meaningful. Although most schools of therapy would agree with this, greater attention must be paid to the ways in which it can be actually achieved.

This view of hypnosis also emphasizes the constructive nature of perceptual and cognitive processes (Minsky, 1986). This constructive process is related to the way in which attention is focused. There is a relationship between hypnotic ability and other measures of absorption (Tellegen, 1974; Rhue, 1989). In this sense, amnesia is not the result of a "barrier" but rather the result of material not reaching the second stage of the attention process (Kissin, 1986). Similarly, the "hidden observer," the dissociative "barrier," or the "alternate" personality of a patient with MPD may be somewhat misleading ways of describing the functions of a single, integrated, individual brain.

Those functions combine fluidly as the result of the integration of external contextual demands and the inherent rhythm of the brain. The ultradian rhythm, as well as being a gate to sleep, serves as a gate (or time of relative ease of access) to a state in which the individual is more receptive to new learning if it is imagery-based, compelling in its personal meaning to produce arousal for state-dependent learning, and rhythmic to permit synchronization. This repatterning of necessity involves both dissociation (of previous experience and related emotional states) and association (or a resynthesis that involves the linking of problem areas with the individual's own creative resources).

Overall, the evidence suggests a subtle but powerful bonding of bodily rhythms through sound and movement, which parallels the degree of rapport and immediacy experienced in the interaction. Although these rhythms are universally present, they vary considerably with the nature of the participants and the setting. The changes that occur in interactional rhythm are far more dramatic when there is a high degree of interpersonal involvement between the participants (Coker, 1987). Erickson's emphasis on utilization of communication at the unconscious level provides a therapeutic link between interpersonal connection and intrapersonal meaning.

The tight functional and neuroanatomic relationship among gesture, facial expression, and prosody (McNeill, 1985) is necessary both for the coordination of interactions and for the elaboration of internal experience. Nonverbal communication establishes a frame of reference in the relationship while simultaneously activating a particular cognitive schema composed of relevant memories, emotional evaluations, and behavioral programs. Interpersonal frames and mental schemata interact in a dynamic way (Tannen, 1987). Shared frames produce the rapport that makes change possible by providing an opportunity for schemata to be altered (Horowitz, 1987). The ability to alter schemata depends on the effective use of metaphor (Haskell, 1987).

Tannen and Wallat (1987) have suggested that there are two distinct types of structures of expectation that we use to interpret communication. They define *frames* as a combination of the verbal and nonverbal cues of the immediate context and *schema* as the preexisting cognitive structure the individual makes use of. The two structures are in constant interaction. The schema helps define the context in which the frame is interpreted. At the same time, alterations in the frame may result in alterations of a particular schema or access of other related or competing schemata (Tannen, 1987). This model provides a useful way of analyzing how patterns of knowledge and expectations, on the one hand, and the shifting way in which context may be defined, on the other, constantly influence each other. Our knowledge is based primarily on social interaction, and in turn our interactions are constantly being influenced by our expectations and previous experience. Erickson achieved rapport both at the level of the frame with his naturalistic language and at the level of the schema with his therapeutic stories. This approach encouraged full involvement in the hypnotic interaction.

Imagery and metaphor are not peripheral but central to normal cognitive processes. Similarly, our unconscious processes reveal themselves (if only gradually) as a rich and highly structured system involving cognitive, perceptual, and motor skills with a structure at least as elaborate and varied as we find in our conscious brain (Kihlstrom,

1987). Similarly, the structure of emotional experience, both conscious and unconscious, appears to involve a multilevel structural transformation of sensation that parallels the structure of other cognitive processes (Lane, 1987).

We have seen that there are rhythms in the autonomic and sensory motor frame activities that are associated with the ultradian changes in the level and nature of potential processes in the brain. Communication rhythms would be pointless if they did not enhance the brain's capacity to interpret and express communication. As is the case with interactions, a flexible rhythm is needed to provide organization through time to a variety of brain functions so that they can synchronize effectively. In order for communication to succeed, synchrony at a number of levels is required to link the individual members physiologically, psychologically, and socially.

There is also a relationship between the nonverbal frame and the schemata of personal experience that each individual uses to interpret events. Grounded in sensory awareness, metaphor is a method for expressing and transforming personal understanding. The construction of metaphor is simultaneously a conscious and unconscious process. The nonverbal frame of the interaction provides the basis for unconscious learning, which is critical in the formation of personal meaning and social expectation. Thus, in a very real sense, it is precisely the same mechanisms that make each of us uniquely individual that provide a means for intense mutual understanding.

It is highly appropriate that this model of hypnotherapy emphasizes the complex but essentially unified nature of brain processes. The most significant advances in clinical hypnosis in the past quarter century have involved a progressive integration with other forms of treatment (Fromm, 1987). At this point in the history of our cumulative clinical knowledge, only an integrated approach offers an opportunity for further advances. Fromm warns, wisely, that the sensational or magical view of hypnosis as a quick panacea will only delay the acceptance of hypnotherapy as a useful tool for treating psychological and physiologic dysfunctions.

There is a continued need to demystify hypnosis and free it from the unreasonable expectations and atavistic fears that have long limited its acceptance (Bowers, 1976). Hypnotic behaviors are clearly phenomena that are similar to other forms of interpersonal behavior that depend on how subjects interpret their situation (Spanos, 1986a). The future of hypnosis depends upon the twin streams of clinical work and laboratory experiment, its advance upon the balance between clinical creativity and careful experimentation (Fromm, 1979; Frankel, 1982). As Frankel has suggested, "the poetry and the science are both essential for survival" (1982).

Erickson's work has had a pervasive influence in many areas of psychotherapy; it represents not a radical departure but a distillation of the essence of effective therapeutic work (Fromm, 1987). There is no more magic in an Ericksonian approach than in any other clinical method. The "magic" lies in the creativity of patient and therapist working in cooperation. That creativity is best served by being balanced with scientific rigor and plain hard work. Erickson spent decades developing his skills, and his trust of his unconscious processes was firmly based.

The work of Milton Erickson has achieved considerable public attention, but it is also important to recognize the many others who have contributed to the development of clinical hypnosis and hypnotherapy. The field is expanding on a far more solid scientific and clinical basis than ever before (Fromm, 1987). Hypnotherapeutic techniques are being integrated clinically with other treatment approaches and are benefiting from a more rigorous scientific methodology that allows us to evaluate claims of efficacy. Similarly, the vigorous debate between the nonstate and state theorists in the experimental literature is stimulating an ongoing development of the underlying concepts and forcing a greater recognition of the connection between hypnotic events and basic cognitive and neurophysiologic processes.

All these processes are linked inextricably in clinical practice. Similarly, an account of brain function requires all three elements: fluid methods of communication based on shared behavioral rhythms of speech, gesture, and facial expression; a compelling but flexible structure of language that has evolved along with the brain in order to be maximally "user-friendly"; and a cognitive structure that blends perceptual experience with imaginative involvement. More simply put, there are elements of music, poetry, and storytelling in Erickson's approach that can enhance learning in the therapeutic encounter.

Perhaps the most significant of Erickson's contributions to new directions in therapy is a reemphasis on careful observation of what actually takes place, of the structure of the interaction, of the words used and how they are perceived. These points may seem obvious, but their importance is virtually impossible to exaggerate. We have a new image of the brain as an organ that has evolved for communication in a highly personal face-to-face context (arising from the rhythms of interaction and relying on subjective experience and metaphor for the creation of meaning). It is fitting that the heart of the Ericksonian contribution turns out to be an indirect suggestion of these possibilities phrased in the terms of a new metaphor.

The evidence suggests that the hypnotic experience is a complex cognitive task involving the interplay of personal, social, and contextual factors (Laurence, 1986b). Perhaps the most therapeutic suggestion of all is that the locus of healing is within the patient-therapist interaction. It is on this that we must focus to continue to expand our knowledge.

REFERENCES

Achmon, J., Granek, M., Golomb, M., & Hart, J. (1989). Behavioral treatment of essential hypertension: A comparison between cognitive therapy and biofeedback of heart rate. *Psychosomatic Medicine, 51,* 152–164.

Acosta, A., & Vila, J. (1990). Emotional imagery: Effect of autonomic response information on physiological arousal. *Cognition and Emotion, 4*(2), 145–160.

Adams, H. E., Feuerstein, M., & Fowler, J. L. (1980). Migraine headache: Review of parameters, etiology, and intervention. *Psychological Bulletin, 87,* 217–237.

Adelmann, P. K., & Zajonc, R. B. (1989). Facial efference and the experience of emotion. *Annual Review of Psychology, 40,* 249–280.

Adey, W. R., Kado, R. T., & Walter, D. O. (1967). Computer analysis of EEG data from Gemini Flight GT-7. *Aerospace Medicine, 38,* 345–359.

Adler, C. S., & Adler, S. M. (1976). Biofeedback-psychotherapy for the treatment of headaches: A five year follow-up. *Headache, 16,* 189–191.

Aldrich, K. J., & Bernstein, D. A. (1987). The effect of time of day on hypnotizability. *International Journal of Clinical and Experimental Hypnosis, 35,* 141–145.

Alladin, A. (1988). Hypnosis in the treatment of severe chronic migraine. In M. Heap (Ed.), *Hypnosis: Current clinical, experimental and forensic practices* (pp. 159–166). London: Croom Helm.

Allen, S. A. (1985). *Hypnotic responsiveness in children: Imaginative and creative correlates.* Unpublished doctoral dissertation, University of Wyoming.

Alman, B. M., & Carney, R. E. (1980). Consequences of direct and indirect suggestions on success of posthypnosis behavior. *American Journal of Clinical Hypnosis, 23,* 112–118.

American Psychiatric Association. (1987). *Diagnostic and statistical manual of mental disorders* (3rd ed., rev.). Washington, DC: Author.

Ancoli, S., Kamiya, J., & Ekman, P. (1980). Psychophysiological differentiation of positive and negative affects. *Biofeedback and Self-regulation, 5,* 356–357.

Anderson, J. A. D., Basker, M. A., & Dalton, R. (1975). Migraine and hypnotherapy. *International Journal of Clinical and Experimental Hypnosis, 23,* 48–58.

Andrade, C., & Srinath, S. (1986). True auditory hallucinations as a conversion symptom. *British Journal of Psychiatry, 148,* 100–102.

Andreasen, N. C. (1985). Posttraumatic stress disorder. In H. I. Kaplan & B. J. Sadock (Eds.), *Comprehensive textbook of psychiatry/IV* (pp. 918–924). 4th ed. Baltimore: Williams & Wilkins.

Andreychuk, T., & Skriver, C. (1975). Hypnosis and biofeedback in the treatment of migraine headache. *International Journal of Clinical and Experimental Hypnosis, 23,* 172–183.

Angus, L. E., & Rennie, D. L. (1988). Therapist participation in metaphor generation: Collaborative and noncollaborative styles. *Psychotherapy, 25,* 552–560.

Antrobus, J. S. (1986). Dreaming: Cortical activation and perceptual thresholds. *Journal of Mind and Behavior, 7,* 193–210.

Antrobus, J. (1987). Cortical hemisphere asymmetry and sleep mentation. *Psychological Review, 94,* 359–368.

Arabian, M. M., & Furedy, J. J. (1983). Individual differences in imagery ability and Pavlovian heart rate decelerative conditioning. *Psychophysiology, 20,* 325–331.

Aravindakshan, K. K., Jenner, F. A., & Souster, L. P. (1988). A study of the effects of hypnotic regression on the auditory evoked response. *International Journal of Clinical and Experimental Hypnosis, 36,* 89–95.

Asaad, G., & Shapiro, B. (1986). Hallucinations: Theoretical and clinical overview. *American Journal of Psychiatry, 143,* 1088–1097.

Askenasy, J. J. M. (1989). Is yawning an arousal defense reflex? *Journal of Psychology, 123*(6), 609–621.

Assal, G., Favre, C., & Anderes, J. P. (1984). Non-reconnaissance d'animaux familiers chez un paysan: Zooagnosie ou prosopagnosie pour les animaux. *Revue Neurologique, 140,* 580–584.

Auerhahn, N. C., & Laub, D. (1984). Annihilation and restoration: Posttraumatic memory as pathway and obstacle to recovery. *International Review of Psychoanalysis, 11,* 327–344.

Baars, B. J. (1988). *A cognitive theory of consciousness.* Cambridge: Cambridge University Press.

Bachelard, G. (1971). *The Poetics of Reverie.* Boston, MA: Beacon Press.

Bakal, D. A. (1982). *The psychobiology of chronic headache.* New York: Springer-Verlag.

Bakan, P. (1969). Hypnotizability, laterality of eye movement and functional brain asymmetry. *Perceptual and Motor Skills, 28,* 927–932.

Bakan, P. (1978). Two streams of consciousness: A typological approach. In K. S. Pope & J. L. Singer (Eds.), *The stream of consciousness: Scientific investigations into the flow of human experience* (pp. 159–184). New York: Plenum Press.

Baker, E. L. (1988). The contributions of Milton Erickson: Reflections on the forest and the trees. *International Journal of Clinical and Experimental Hypnosis, 36,* 125–127.

Baker, R. A., & Patrick, B. S. (1987). Hypnosis and memory: The effects of emotional arousal. *American Journal of Clinical Hypnosis, 29,* 177–184.

Balthazard, C. G., & Woody, E. Z. (1985). The "stuff" of hypnotic performance: A review of psychometric approaches. *Psychological Bulletin, 98,* 283–296.

Bander, R., & Grinder, J. (Eds.). (1975). *Patterns of the hypnotic techniques of Milton H. Erickson, M.D.* (Vol. 1). Cupertino, CA: Meta Publications.

Bandura, A., Cioffi, D., Taylor, C. B., & Brouillard, M. E. (1988). Perceived self-efficacy in coping with cognitive stressors and opioid activation. *Journal of Personality and Social Psychology, 55,* 479–488.

Banks, A. (1985). Hypnotic suggestion for the control of bleeding in the angiography suite. *Ericksonian Monographs, 1,* 76–88.

Banquet, J. P. (1973). Spectral analysis of the EEG in meditation. *Electroencephalography and Clinical Neurophysiology, 35,* 143–151.

Bányai, E. I., Mészáros, I., & Csókay, L. (1985). Interaction between hypnotist and subject: A social psychophysiological approach (preliminary report). In D. Waxman, P. Mizra, M. Gibson, & M. Baker (Eds.), *Modern trends in hypnosis* (pp. 97–108). New York: Plenum Press.

Barabasz, A. F., & Lonsdale, C. (1983). Effects of hypnosis on P_{300} olfactory-evoked potential amplitudes. *Journal of Abnormal Psychology, 92,* 520–523.

Barabasz, A. F., & Barabasz, M. (1989). Effects of restricted environmental stimulation: Enhancement of hypnotizability for experimental and chronic pain control. *International Journal of Clinical and Experimental Hypnosis, 37,* 217–231.

Barber, J. (1977). Rapid induction analgesia: A clinical report. *American Journal of Clinical Hypnosis, 19,* 138–147.

Barber, T. X. (1984). Changing unchangeable bodily processes by (hypnotic) suggestions: A new look at hypnosis, cognitions, imagining, and the mind-body problem. *Advances, 1,* 7–40.

Bargh, J. A. (1982). Attention and automaticity in the processing of self-relevant information. *Journal of Personality and Social Psychology, 43,* 425–436.

Barker, J., & Mayer, D. (1977). Evaluation of the efficacy and neural mechanism of a hypnotic analgesia procedure in experimental and clinical dental pain. *Pain, 4,* 41–48.

Barnes, P. J. (1987). Mechanisms of asthma. *Medicine International, 37,* 1522–1525.

Bartis, S. P., & Zamansky, H. S. (1986). Dissociation in posthypnotic amnesia: Knowing without knowing. *American Journal of Clinical Hypnosis, 29,* 103–108.

Barton, J. (1984). *Playing Shakespeare.* New York: Methuen.

Bass, C., Cawley, R., Wade, C., Ryan, K. C., Gardner, W. N., Hutchison, D. C. S., & Jackson, G. (1983, March 19). Unexplained breathlessness and psychiatric morbidity in patients with normal and abnormal coronary arteries. *Lancet,* pp. 605–609.

Bateson, G. (1972). *Steps to an ecology of mind.* New York: Ballantine.

Bateson, G., & Bateson, M. C. (1987). *Angels fear: Towards an epistemology of the sacred.* New York: Macmillan.

Battig, W. F. (1979). Are the important "individual differences" between or within individuals? *Journal of Research in Personality, 13,* 546–558.

Beahrs, J. O. (1971). The hypnotic psychotherapy of Milton H. Erickson. *American Journal of Clinical Hypnosis, 14*(2), 73–90.

Beahrs, J. O. (1982). *Unity and multiplicity: Multilevel consciousness of self in hypnosis, psychiatric disorder and mental health.* New York: Brunner/Mazel.

Beahrs, J. O. (1988). [Review of R. P. Kluft (Ed.), *Childhood antecedents of multiple personality,* and B. G. Braun (Ed.), *Treatment of multiple personality disorder*]. *American Journal of Clinical Hypnosis, 30,* 227–231.

Beair, K., Peterson, C., & Whitmire, R. (1984). *Unconscious acquisition of cognitive algorithms.* Unpublished manuscript, University of Tulsa.

Beatty, J., Greenberg, A., Diebler, W. P., & O'Hanlon, J. F. (1974). Operant control of occipital theta rhythm affects performance in a radar monitoring task. *Science, 183,* 871–873.

Beck, B. E. F. (1987). Metaphors, cognition, and artificial intelligence. In R. E. Haskell (Ed.), *Cognition and symbolic structures: The psychology of metaphoric transformation* (pp. 9–30). Norwood, NJ: Ablex.

Beebe, B. (1982). Rhythmic communication in the mother-infant dyad. In M. Davis (Ed.), *Interaction rhythms: Periodicity in communicative behavior* (pp. 79–100). New York: Human Sciences Press.

Begleiter, H., Porjesz, B., Yerre, C., & Kissin, B. (1973). Evoked potential correlates of expected stimulus intensity. *Science, 179,* 814–816.

Benedikt, R. A., & Kolb, L. C. (1986). Preliminary findings on chronic pain and posttraumatic stress disorder. *American Journal of Psychiatry, 143,* 908–910.

Bengtsson, U. (1984). Emotions and asthma. I. *European Journal of Respiratory Diseases Supplement, 136*(65), 123–129.

Benowitz, L. I., Bear, D. M., Rosenthal, R., Mesulam, M. M., Zaidel, E., & Sperry, R. W. (1983). Hemispheric specialization in nonverbal communication. *Cortex, 19,* 5–11.

Berlin, B., Breedlove, D. E., & Raven, P. H. (1974). *Principles of Tzeltal plant classification.* New York: Academic Press.

Bernardi, L., Galeazzi, L., & Bardelli, R. (1982, August). *Hypnotic responsivity of cold PressorTest in normal and hypertensive subjects.* Paper presented at the International Society of Hypnosis, 9th International Congress of Hypnosis and Psychosomatic Medicine, Glasgow, Scotland.

Bernheim, H. (1886). *Suggestive therapeutics: A treatise on the nature and uses of hypnotism.* (C. A. Herter, Trans.). Westport, CT: Associated Booksellers, 1957.

Bernstein, E. M., & Putnam, F. W. (1986). Development, reliability, and validity of a dissociation scale. *Journal of Nervous and Mental Disease, 174,* 727–735.

Bhatnagar, S., & Andy, O. J. (1983). Language in the nondominant right hemisphere. *Archives of Neurology, 40,* 728–731.

Blank, G. D. (1988). Metaphors in the lexicon. *Metaphor and Symbolic Activity, 3,* 21–36.

Bliss, E. L., & Jeppsen, E. A. (1985). Prevalence of multiple personality among inpatients and outpatients. *American Journal of Psychiatry, 142,* 250–251.

Bliss, E. L. (1986). *Multiple personality, allied disorders, and hypnosis.* New York: Oxford University Press.

Blocker, H. G. (1979). *Philosophy and art.* New York: Charles Scribner's Sons.

Bloom, F. (1986). Chemical signalling in the spatial, temporal continuum. In L. Iversen & E. Goodman (Eds.), *Fast and slow chemical signalling in the nervous system* (pp. 295–308). New York: Oxford University Press.

Bolinger, D. (1986). *Intonation and its parts: Melody in spoken English.* Stanford, CA: Stanford University Press.

Borod, J. C., & Caron, H. S. (1980). Facedness and emotion related to lateral dominance, sex, and expression type. *Neuropsychologia, 18,* 237–241.

Borod, J. C., Koff, E., Lorch, M. P., & Nicholas, M. (1986). The expression and perception of facial emotion in brain-damaged patients. *Neuropsychologia, 24,* 169–180.

Borod, J. C., St. Clair, J., Koff, E., & Alpert, M. (1990a). Perceiver and poser asymmetries in processing facial emotion. *Brain and Cognition, 13,* 167–177.

Borod, J. C., & van Gelder, R. S. (1990b). Facial asymmetry [editorial]. *International Journal of Psychology, 25,* 135–139.

Bourguignon, E. (1973). Introduction: A framework for the comparative study of altered states of consciousness. In E. Bourguignon (Ed.), *Religion, altered states of consciousness, and social change* (pp. 3–35). Columbus: Ohio State University Press.

Bourguignon, E. (1989). Trance and shamanism: What's in a name? *Journal of Psychoactive Drugs, 21,* 9–15.

Boutelle, R. C., Epstein, S., & Ruddy, M. (1987). The relation of essential hypertension to feelings of anxiety, depression and anger. *Psychiatry, 50,* 206–217.

Bower, G. H. (1981). Emotional mood and memory. *American Psychologist, 36,* 129–148.

Bowers, K. (1976). *Hypnosis for the seriously curious.* New York: Norton.

Bowers, K. S., & LeBaron, S. (1986). Hypnosis and hypnotizability: Implications for clinical intervention. *Hospital and Community Psychiatry, 37,* 457–467.

Bowers, K. S. (1987). Revisioning the unconscious. *Canadian Psychology, 28,* 93–104.

Bowers, K. S., & Hilgard, E. R. (1988). Some complexities in understanding memory. In H. M. Pettinati (Ed.), *Hypnosis and memory* (pp. 3–18). New York: Guilford Press.

Bowlby, J. (1969). *Attachment and loss: Vol. 1. Attachment.* London: Hogarth Press.

Bradshaw, J. L., & Nettleton, N. C. (1981). The nature of hemispheric specialization in man. *Behavioral and Brain Sciences, 4,* 51–92.

Bramwell, J. M. (1903). *Hypnotism, its history, practice and theory.* Philadelphia: J. B. Lippincott.

Braun, B. G. (1983). Neurophysiologic changes in multiple personality due to integration: A preliminary report. *American Journal of Clinical Hypnosis, 26,* 84–92.

Braun, B. G. (1984). Hypnosis creates multiple personality: Myth or reality? *International Journal of Clinical and Experimental Hypnosis, 32,* 191–197.

Braun, B. G. (1986a). Introduction. In B. G. Braun (Ed.), *Treatment of multiple personality disorder* (pp. xi–xxi). Washington, DC: American Psychiatric Press.

Braun, B. G. (1986b). Issues in the psychotherapy of multiple personality disorder. In B. G. Braun (Ed.), *Treatment of multiple personality disorder* (pp. 1–28). Washington, DC: American Psychiatric Press.

Brazelton, T. B., & Cramer, B. G. (1990). *The earliest relationship: Parents, infants, and the drama of early attachment.* Reading, MA: Addison-Wesley.

Bregman, N. J., & McAllister, H. A. (1981). Effects of suggestion on increasing or decreasing skin temperature control. *International Journal of Neuroscience, 14,* 205–210.

Brende, J. O. (1982). Electrodermal responses in post-traumatic syndromes: A pilot study of cerebral hemisphere functioning in Vietnam veterans. *Journal of Nervous and Mental Disease, 170,* 352–361.

Brett, E. A., & Ostroff, R. (1985). Imagery and posttraumatic stress disorder: An overview. *American Journal of Psychiatry, 142,* 417–424.

Broadbent, D. E. (1977). The hidden preattentive processes. *American Psychologist, 32,* 109–118.

Bronowski, J. (1971). *The identity of man.* Garden City, NY: Natural History Press.

Brooks, L. (1968). Spatial and verbal components of the act of recall. *Canadian Journal of Psychology, 22,* 349–368.

Brooks, L. (1978). Nonanalytic concept formation and memory for instances. In E. Rosch & B. B. Lloyd (Eds.), *Cognition and categorization.* Hillsdale, NJ: Erlbaum.

Broughton, R. J. (1985). Three central issues concerning ultradian rhythms. *Experimental Brain Research, Suppl. 12,* 218–233.

Brown, D. B. (1971). Awareness of EEG-subjective activity relationships detected within a closed feedback system. *Psychophysiology, 7,* 451–464.

Brown, D. P., & Fromm, E. (1986). *Hypnotherapy and hypnoanalysis.* Hillsdale, NJ: Erlbaum.

Brown, D. P., & Fromm, E. (1987). *Hypnosis and behavioral medicine.* Hillsdale, NJ: Erlbaum.

Bruce, V., & Young, A. (1986). Understanding face recognition. *British Journal of Psychology, 77,* 305–327.

Bruyn, G. W. (1980). The biochemistry of migraine. *Headache, 20,* 235–246.

Burges Watson, I. P., Hoffman, L., & Wilson, G. V. (1988). The neuropsychiatry of post-traumatic stress disorder. *British Journal of Psychiatry, 152,* 164–173.

Burgoon, J. D., & Hale, J. L. (1988). Nonverbal expectancy violations: Model elaboration and application to immediacy behaviors. *Communication Monographs, 55,* 58–79.

Burney, P. G. J. (1986, August 9). Asthma mortality in England and Wales: Evidence for a further increase, 1974–84. *Lancet,* pp. 323–326.

Burstein, A. (1986). Two cases of lifelike visualizations based on imagination in posttraumatic stress disorder. *American Journal of Psychiatry, 143,* 939.

Butler, S. (1912). *The notebooks of Samuel Butler.* E.-P. Breuer (Ed.). Lanham, MD: University Press of America, 1984.

Campbell, J. (1984). *Historical atlas of world mythology.* New York: Harper & Row.

Campbell, J. (1986). *Winston Churchill's afternoon nap: A wide-awake inquiry into the human nature of time.* New York: Simon & Schuster.

Campbell, R. (1978). Asymmetries in interpreting and expressing a posed facial expression. *Cortex, 14,* 327–342.

Cappo, B. M., & Holmes, D. S. (1984). The utility of prolonged respiratory exhalation for reducing physiological and psychological arousal in nonthreatening and threatening situations. *Journal of Psychosomatic Research, 28,* 265–273.

Carey, M. P., & Burish, T. G. (1988). Etiology and treatment of the psychological side effects associated with cancer chemotherapy: A critical review and discussion. *Psychological Bulletin, 104,* 307–325.

Carlson, E. B., & Putnam, F. W. (1989). Integrating research on dissociation and hypnotizability: Are there two pathways to hypnotizability? *Dissociation, 2*(1): 32–38.

Carroll, D., Marzillier, J. S., & Merian, S. (1982). Psychophysiological changes accompanying different types of arousing and relaxing imagery. *Psychophysiology, 19,* 75–82.

Cassirer, E. (1944). *An essay on man.* New Haven: Yale University Press.

Caughey, J. (1984). *Imaginary social worlds: A cultural approach.* Lincoln: University of Nebraska Press.

Chapple, E. D. (1979). *The biological foundations of individuality and culture.* Huntington, NY: Robert Krieger. (Originally published as *Culture and Biological Man,* 1970).

Chapple, E. D. (1982). Movement and sound: The musical language of body rhythms in interaction. In M. Davis (Ed.), *Interaction rhythms: Periodicity in communicative behavior* (pp. 31–51). New York: Human Sciences Press.

Charney, D. S., Krystal, J. H., & Southwick, S. M. (1990, May). Animal models for PTSD. Abstract for a paper presented at the Annual Meeting of the American Psychiatric Association, New York.

Charney, E. J. (1966). Psychosomatic manifestations of rapport in psychotherapy. *Psychosomatic Medicine, 28,* 305–315.

Chase, M. H., & Morales, F. R. (1983). Subthreshold excitatory activity and motoneuron discharge during REM periods of active sleep. *Science, 221,* 1195–1198.

Chaves, J. F., & Brown, J. M. (1987). Spontaneous cognitive strategies for the control of clinical pain and stress. *Journal of Behavioral Medicine, 10,* 263–276.

Chavoix, C., Desi, M., & de Bonis, M. (1987). Relationship between mood state and information processing of negative versus positive emotional stimuli in brain-damaged patients. *Psychopathology, 20,* 34–41.

Chen, A. C. N., Dworkin, S. F., & Bloomquist, D. S. (1981). Cortical power spectrum analysis of hypnotic pain control in surgery. *International Journal of Neuroscience, 13,* 127–136.

Chen, A. C. N., Dworkin, S. F., & Drangsholt, M. T. (1983). Cortical power spectral analysis of acute pathophysiological pain. *International Journal of Neuroscience, 18,* 269–278.

Chu, J. A., & Dill, D. L. (1990). Dissociative symptoms in relation to childhood physical and sexual abuse. *American Journal of Psychiatry, 147,* 887–892.

Cicourel, A. V. (1987). The interpenetration of communicative contexts: Examples from medical encounters. *Social Psychology Quarterly, 50,* 217–226.

Cikurel, K., & Gruzelier, J. (1990). The effect of an active-alert hypnotic induction on lateral asymmetry in haptic processing. *British Journal of Experimental and Clinical Hypnosis, 7,* 17–25.

Claghorn, J. L., Mathew, R. J., Largen, J. W., & Meyer, J. S. (1981). Directional effects of skin temperature self-regulation on regional cerebral blood flow in normal subjects and migraine patients. *American Journal of Psychiatry, 138,* 1182–1187.

Clanchy, M. T. (1979). *From memory to written record: England, 1066–1307.* Cambridge, MA: Harvard University Press.

Clark, M. S., & Isen, A. M. (1982). Toward understanding the relationship between feeling states and social behavior. In S. Hastorf & A. Isen (Eds.), *Cognitive social psychology.* New York: Elsevier North-Holland.

Clarke, P. S., & Gibson, J. R. (1980). Asthma, hyperventilation and emotion. *Australian Family Physician, 9,* 715–719.

Clement, C. A., & Falmagne, R. J. (1986). Logical reasoning, world knowledge, and mental imagery: Interconnections in cognitive processes. *Memory and Cognition, 14,* 299–307.

Cluff, R. A. (1984). Chronic hyperventilation and its treatment by phys-iotherapy. *Journal of the Royal Society of Medicine, 77,* 855–862.

Clynes, M. (1984). Music beyond the score. *Somatics, 5,* 4–14.

Clynes, M. (1986). Generative principles of musical thought: Integration of micro-structure with structure. *CCAI, 3,* 185–223.

Cohen, J., & Sedlacek, K. (1983). Attention and autonomic self-regulation. *Psychosomatic Medicine, 45,* 243–257.

Cohen, R. A., Williamson, D. A., Monguillot, J. E., Hutchinson, P. C., Gottlieb, J., & Waters, W. F. (1983). Psychophysiological response patterns in vascular and muscle-contraction headaches. *Journal of Behavioral Medicine, 6,* 93–107.

Cohen, R. A., & Waters, W. F. (1985). Psychophysiological correlates of levels and stages of cognitive processing. *Neuropsychologia, 23,* 243–256.

Coker, D. A., & Burgoon, J. K. (1987). The nature of conversational involve-ment and nonverbal encoding patterns. *Human Communication Research, 13,* 463–494.

Coles, M. G. H., Pellegrini, A. M., & Wilson, G. V. (1982). The cardiac cycle time effect: Influence of respiration phase and information processing require-ments. *Psychophysiology, 19,* 648–657.

Colgan, S. M., Faragher, E. B., & Whorwell, P. J. (1988, June 11). Controlled trial of hypnotherapy in relapse prevention of duodenal ulceration. *Lancet,* pp. 1299–1300.

Collins, S. M. (1988). The irritable bowel syndrome. *Canadian Medical Associa-tion Journal, 138,* 309–315.

Collison, D. R. (1975). Which asthmatic patients should be treated with hypno-therapy? *Medical Journal of Australia, 1,* 776–781.

Colquhoun, P. (1981). Rhythms in performance. In J. Aschoff (Ed.), *Handbook of behavioral neurobiology: Vol. 4. Biological rhythms* (pp. 333–348). New York: Plenum Press.

Condon, W. S. (1982). Cultural microrhythms. In M. Davis (Ed.), *Interaction rhythms: Periodicity in communicative behavior* (pp. 53–77). New York: Human Sciences Press.

Conn, L., & Mott, T. (1984). Plethysmographic demonstration of rapid vaso-dilation by direct suggestion: A case of Raynaud's disease treated by hypno-sis. *American Journal of Clinical Hypnosis, 26,* 166–170.

Connor, J. A. (1985). Neural pacemakers and rhythmicity. *Annual Review of Physiology, 47,* 17–28.

Conway, A. V., Freeman, L. J., & Nixon, P. G. F. (1988). Hypnotic examination of trigger factors in the hyperventilation syndrome. *American Journal of Clinical Hypnosis, 30,* 296–304.

Coons, P. M., Milstein, V., & Marley, C. (1982). EEG studies of two multiple personalities and a control. *Archives of General Psychiatry, 39,* 823–825.

Coons, P. M., & Milstein, V. (1986). Psychosexual disturbances in multiple personality: Characteristics, etiology, and treatment. *Journal of Clinical Psychiatry, 47,* 106–110.

Corby, J. C., Roth, W. T., Zarcone, V. P., Jr., & Kopell, B. S. (1978). Psychophysiological correlates of the practice of tantric yoga meditation. *Archives of General Psychiatry, 35,* 571–577.

Corrigan, M. H., Garbutt, J. C., Gillette, G. M., Mason, G., Carson, S., & Golden, R. N. (1990, May). Serotonin and victims of childhood sexual abuse. Abstract for a paper presented at the Annual Meeting of the American Psychiatric Association, New York.

Corteen, R. S., & Wood, B. (1972). Autonomic responses to shock-associated words in unattended channel. *Journal of Experimental Psychology, 94,* 308–313.

Corteen, R. S., & Dunn, D. (1974). Shock-associated words in a nonattended message: A test for momentary awareness. *Journal of Experimental Psychology, 102,* 1143–1144.

Cotanch, P., Hockenberry, M., & Herman, S. (1985). Self-hypnosis antiemetic therapy in children receiving chemotherapy. *Oncology Nursing Forum, 12,* 41–46.

Council, J. R., Kirsch, I., & Hafner, L. P. (1986). Expectancy versus absorption in the prediction of hypnotic responding. *Journal of Personality and Social Psychology, 50,* 182–189.

Crawford, H. J. (1982a). Hypnotizability, daydreaming styles, imagery vividness, and absorption: A multidimensional study. *Journal of Personality and Social Psychology, 42,* 915–926.

Crawford, H. J., & Allen, S. N. (1982b, August). *Visual memory processing during hypnosis: Does it differ from waking?* Paper presented at the International Society of Hypnosis, 9th International Congress of Hypnosis and Psychosomatic Medicine, Glasgow, Scotland.

Crawford, H. J., & Allen, S. N. (1983a). Enhanced visual memory during hypnosis as mediated by hypnotic responsiveness and cognitive strategies. *Journal of Experimental Psychology: General, 112,* 662–685.

Crawford, H. J., Crawford, K., & Koperski, B. J. (1983b). Hypnosis and lateral cerebral function as assessed by dichotic listening. *Biological Psychiatry, 18,* 415–427.

Crawford, H. J., Kitner-Triolo, M., Clarke, S., & Brown, A. M. (1988, November). *EEG activation patterns accompanying induced happy and sad moods: Moderating effects of hypnosis and hypnotic responsiveness level.* Paper presented at the Annual Meeting of the Society for Clinical and Experimental Hypnosis, Asheville, NC.

Crawford, H. J. (1989a). Cognitive and psychological flexibility: Multiple pathways to hypnotic responsiveness. In V. A. Gheorghiu, P. Netter, H. J. Eysenck, & R. Rosenthal (Eds.), *Suggestion and suggestibility: Theory and research* (pp. 155–167). New York: Springer-Verlag.

Crawford, H. J., & Brown, A. (1989b). *Intensity of emotions: Differences between low and high hypnotizables.* Unpublished manuscript.

Crawford, H. J., Clarke, S. N., Kitner-Triolo, M., & Olesko, B. (1989c, August). *EEG correlates of emotions: Moderated by hypnosis and hypnotic level.* Paper presented at the American Psychological Association annual meeting, New Orleans, LA.

Crawford, H. J. (1990). Cognitive and psychophysiological correlates of hypnotic responsiveness and hypnosis. In M. L. Fass & D. Brown (Eds.), *Creative mastery in hypnosis and hypnoanalysis: A festschrift for Erika Fromm* (pp. 47–54). Hillsdale, NJ: Erlbaum.

Crick, F., & Mitchison, G. (1983). The function of dream sleep. *Nature, 304,* 111–114.

Crowley, R. (1980). Effects of indirect hypnosis (rapid induction analgesia) for relief of acute pain associated with minor podiatric surgery. *Dissertation Abstracts International, 40,* 4549.

Cruttenden, A. (1986). *Intonation.* Cambridge: Cambridge University Press.

Csikszentmihalyi, M. (1988). Motivation and creativity: Toward a synthesis of structural and energistic approaches to cognition. *New Ideas in Psychology, 6,* 159–176.

Czyzewska, M. (1984). *Unconscious social information processing.* Unpublished doctoral dissertation, University of Warsaw, Poland.

Dabbs, J. M., Jr. (1969). Similarity of gestures and interpersonal influence. *Proceedings of the 77th Annual Convention of the American Psychological Association, 4,* 337–338.

Dance, K. A., & Neufeld, R. W. J. (1988). Aptitude-treatment interaction research in the clinical setting: A review of attempts to dispel the "patient uniformity" myth. *Psychological Bulletin, 104,* 192–213.

Dane, F. C., & Thompson, J. K. (1985). Asymmetrical facial expressions: A different interpretation. *Cortex, 21,* 301–303.

Daniel, R. S. (1967). Alpha and theta EEG in vigilance. *Perceptual and Motor Skills, 25,* 697–703.

Darwin, C. (1872). *The expression of the emotions in man and animals.* Chicago: University of Chicago Press, 1965.

Davidson, R. J., Schwartz, G. E., Saron, C., Bennett, J., & Goleman, D. J. (1974). Frontal versus parietal EEG asymmetry during positive and negative affect. *Psychophysiology, 16,* 202–203.

Davidson, R. J., & Schwartz, G. E. (1977). The influence of musical training on patterns of EEG asymmetry during musical and non-musical self-generation tasks. *Psychophysiology, 14,* 58–63.

Davis, M. (Ed.). (1982). *Interaction rhythms: Periodicity in communicative behavior.* New York: Human Sciences Press.

Davis, M. (1984). Nonverbal behavior and psychotherapy process research. In A. Wolfgang (Ed.), *Nonverbal behavior: Perspectives, applications, intercultural insights* (pp. 203–228). Lewiston, NY: C. J. Hogrefe.

Davis, M. H., Saunders, D. R., Creer, T. L., & Chai, H. (1973). Relaxation training facilitated by biofeedback apparatus as a supplemental treatment in bronchial asthma. *Journal of Psychosomatic Research, 17,* 121–128.

Deanfield, J. E., Shea, M., Kensett, M., Horlock, P., Wilson, R. A., de Landsheere, C. M., & Selwyn, A. P. (1984, November 3). Silent myocardial ischaemia due to mental stress. *Lancet,* pp. 1001–1005.

DeBenedittis, G., & Sironi, V. A. (1986). Depth cerebral electrical activity in man during hypnosis. *International Journal of Clinical and Experimental Hypnosis, 34,* 63–70.

DeBenedittis, G., & Sironi, V. A. (1988). Arousal effects of electrical deep brain stimulation in hypnosis. *International Journal of Clinical and Experimental Hypnosis, 36,* 96–106.

DeBenedittis, G., Panerai, A. A., & Villamira, M. A. (1989). Effects of hypnotic analgesia and hypnotizability on experimental ischemic pain. *International Journal of Clinical and Experimental Hypnosis, 37,* 55–69.

DeCasper, A., & Prescott, P. (1984). Human newborns' perception of male voices: Preference, discrimination, and reinforcing value. *Developmental Psychobiology, 17,* 482–491.

DeCasper, A., & Spence, M. (1986). Prenatal maternal speech influences newborns' perception of speech sounds. *Infant Behavior and Development, 9,* 133–150.

Delmonte, M. M. (1984a). Electrocortical activity and related phenomena associated with meditation practice: A literature review. *International Journal of Neuroscience, 24,* 217–231.

Delmonte, M. M. (1984b). Meditation: Similarities with hypnoidal states and hypnosis. *International Journal of Psychosomatics, 31,* 24–34.

Demes, B. (1987). Another look at an old face: Biomechanics of the Neanderthal facial skeleton reconsidered. *Journal of Human Evolution, 16,* 297–303.

Dennett, D. C. (1984). *Elbow room: The varieties of free will worth wanting.* Cambridge, MA: MIT Press.

DePascalis, V., & Palumbo, G. (1986). EEG alpha asymmetry: Task difficulty and hypnotizability. *Perceptual and Motor Skills, 62,* 139–150.

DePascalis, V., Silveri, A., & Palumbo, G. (1988). EEG asymmetry during covert mental activity and its relationship with hypnotizability. *International Journal of Clinical and Experimental Hypnosis, 36,* 38–52.

Deputte, B. (1978). *Study of yawning in two species of Cercopithecidae,* Cercocebus albigena albigena *GRAY and* Macaca fascicularis *RAFFLES: Research on causal and functional factors: A consideration of socio-bioenergetic factors.* Unpublished doctoral dissertation, University of Rennes, France.

Deutsch, D. (Ed.). (1982). *The psychology of music.* New York: Academic Press.

Devenport, L. D., Devenport, J. A., & Holloway, F. A. (1981). Reward-induced stereotypy: Modulation by the hippocampus. *Science, 212,* 1288–1289.

Devereux, R. B., Pickering, T. G., Harshfield, G. A., Kleinert, H. D., Denby, L., Clark, L., Pregibon, D., Jason, M., Kleiner, B., Borer, J. S., & Laragh, J. H.

(1983). Left ventricular hypertrophy in patients with hypertension: Importance of blood pressure response to regularly recurring stress. *Circulation, 68,* 470–476.

DeWitt, G. W., & Averill, J. R. (1976). Lateral eye movements, hypnotic susceptibility and field independence-dependence. *Perceptual and Motor Skills, 43,* 1179–1184.

Diamond, M. J. (1982). Modifying hypnotic experience by means of indirect hypnosis and hypnotic skill training: An update (1981). *Research Communications in Psychology, Psychiatry and Behavior, 7,* 233–239.

Diamond, M. J. (1987). The interactional basis of hypnotic experience: On the relational dimensions of hypnosis. *International Journal of Clinical and Experimental Hypnosis, 35,* 95–115.

Dimond, S. J. (1979). Performance by split brain humans on lateralised vigilance tests. *Cortex, 15,* 43–50.

Dobkin de Rios, M., & Winkelman, M. (1989). Shamanism and altered states of consciousness: An introduction. *Journal of Psychoactive Drugs, 21,* 1–7.

Dolce, G., & Waldeier, H. (1974). Spectral and multivariate analysis of EEG changes during mental activity in man. *Electroencephalography and Clinical Neurophysiology, 36,* 577–584.

Domangue, B. B., Margolis, C. G., Lieberman, D., & Kaji, H. (1985). Biochemical correlates of hypnoanalgesia in arthritic pain patients. *Journal of Clinical Psychiatry, 46,* 235–238.

Donohew, L., Sypher, H. E., & Cook, P. L. (1988). Communication and affect. *American Behavioral Scientist, 31,* 287–295.

Dowling, W. J., & Harwood, D. L. (1986). *Music cognition.* Orlando, FL: Academic Press.

Draguitinovich, S., & Sheehan, P. W. (1986). Hypnotic susceptibility and cortical modulation of stimulus intensity. *Australian Journal of Clinical and Experimental Hypnosis, 14,* 1–14.

Dywan, J., & Bowers, K. (1983). The use of hypnosis to enhance recall. *Science, 222,* 184–185.

Eason, R. G. (1984). Selective attention effects on retinal and forebrain responses in humans: A replication and extension. *Bulletin of the Psychonomic Society, 22,* 341–344.

Ebbesen, E. B., & Konecni, V. J. (1980). On the external validity of decision-making research: What do we know about decisions in the real world? In T. S. Wallsten (Ed.), *Cognitive processes in choice and decision behavior* (pp. 21–45). Hillsdale, NJ: Erlbaum.

Eccles, R., & Lee, R. L. (1981). The influence of the hypothalamus on the sympathetic innervation of the nasal vasculature of the cat. *Acta Otolaryngology, 91,* 127–134.

Edelman, G. M. (1987). *Neural Darwinism.* New York: Basic Books.

Edelman, G. M. (1989). *The remembered present: A biological theory of consciousness.* New York: Basic Books.

Edelson, J., & Fitzpatrick, J. L. (1989). A comparison of cognitive-behavioral and hypnotic treatments of chronic pain. *Journal of Clinical Psychology, 45,* 316–323.

Edmonston, W. E., Jr. (1986). *The induction of hypnosis.* New York: John Wiley.

Eikelboom, R., & Stewart, J. (1982). Conditioning of drug-induced physiological responses. *Psychological Review, 89,* 507–528.

Eisenberg, J. F. (1981). *The mammalian radiations: An analysis of trends in evolution, adaptation, and behavior.* Chicago: University of Chicago Press. (Paperback ed., 1983)

Ekman, P. (1972). Universals and cultural differences in facial expressions of emotion. In J. Cole (Ed.), *Nebraska Symposium on Motivation, 1971* (Vol. 19). Lincoln: University of Nebraska Press.

Ekman, P. (1980). Asymmetry in facial expression. *Science, 209,* 833–834.

Ekman, P., Hager, J. C., & Friesen, W. V. (1981). The symmetry of emotional and deliberate facial actions. *Psychophysiology, 18,* 101–106.

Ekman, P. (Ed.). (1982). *Emotion in the human face.* (2nd ed.). Cambridge: Cambridge University Press.

Ekman, P., Levenson, R. W., & Friesen, W. V. (1983). Autonomous nervous system activity distinguishes among emotions. *Science, 221,* 1208–1210.

Ellenberger, H. (1970). *The discovery of the unconscious.* New York: Basic Books.

Elmore, A. M., & Tursky, B. (1981). A comparison of two psychophysiological approaches to the treatment of migraine. *Headache, 21,* 93–101.

Elson, B. D., Hauri, P., & Cunis, D. (1977). Physiological changes in yoga meditation. *Psychophysiology, 14,* 52–57.

Emde, R. N., Gaensbauer, T. J., & Harmon, R. J. (1976). Emotional expression in infancy: A biobehavioral study. *Psychological Issues Monograph, 37* (Series 10).

Engel, B. T. (1986). An essay on the circulation as behavior. *Behavioral and Brain Sciences, 9,* 285–318.

Engel, S. (1988). Metaphors: How are they different for the poet, the child and the everyday adult? *New Ideas in Psychology, 6,* 333–341.

Engstrom, D. R. (1976). Hypnotic susceptibility, EEG-alpha, and self-regulation. In G. E. Schwartz & D. Shapiro (Eds.), *Consciousness and self-regulation: Advances in research* (Vol. 1, pp. 173–221). New York: Plenum Press.

Epstein, A. W., & Simmons, N. N. (1983). Aphasia with reported loss of dreaming. *American Journal of Psychiatry, 140,* 108–109.

Erickson, M. H., Rossi, E. L., & Rossi, S. I. (1976). *Hypnotic realities: The induction of clinical hypnosis and forms of indirect suggestion.* New York: Irvington.

Erickson, M. H., & Rossi, E. L. (1979). *Hypnotherapy: An exploratory casebook.* New York: Irvington.

Erickson, M. H. (1980a). *The collected papers of Milton H. Erickson on hypnosis: Vol. 1. The nature of hypnosis and suggestion* (E. L. Rossi, Ed.). New York: Irvington.

Erickson, M. H. (1980b). *The collected papers of Milton H. Erickson on hypnosis: Vol.*

3. *Hypnotic investigation of psychodynamic processes* (E. L. Rossi, Ed.). New York: Irvington.

Erickson, M. H. (1980c). *The collected papers of Milton H. Erickson on hypnosis: Vol. 4. Innovative hypnotherapy* (E. L. Rossi, Ed.). New York: Irvington.

Erickson, M. H., & Rossi, E. L. (1981). *Experiencing hypnosis: Therapeutic approaches to altered states.* New York: Irvington.

Erickson, M. H. (1983). *The seminars, workshops, and lectures of Milton H. Erickson: Vol. 1. Healing in hypnosis* (E. L. Rossi, M. O. Ryan, F. A. Sharp, Eds.). New York: Irvington.

Ericsson, K. A., & Chase, W. G. (1982). Exceptional memory. *American Scientist, 70,* 607–615.

Ervin, F. R., Palmour, R. M., Pearson Murphy, B. E., Prince, R., & Simons, R. C. (1988). The psychobiology of trance. II. Physiological and endocrine correlates. *Transcultural Psychiatric Research Review, 25,* 267–284.

Etcoff, N. L. (1984). Perceptual and conceptual organization of facial emotions: Hemispheric differences. *Brain and Cognition, 3,* 385–412.

Ettlinger, G. (1984). Humans, apes and monkeys: The changing neuropsychological viewpoint. *Neuropsychologia, 22,* 685–696.

Evans, F. (1972). Hypnosis and sleep: Techniques for exploring cognitive activity during sleep. In E. Fromm & R. Shor (Eds.), *Hypnosis: Research developments and perspectives* (pp. 43–83). Chicago: Aldine-Atherton.

Evans, M. B. (1988). The role of metaphor in psychotherapy and personality change: A theoretical reformulation. *Psychotherapy, 25,* 543–551.

Ewer, T. C., & Stewart, D. E. (1986). Improvement in bronchial hyperresponsiveness in patients with moderate asthma after treatment with a hypnotic technique: A randomised controlled trial. *British Medical Journal, 293,* 1129–1132.

Farah, M. J., Gazzaniga, M. S., Holtzman, J. D., & Kosslyn, S. M. (1985). A left hemisphere basis for visual mental imagery? *Neuropsychologia, 23,* 115–118.

Fauconnier, G. (1985). *Mental spaces.* Cambridge, MA: MIT Press.

Fernald, A. (1984). The perceptual and affective salience of mothers' speech to infants. In L. Feagans et al. (Eds.), *The origins and growth of communication* (pp. 5–29). Norwood, NJ: Ablex.

Field, T. M., Woodson, R., Greenberg, R., & Cohen, D. (1982). Discrimination and imitation of facial expressions by neonates. *Science, 218,* 179–181.

Field, T. M. (1985). Attachment as psychobiological attunement: Being on the same wavelength. In M. Reite & T. Field (Eds.), *The psychobiology of attachment and separation* (pp. 415–454). New York: Academic Press.

Fields, H. L., & Levine, J. D. (1981). Biology of placebo analgesia. *American Journal of Medicine, 70,* 745–746.

Fillmore, C. (1974). Pragmatics and the description of discourse. In S. Schmidt (Ed.), *Pragmatik II* (pp. 83–104). Munich: Fink.

Finer, B. (1982, August). *Endorphins under hypnosis in chronic pain patients: Some experimental findings.* Paper presented at the International Society of Hypnosis, 9th International Congress of Hypnosis and Psychosomatic Medicine, Glasgow, Scotland.

Fischer, R., & Landon, G. (1972). On the arousal state-dependent recall of "subconscious" experience: Stateboundness. *British Journal of Psychiatry, 120,* 159–172.

Fiske, S. (1981). Social cognition and affect. In J. Harvey (Ed.), *Cognition, social behavior, and the environment.* Hillsdale, NJ: Erlbaum.

Fiske, S. (1982). Schema-triggered affect: Applications to social perception. In M. S. Clark & S. T. Fiske (Eds.), *Affect and cognition: The 17th Annual Carnegie Symposium on Cognition.* Hillsdale, NJ: Erlbaum.

Fleminger, J. J., McClure, G. M., & Dalton, R. (1980). Lateral response to suggestion in relation to handedness and the side of psychogenic symptoms. *British Journal of Psychiatry, 136,* 562–566.

Flor, H., & Turk, D. C. (1989). Psychophysiology of chronic pain: Do chronic pain patients exhibit symptom-specific psychophysiological responses? *Psychological Bulletin, 105,* 215–239.

Fogel, A., & Thelen, E. (1987). Development of early expressive and communicative action: Reinterpreting the evidence from a dynamic systems perspective. *Developmental Psychology, 23,* 747–761.

Ford, A. (1954). Bioelectric potentials and mental effort. II. Frontal lobe effects. *Journal of Comparative and Physiological Psychology, 47,* 28–30.

Ford, M. R. (1985). Interpersonal stress and style as predictors of biofeedback/relaxation training outcome: Preliminary findings. *Journal of Biofeedback and Self-Regulation, 10,* 223–239.

Fowler, C. A., Wolford, G., Slade, R., & Tassinary, L. (1981). Lexical access with and without awareness. *Journal of Experimental Psychology: General, 110,* 341–362.

Frankel, F. H. (1982, August). *Hypnosis: Both poetry and science.* Paper presented at the International Society of Hypnosis, 9th International Congress of Hypnosis and Psychosomatic Medicine, Glasgow, Scotland.

Frankel, F. H. (1987). Significant developments in medical hypnosis during the past 25 years. *International Journal of Clinical and Experimental Hypnosis, 35,* 231–247.

Frankel, F. H. (1988). The clinical use of hypnosis in aiding recall. In H. M. Pettinati (Ed.), *Hypnosis and memory* (pp. 247–264). New York: Guilford Press.

Frankel, F. H. (1990). Hypnotizability and dissociation. *American Journal of Psychiatry, 147,* 823–829.

Franklin, J., Donohew, L., Dhoundiyal, V., & Cook, P. L. (1988). Attention and our ancient past: The scaly thumb of the reptile. *American Behavioral Scientist, 31,* 312–326.

Frecska, E., & Kulcsar, Z. (1989). Social bonding in the modulation of the physiology of ritual trance. *Ethos, 17,* 70–87.

Freeman, L. J., Conway, A., & Nixon, P. G. F. (1986). Physiological responses to psychological challenge under hypnosis in patients considered to have the hyperventilation syndrome. *Journal of the Royal Society of Medicine, 79,* 76–83.

Freud, S. (1888). Hypnotism and suggestion. In J. Strachey (Ed. and Trans.), *Sigmund Freud: Collected Papers* (Vol. 5, pp. 11–24). New York: Basic Books, 1959.

Freud, S. (1893). A case of successful treatment by hypnotism. In J. Strachey (Ed. and Trans.), *Sigmund Freud: Collected Papers* (Vol. 5, pp. 33–46). New York: Basic Books, 1959.

Frichton, J. R., & Roth, P. (1985). The effects of direct and indirect hypnotic suggestions for analgesia in high and low susceptible subjects. *American Journal of Clinical Hypnosis, 27,* 226–231.

Frick, R. W. (1985). Communicating emotion: The role of prosodic features. *Psychological Bulletin, 97,* 412–429.

Friedman, H., & Taub, H. (1977). The use of hypnosis and biofeedback procedures for essential hypertension. *International Journal of Clinical and Experimental Hypnosis, 25,* 335–347.

Friedman, H., & Taub, H. (1978). A six month follow-up of the use of hypnosis and biofeedback procedures in essential hypertension. *American Journal of Clinical Hypnosis, 20,* 184–188.

Friedman, H., & Taub, H. A. (1984). Brief psychological training procedures in migraine treatment. *American Journal of Clinical Hypnosis, 26,* 187–200.

Friedman, M. J. (1988). Toward rational pharmacotherapy for posttraumatic stress disorder: An interim report. *American Journal of Psychiatry, 145,* 281–285.

Friedrich, P. (1979). Poetic language and the imagination: Reformulation of the Sapir Hypothesis. In *Language, context, and the imagination* (pp. 441–512). Stanford, CA: Stanford University Press.

Frijda, N. H. (1986). *The emotions.* Cambridge: Cambridge University Press.

Frischholz, E. J. (1985). The relationship among dissociation, hypnosis, and child abuse in the development of multiple personality disorder. In R. P. Kluft (Ed.), *Childhood antecedents of multiple personality* (pp. 100–126). Washington, DC: American Psychiatric Press.

Fromm, E., & Shor, R. E. (Eds.). (1979). *Hypnosis: Developments in research and new perspectives* (2nd ed.). New York: Aldine.

Fromm, E., Brown, D. P., Hurt, S. W., Oberlander, J. Z., Boxer, A. M., & Pfeifer, G. (1981). The phenomena and characteristics of self-hypnosis. *International Journal of Clinical and Experimental Hypnosis, 29,* 189–246.

Fromm, E. (1987). Significant developments in clinical hypnosis during the past 25 years. *International Journal of Clinical and Experimental Hypnosis, 35,* 215–230.

Fromm-Reichman, F. (1950). *Psychoanalysis and psychotherapy.* Chicago: University of Chicago Press.

Frumkin, L. R., Ripley, H. S., & Cox, G. B. (1978). Changes in cerebral hemispheric lateralization with hypnosis. *Biological Psychiatry, 13,* 741–750.

Fussell, P. (1979). *Poetic meter and poetic form* (rev. ed.). New York: Random House.

Gabel, S. (1988). The right hemisphere in imagery, hypnosis, rapid eye movement sleep and dreaming: Empirical studies and tentative conclusions. *Journal of Nervous and Mental Disease, 176,* 323–331.

Galbraith, G. C., London, P., Leibovitz, M. P., Cooper, L. M., & Hart, J. T. (1970). EEG and hypnotic susceptibility. *Journal of Comparative and Physiological Psychology, 72,* 125–131.

Gale, A., Christie, B., & Penfold, V. (1971a). Stimulus complexity and the occipital EEG. *British Journal of Psychology, 62,* 527–531.

Gale, A., Coles, M., & Boyd, E. (1971b). Variations in visual input and the occipital EEG: II. *Psychonomic Science, 23,* 99–100.

Gale, A., Spratt, G., Christie, B., & Smallbone, A. (1975). Stimulus complexity, EEG abundance gradients and detection efficiency in a visual recognition task. *British Journal of Psychology, 66,* 289–298.

Galeazzi, L., & Bernardi, L. (1982, August). *Cerebral rheographic variations by hypnosis.* Paper presented at the International Society of Hypnosis, 9th International Congress of Hypnosis and Psychosomatic Medicine, Glasgow, Scotland.

Gardiner, J. M. (1989). A generation effect in memory without awareness. *British Journal of Psychology, 80,* 163–168.

Gautier, J.-P., & Gautier, A. (1977). Communication in Old World monkeys. In T. A. Sebeok (Ed.), *How animals communicate* (pp. 890–964). Bloomington: Indiana University Press.

Gazzaniga, M. S. (1985). *The social brain: Discovering the networks of the mind.* New York: Basic Books.

Gehm, T., Appel, J., & Apsel, D. (1989). Slight manipulations with great effects: On the suggestive impact of vocal parameter change. In V. A. Gheorghiu, P. Netter, H. J. Eysenck, & R. Rosenthal (Eds.), *Suggestion and Suggestibility: Theory and research* (pp. 351–359). New York: Springer-Verlag.

Gentner, D., & Gentner, D. R. (1982). Flowing waters or teeming crowds: Mental models of electricity. In D. Gentner & A. L. Stevens (Eds.), *Mental models.* Hillsdale, NJ: Erlbaum.

Gerrig, R. J., & Gibbs, R. W., Jr. (1988). Beyond the lexicon: Creativity in language production. *Metaphor and Symbolic Activity, 3,* 1–19.

Geschwind, N., & Galaburda, A. M. (1987). *Cerebral lateralization: Biological mechanisms, associations, and pathology.* Cambridge, MA: MIT Press.

Gevins, A. S., Schaffer, R. E., Doyle, J. C., Cutillo, B. A., Tannehill, R. S., & Bressler, S. L. (1983). Shadows of thought: Shifting lateralization of human brain electrical patterns during brief visuomotor task. *Science, 220,* 97–99.

Gfeller, J. D., Lynn, S. J., & Pribble, W. E. (1987). Enhancing hypnotic susceptibility: Interpersonal and rapport factors. *Journal of Personality and Social Psychology, 52,* 586–595.

Ghiglieri, M. P. (1987). Sociobiology of the great apes and the hominid ancestor. *Journal of Human Evolution, 16,* 319–357.

Gibbs, R. W., Jr., & Gerrig, R. J. (1989). Context and metaphor comprehension: Introduction. *Metaphor and Symbolic Activity, 4,* 123–124.

Giller, E. L., Kosten, T. R., Wahby, V., & Mason, J. W. (1989, May). *Psychoendocrinology of PTSD.* Paper presented at the Annual Meeting of the American Psychiatric Association, San Francisco.

Gillett, P. L., & Coe, W. C. (1984). The effects of rapid induction analgesia (RIA), hypnotic susceptibility, and severity of discomfort on reducing dental pain. *American Journal of Clinical Hypnosis, 27,* 81–90.

Gilligan, S. G. (1987). *Therapeutic trances: The cooperation principle in Ericksonian hypnotherapy.* New York: Brunner/Mazel.

Glantz, S. A. (1980). Biostatistics: How to detect, correct and prevent errors in the medical literature. *Circulation, 61,* 1–7.

Glass, L., & Mackey, M. C. (1988). *From clocks to chaos: The rhythms of life.* Princeton: Princeton University Press.

Globus, G. G., Phoebus, E., & Moore, C. (1970). REM "sleep" manifestations during waking. *Psychophysiology, 7,* 308.

Goldstein, A., & Hilgard, E. R. (1975). Lack of influence of the morphine antagonist naloxone on hypnotic analgesia. *Proceedings of the National Academy of Sciences, 72,* 2041–2043.

Goodall, J. (1986). *The chimpanzees of Gombe.* Cambridge, MA: Belknap Press of Harvard University Press.

Goodman, D., & Kelso, J. A. S. (1980). Are movements prepared in parts? Not under compatible (natural) conditions. *Journal of Experimental Psychology: General, 109,* 475–495.

Goodwin, J. M. (1989, May). *Somatic symptoms in post-incest syndromes.* Paper presented at the Annual Meeting of the American Psychiatric Association, San Francisco.

Gopher, D., & Lavie, P. (1980). Short-term rhythms in the performance of a simple motor task. *Journal of Motor Behavior, 12,* 207–219.

Gorassini, D. R., & Spanos, N. P. (1986). A social-cognitive skills approach to the successful modification of hypnotic susceptibility. *Journal of Personality and Social Psychology, 50,* 1004–1012.

Gordon, D. (1978). *Therapeutic metaphors: Helping others through the looking glass.* Cupertino, CA: Meta Publications.

Gordon, H. W., Frooman, B., & Lavie, P. (1982). Shift in cognitive asymmetries between wakings from REM and NREM sleep. *Neuropsychologia, 20,* 99–103.

Gorman, J. M., Askanazi, J., Liebowitz, M. R., Fyer, A. J., Stein, J., Kinney, J. M., & Klein, D. F. (1984). Response to hyperventilation in a group of patients with panic disorder. *American Journal of Psychiatry, 141,* 857–861.

Gorman, J. M., Fyer, M. R., Goetz, R., Askanazi, J., Liebowitz, M. R., Fyer, A. J.,

Kinney, J., & Klein, D. F. (1988). Ventilatory physiology of patients with panic disorder. *Archives of General Psychiatry, 45,* 31–39.

Graham, J. A., & Argyle, M. (1975). A cross-cultural study of the communication of extra verbal meaning by gestures. *International Journal of Psychology, 10,* 57–67.

Grau, J. W. (1987). Activation of the opioid and nonopioid analgesic systems: Evidence for a memory hypothesis and against the coulometric hypothesis. *Journal of Experimental Psychology: Animal Behavior Processes, 13,* 215–225.

Greeley, A. M. (1987). Hallucinations among the widowed. *Social Science Reviews, 71,* 258–265.

Green, B. L., Wilson, J. P., & Lindy, J. D. (1985). Conceptualizing post-traumatic stress disorder: A psychosocial framework. In C. R. Figley (Ed.), *Trauma and its wake: The study and treatment of post-traumatic stress disorder* (pp. 53–69). New York: Brunner/Mazel.

Greenberg, M. S., & Farah, M. J. (1986). The laterality of dreaming. *Brain and Cognition, 5,* 307–321.

Grevert, P., Albert, L. H., & Goldstein, A. (1983). Partial antagonism of placebo analgesia by naloxone. *Pain, 16,* 129–143.

Gross, H. (Ed.). (1979). *The structure of verse: Modern essays on prosody* (rev. ed.). New York: Ecco Press.

Grossman, P. (1983). Respiration, stress, and cardiovascular function. *Psychophysiology, 20,* 284–300.

Grüsser, O.-J. (1984). Face recognition within the reach of neurobiology and beyond it. *Human Neurobiology, 3,* 183–190.

Gruzelier, J. H., & Brow, T. D. (1985). Psychophysiological evidence for a state theory of hypnosis and susceptibility. *Journal of Psychosomatic Research, 29,* 287–302.

Gruzelier, J. H., & Eves, F. (1987a). Rate of habituation of electrodermal orienting responses: A comparison of instructions to stop responding, count stimuli, or relax and remain indifferent. *International Journal of Psychophysiology, 5,* 289–292.

Gruzelier, J., Thomas, M., Brow, T., Conway, A., Golds, J., Jutai, J., Liddiard, D., McCormack, K., Perry, A., & Rhonder, J. (1987b). Involvement of the left hemisphere in hypnotic induction: Electrodermal, haptic, electrocortical and divided visual field evidence. *Advances in Biological Psychiatry, 16,* 6–17.

Gruzelier, J. (1988). The neuropsychology of hypnosis. In M. Heap (Ed.), *Hypnosis: Current clinical, experimental and forensic practices* (pp. 68–76). London: Croom Helm.

Gudjonsson, G. H. (1989). Theoretical and empirical aspects of interrogative suggestibility. In V. A. Gheorghiu, P. Netter, H. J. Eysenck, & R. Rosenthal (Eds.), *Suggestion and suggestibility: Theory and research* (pp. 135–143). New York: Springer-Verlag.

Guerra, G., & Guantieri, G. (1982, August). *Hypnosis and plasmatic B-endorphins.*

Paper presented at the International Society of Hypnosis, 9th International Congress of Hypnosis and Psychosomatic Medicine, Glasgow, Scotland.

Gundel, A., & Witthoft, H. (1983). Circadian rhythm in the EEG of man. *International Journal of Neuroscience, 19,* 287–292.

Gundel, A. (1984). Circadian rhythms in the waking EEG. In A. Reinberg et al. (Eds.), *Annual review of chronopharmacology. Proceedings of the First International Montreux Conference of Biological Rhythms and Medication.* Oxford: Pergamon Press.

Gur, R. C., Gur, R. E., & Obrist, W. D. (1982). Sex and handedness differences in cerebral blood flow during rest and cognitive activity. *Science, 217,* 659–661.

Gur, R. E., & Reyher, J. (1973). The relationship between style of hypnotic induction and direction of lateral eye movement. *Journal of Abnormal Psychology, 82,* 499–505.

Gur, R. E., Gur, R. C., & Harris, L. J. (1975). Hemispheric activation as measured by the subjects' conjugate lateral eye movements is influenced by experimenter location. *Neuropsychologia, 13,* 35–44.

Hager, J. C. (1982). Asymmetries in facial expression. In P. Ekman (Ed.), *Emotion in the human face* (2nd ed., pp. 318–352). Cambridge: Cambridge University Press.

Haley, J. (1973). *Uncommon therapy: The psychiatric techniques of Milton H. Erickson, M.D.* New York: W. W. Norton.

Hall, J. (1978). Gender effects in decoding nonverbal cues. *Psychological Bulletin, 85,* 845–857.

Hallin, R. G., & Wiesenfeld-Hallin, Z. (1983). Does sympathetic activity modify afferent inflow at the receptor level in man? *Journal of the Autonomic Nervous System, 7,* 391–397.

Hammond, D. C. (1988). "Will the real Milton Erickson please stand up?" *International Journal of Clinical and Experimental Hypnosis, 36,* 173–181.

Hammond, K. R., Hamm, R. M., Grassia, J., & Pearson, T. (1984). *The relative efficacy of intuitive and analytical cognition.* Boulder, CO: Center for Research on Judgment and Policy.

Hamner, M. B., Hitri, A., & Appelbaum, B. (1989, May). *Plasma beta-endorphins in PTSD.* Paper presented at the Annual Meeting of the American Psychiatric Association, San Francisco.

Hamner, M. B., & Diamond, B. I. (1990a, May). *Elevated plasma dopamine levels in PTSD.* Paper presented at the Annual Meeting of the American Psychiatric Association, New York.

Hamner, M. B., Diamond, B. I., & Hitri, A. (1990b, May). *Plasma catecholamine response to exercise in PTSD.* Paper presented at the Annual Meeting of the American Psychiatric Association, New York.

Hansch, E. C., & Pirozzolo, F. J. (1980). Task relevant effects on the assessment of cerebral specialization for facial emotion. *Brain and Language, 10,* 51–59.

Harrigan, J. A., Kues, J. R., Ricks, D. F., & Smith, R. (1984). Moods that predict coming migraine headaches. *Pain, 20,* 385–396.

Harrist, R. S., Gordon, D. M., Mann, C. A., Nash, M. R., & Lubar, J. F. (1988, November). *Changes in EEG in hypnosis.* Paper presented at the Annual Meeting of the Society for Clinical and Experimental Hypnosis, Asheville, NC.

Hart, B. B. (1988). Applications to psychological therapies: Overview. In M. Heap (Ed.), *Hypnosis: Current clinical, experimental and forensic practices* (pp. 201–207). London: Croom Helm.

Hartse, K. M., Roth, T., & Zorick, F. J. (1982). Daytime sleepiness and daytime wakefulness: The effect of instruction. *Sleep, 5*(Suppl. 2), 107–118.

Harvey, R. F., Hinton, R. A., Gunary, R. M., & Barry, R. E. (1989, February 25). Individual and group hypnotherapy in treatment of refractory irritable bowel syndrome. *Lancet,* pp. 424–425.

Hasegawa, M., & Kern, E. (1977). The human nasal cycle. *Mayo Clinic Proceedings, 52,* 28–34.

Hasher, L., & Zacks, R. T. (1984). Automatic processing of fundamental information: The case of frequency of occurrence. *American Psychologist, 39,* 1372–1388.

Haskell, R. E. (Ed.). (1987). *Cognition and symbolic structures: The psychology of metaphoric transformation.* Norwood, NJ: Ablex.

Haskell, R. E. (1989). Analogical transforms: A cognitive theory of the origin and development of equivalence transformations. *Metaphor and Symbolic Activity, 4,* 247–277.

Haslum, M. N., & Gale, A. (1973). Inter-modal and intra-subject consistency in EEG correlates of vigilance. *Biological Psychology, 1,* 139–150.

Hassler, R. (1978). Interaction of reticular activating system for vigilance and the truncothalamic and pallidal systems for directing awareness and attention under striatal control. In P. A. Buser & A. Rogeul-Buser (Eds.), *Cerebral correlates of consciousness* (pp. 111–130). Amsterdam: Elsevier/North Holland.

Havelock, E. A. (1963). *Preface to Plato.* Cambridge, MA: Belknap Press of Harvard University Press.

Havelock, E. A. (1982). *The literate revolution in Greece and its cultural consequences.* Princeton: Princeton University Press.

Havelock, E. A. (1986). *The muse learns to write: Reflections on orality and literacy from antiquity to the present.* New Haven: Yale University Press.

Hayden, G. F., Kramer, M. S., & Horwitz, R. I. (1982). The case-control study. *Journal of the American Medical Association, 247,* 326–331.

Hayes, D. P., & Cobb, L. (1982). Cycles of spontaneous conversation under long-term isolation. In M. Davis (Ed.), *Interaction rhythms: Periodicity in communicative behavior* (pp. 319–339). New York: Human Sciences Press.

Hebert, R., & Lehmann, D. (1977). Theta bursts: An EEG pattern in normal subjects practising the transcendental meditation technique. *Electroencephalography and Clinical Neurophysiology, 42,* 397–405.

Heilman, K. M., Bowers, D., Valenstein, E., & Watson, R. T. (1986). The right hemisphere: Neuropsychological functions. *Journal of Neurosurgery, 64*, 693–704.

Helstrup, T. (1988). The influence of verbal and imagery strategies on processing figurative language. *Scandinavian Journal of Psychology, 29*, 65–84.

Hendin, H., & Pollinger Haas, A. (1984). Combat adaptations of Vietnam veterans without posttraumatic stress disorders. *American Journal of Psychiatry, 141*, 956–960.

Hendler, C. S., & Redd, W. H. (1986). Fear of hypnosis: The role of labeling in patients' acceptance of behavioral intervention. *Behavior Therapy, 17*, 2–13.

Herbert, W. (1983). The three brains of Eve: EEG data. *Science, 121*, 356.

Heyneman, N. E., Fremouw, W. J., Gano, D., Kirkland, F., & Heiden, L. (1990). Individual differences and the effectiveness of different coping strategies for pain. *Cognitive Therapy and Research, 14*, 63–77.

Hilgard, E. R., & Hilgard, J. R. (1975). *Hypnosis in the relief of pain*. Los Altos, CA: William Kaufman.

Hilgard, E. R. (1976). Neodissociation theory of multiple cognitive controls. In G. E. Schwartz & D. Shapiro (Eds.), *Consciousness and self-regulation*. New York: Plenum Press.

Hilgard, E. R. (1977). *Divided consciousness: Multiple controls in human thought and action*. New York: John Wiley.

Hilgard, E. R. (1982). Hypnotic susceptibility and implications for measurement. *International Journal of Clinical and Experimental Hypnosis, 30*, 394–403.

Hilgard, E. R. (1984). [Review of E. L. Rossi (Ed.), *The collected papers of Milton H. Erickson on hypnosis, by Milton H. Erickson*]. *International Journal of Clinical and Experimental Hypnosis, 32*, 257–265.

Hilgard, E. R. (1988). Milton Erickson as playwright and director. *International Journal of Clinical and Experimental Hypnosis, 36*, 128–140.

Hilgard, J. R. (1979). *Personality and hypnosis: A study of imaginative involvement* (2nd ed.). Chicago: University of Chicago Press.

Hilgard, J. R., & LeBaron, S. (1982). Relief of anxiety and pain in children and adolescents with cancer: Quantitative measures and clinical observations. *International Journal of Clinical and Experimental Hypnosis, 30*, 417–442.

Hillyard, S. A., & Woods, D. L. (1979). Electrophysiological analysis of human brain function. In M. S. Gazzaniga (Ed.), *Handbook of behavioral neurobiology: Vol. 2. Neuropsychology* (pp. 345–378). New York: Plenum Press.

Hink, R. F., & Hillyard, S. A. (1978). Electrophysiological measures of attentional processes in man as related to the study of schizophrenia. *Journal of Psychiatric Research, 14*, 155–165.

Hobson, J. A., & McCarley, R. W. (1977). The brain as a dream state generator: An activation-synthesis hypothesis of the dream process. *American Journal of Psychiatry, 134*, 1335–1348.

Hobson, J. A., Lydic, R., & Baghdoyan, H. A. (1986). Evolving concepts of sleep cycle generation: From brain centers to neuronal populations. *Behavioral and Brain Sciences, 9,* 371–448.

Hobson, J. A. (1988). *The dreaming brain.* New York: Basic Books.

Hofer, M. A. (1981). *The roots of human behavior.* San Francisco: W. H. Freeman.

Hofer, M. A. (1984). Relationships as regulators: A psychobiologic perspective on bereavement. *Psychosomatic Medicine, 46,* 183–197.

Hofstadter, D. R. (1979). *Gödel, Escher, Bach: An eternal golden brain.* New York: Basic Books.

Hogan, M., MacDonald, J., & Olness, K. (1982, August). *Effect of hypnosis on brainstem auditory evoked response.* Paper presented at the International Society of Hypnosis, 9th International Congress of Hypnosis and Psychosomatic Medicine, Glasgow, Scotland.

Holloway, F. (1978). State-dependent retrieval based on time of day. In B. Ho, D. Richards, & D. Chute (Eds.), *Drug discrimination and state-dependent learning* (pp. 319–343). New York: Academic Press.

Holmes, J. D., Hekmat, H., & Mozingo, B. S. (1983). Cognitive and behavioral regulation of pain: The facilitative effects of analgesic suggestions. *Psychological Record, 33,* 151–159.

Holroyd, J. C., Nuechterlein, K. H., Shapiro, D., & Ward, F. (1982). Individual differences in hypnotizability and effectiveness of hypnosis and biofeedback. *International Journal of Clinical and Experimental Hypnosis, 30,* 45–65.

Holtzman, J. D., & Gazzaniga, M. S. (1982). Dual task interactions due exclusively to limits in processing resources. *Science, 218,* 1325–1327.

Hopkins, M. B., Jordan, J. M., & Lundy, R. M. (1988, November). *A procedure for testing the effect of hypnosis and imagery on bleeding time.* Paper presented at the Annual Meeting of the Society for Clinical and Experimental Hypnosis, Asheville, NC.

Horne, J. A., & Whitehead, M. (1976). Ultradian and other rhythms in human respiration rate. *Experientia, 32,* 1165–1167.

Horowitz, M. J. (1986). *Stress response syndromes* (2nd ed.). Northvale, NJ: Jason Aronson.

Horowitz, M. J. (1987). *States of mind: Configurational analysis of individual psychology* (2nd ed.). New York: Plenum Medical Book.

Horton, D. J., Suda, W. L., Kinsman, R. A., Souhrada, J., & Spector, S. L. (1977). *Bronchoconstrictive suggestion in asthma: A role for airways in hyperactivity and emotions.* Unpublished manuscript. National Jewish Hospital and Research Center, Tel Aviv, Israel.

Horvath, T., Friedman, J., & Meares, R. (1980). Attention in hysteria: A study of Janet's hypothesis by means of habituation and arousal measures. *American Journal of Psychiatry, 137,* 217–220.

Howell, P., Cross, I., & West, R. (Eds.). (1985). *Musical structure and cognition.* Orlando, FL: Academic Press.

Hoyt, I. P., Nadon, R., Register, P. A., Chorny, J., Fleeson, W., Grigorian, E. M.,

& Otto, L. (1989). Daydreaming, absorption, and hypnotizability. *International Journal of Clinical and Experimental Hypnosis, 37,* 332–342.

Humphrey, N. (1984). *Consciousness regained: Chapters in the development of mind.* Oxford: Oxford University Press.

Hunn, E. S. (1977). *Tzeltal folk zoology: The classification of discontinuities in nature.* New York: Academic Press.

Hutchings, D. F., & Reinking, R. H. (1976). Tension headaches: What form of therapy is most effective? *Biofeedback and Self-Regulation, 1,* 183–190.

Hyman, S. E. (1988a). Recent developments in neurobiology: Part I. Synaptic transmission. *Psychosomatics, 29,* 157–165.

Hyman, S. E. (1988b). Recent developments in neurobiology: Part II. Neurotransmitter receptors and psychopharmacology. *Psychosomatics, 29,* 254–262.

Ikemi, A., Tomita, S., Kuroda, M., Hayashida, Y., & Ikemi, Y. (1986). Self-regulation method: Psychological, physiological and clinical considerations: An overview. *Psychotherapy and Psychosomatics, 46,* 184–195.

Ikemi, A. (1988). Psychophysiological effects of self-regulation method: EEG frequency analysis and contingent negative variations. *Psychotherapy and Psychosomatics, 49,* 230–239.

Ishihara, T., & Yoshii, N. (1972). Multivariate analytic study of EEG and mental activity in juvenile delinquents. *Electroencephalography and Clinical Neurophysiology, 33,* 71–80.

Ishihara, T., & Yoshii, N. (1973). Theta rhythm in the mid-frontal region during mental work. *Electroencephalography and Clinical Neurophysiology, 35,* 701.

Izard, C. E. (1990). Facial expressions and the regulation of emotions. *Journal of Personality and Social Psychology, 58,* 487–498.

Jackson, J. A., Gass, G. C., & Camp, E. M. (1979). The relationship between posthypnotic suggestion and endurance in physically trained subjects. *International Journal of Clinical and Experimental Hypnosis, 27,* 278–293.

James, L., Singer, A., Zurynski, Y., Gordon, E., Kraiuhin, C., Harris, A., Howson, A., & Meares, R. (1987). Evoked response potentials and regional cerebral blood flow in somatization disorder. *Psychotherapy and Psychosomatics, 47,* 190–196.

James, W. (1890). *The principles of psychology.* Cambridge, MA: Harvard University Press, 1983.

Jarvis, M. J., & Ettlinger, G. (1978). Cross-modal performance in monkeys and apes: Is there a substantial difference? In D. J. Chivers & J. Herbert (Eds.), *Recent advances in primatology* (Vol. 1, pp. 953–956). New York: Academic Press.

Jay, S. M., Elliott, C., & Varni, J. W. (1986). Acute and chronic pain in adults and children with cancer. *Journal of Consulting and Clinical Psychology, 54,* 601–607.

Jeannerod, M. (1985). *The brain machine: The development of neurophysiological thought* (D. Urion, Trans.). Cambridge, MA: Harvard University Press.

Jellinek, M. S., Goldenheim, P. D., & Jenike, M. A. (1985). The impact of grief on ventilatory control. *American Journal of Psychiatry, 142,* 121–123.

Jerison, H. (1975). The evolution of brain and intelligence: A current anthropology book review. *Current Anthropology, 16,* 403–426.

Jessup, B. A., Neufeld, R. W. J., & Merskey, H. (1979). Biofeedback therapy for headache and other pain: An evaluative review. *Pain, 7,* 225–270.

Johanson, D. C., & Edey, M. A. (1981). *Lucy: The beginnings of humankind.* New York: Simon & Schuster.

Johnson, L. S. (1981). Current research in self-hypnotic phenomenology: The Chicago paradigm. *International Journal of Clinical and Experimental Hypnosis, 29,* 247–258.

Johnson, M. (1987). *The body in the mind: The bodily basis of meaning, imagination, and reason.* Chicago: University of Chicago Press.

Jolly, A. (1983). *The evolution of primate behavior* (2nd ed.). New York: Macmillan.

Joralemon, D. (1984). The role of hallucinogenic drugs and sensory stimuli in Peruvian ritual healing. *Culture, Medicine and Psychiatry, 8,* 399–430.

Josiassen, R. C., Shagass, C., Roemer, R. A., Slepner, S., & Czartorysky, B. (1990). Early cognitive components of somatosensory event-related potentials. *International Journal of Psychophysiology, 9,* 139–149.

Juurmaa, J., & Lehtinen-Railo, S. (1988). Cross-modal transfer of forms between vision and touch. *Scandinavian Journal of Psychology, 29,* 95–110.

Kahneman, D., & Tversky, A. (1982). The simulation heuristic. In D. Kahneman et al. (Eds.), *Judgment under uncertainty: Heuristics and biases.* New York: Cambridge University Press.

Kandel, E., & Schwartz, J. (1982). Molecular biology of learning: Modulation of transmitter release. *Science, 218,* 433–443.

Kane, F. J., Jr., Harper, R. G., & Wittels, E. (1988). Angina as a symptom of psychiatric illness. *Southern Medical Journal, 81,* 1412–1416.

Kaplan, J. R., Manuck, S. B., Clarkson, T. B., Lusso, F. M., Taub, D. M., & Miller, E. W. (1983). Social stress and atherosclerosis in normocholesterolemic monkeys. *Science, 220,* 733–735.

Karlin, R. A., Goldstein, L., Cohen, A., & Morgan, D. (1980, September). *Quantitated EEG, hypnosis and hypnotizability.* Paper presented at the Annual Meeting of the American Psychological Association, Montreal, Canada.

Karlin, R. A., Goldstein, L., Cohen, A., Morgan, D., & Berman, A. (1981). *Attention, imagination and brain function.* Paper presented at American Association for the Study of Mental Imagery, Yale University, New Haven, CT.

Karmiloff-Smith, A. (1986). From meta-processes to conscious access: Evidence from children's metalinguistic and repair data. *Cognition, 23,* 95–147.

Katkin, E. S. (1985). Blood, sweat, and tears: Individual differences in autonomic self-perception. *Psychophysiology, 22,* 125–137.

Katz, R. (1982). *Boiling energy: Community healing among the Kalahari Kung.* Cambridge, MA: Harvard University Press.

Katz, R. J. (1980). The temporal structure of motivation. III. Identification and ecological significance of ultradian rhythms of intracranial reinforcement. *Behavioral and Neural Biology, 30,* 148–159.

Kay, P., & McDaniel, C. (1978). The linguistic significance of the meanings of basic color terms. *Language, 54,* 610–646.

Kendon, A. (1982). Coordination of action and framing in face-to-face interaction. In M. Davis (Ed.), *Interaction rhythms: Periodicity in communicative behavior* (pp. 351–363). New York: Human Sciences Press.

Kendon, A. (1984). Did gesture have the happiness to escape the curse at the confusion of Babel? In A. Wolfgang (Ed.), *Nonverbal behavior: Perspectives, applications, intercultural insights* (pp. 75–114). Toronto: C. J. Hogrefe.

Kennedy, B., Ziegler, M., & Shannahoff-Khalsa, D. (1986). Alternating lateralization of plasma catecholamines and nasal patency in humans. *Life Sciences, 38,* 1203–1214.

Kenny, M. G. (1986). *The passion of Ansel Bourne: Multiple personality in American culture.* Washington, DC: Smithsonian Institution Press.

Kerr, N. H. (1987). Locational representation in imagery: The third dimension. *Memory and Cognition, 15,* 521–530.

Kihlstrom, J. F., Brenneman, H. A., Pistole, D. D., & Shor, R. E. (1985). Hypnosis as a retrieval cue in posthypnotic amnesia. *Journal of Abnormal Psychology, 94,* 264–271.

Kihlstrom, J. F. (1987). The cognitive unconscious. *Science, 237,* 1445–1452.

Kingsbury, S. J. (1988). Hypnosis in the treatment of posttraumatic stress disorder: An isomorphic intervention. *American Journal of Clinical Hypnosis, 31,* 81–90.

Kinney, J. M., & Sachs, L. B. (1974). Increasing hypnotic susceptibility. *Journal of Abnormal Psychology, 83,* 145–150.

Kinsbourne, M., & Bruce, R. (1987). Shift in visual laterality within blocks of trials. *Acta Psychologica, 66,* 139–155.

Kirmayer, L. J. (1988). Word magic and the rhetoric of common sense: Erickson's metaphors for mind. *International Journal of Clinical and Experimental Hypnosis, 36,* 157–172.

Kirsch, I., Council, J. R., & Mobayed, C. (1987). Imagery and response expectancy as determinants of hypnotic behavior. *British Journal of Experimental and Clinical Hypnosis, 4,* 25–31.

Kissin, B. (1986). *Psychobiology of human behavior: Vol. 1. Conscious and unconscious programs in the brain.* New York: Plenum Medical Book.

Klein, G. A., & Brezovic, C. P. (1986). Design engineers and the design process: Decision strategies and human factors literature. In *Proceedings of the 30th Annual Meeting of the Human Factors Society* (Vol. 2, pp. 771–775). Dayton, OH: Human Factors Society.

Klein, G. A. (1987). Applications of analogical reasoning. *Metaphor and Symbolic Activity, 2,* 201–218.

Klein, K. B., & Spiegel, D. (1989). Modulation of gastric acid secretion by hypnosis. *Gastroenterology, 96,* 1383–1387.

Klein, R. M., & Armitage, R. (1979). Rhythms in human performance: 1½ hour oscillations in cognitive style. *Science, 204,* 1326–1328.

Klein, R., Pilon, D., Prosser, S., & Shannahoff-Khalsa, D. (1986). Nasal airflow asymmetries and human performance. *Biological Psychology, 23,* 127–137.

Kleinke, C. L. (1986). Gaze and eye contact: A research review. *Psychological Bulletin, 100,* 78–100.

Kleitman, N. (1961). The nature of dreaming. In G. E. W. Wolstenholme & M. O'Connor (Eds.), *The nature of sleep* (p. 349). London: Churchill.

Kleitman, N. (1982). Basic rest-activity cycle—22 years later. *Sleep, 5,* 311–317.

Kluft, R. P. (1984). Treatment of multiple personality disorder: A study of 33 cases. In B. G. Braun (Ed.), *Symposium on multiple personality, psychiatric clinics of North America, 7,* 9–29.

Kluft, R. P. (1985). The natural history of multiple personality disorder. In R. P. Kluft (Ed.), *Childhood antecedents of multiple personality.* Washington, DC: American Psychiatric Press.

Kluft, R. (1987). Making the diagnosis of multiple personality disorder. In F. Flach (Ed.), *Diagnostics and psychopathology.* New York: W. W. Norton.

Knutsson, E., & Mårtensson, A. (1985). Isokinetic measurements of muscle strength in hysterical paresis. *Electroencephalography and Clinical Neurophysiology, 61,* 370–374.

Koe, G. G., & Oldridge, O. A. (1987). An experimental investigation of the interaction between hypnotic responsiveness and type of esteem suggestion on self-concept. *American Journal of Clinical Hypnosis, 30,* 44–50.

Kolb, L. C. (1987). A neuropsychological hypothesis explaining posttraumatic stress disorders. *American Journal of Psychiatry, 144,* 989–995.

Kolb, L. C. (1988). Recovery of memory and repressed fantasy in combat-induced post-traumatic stress disorder of Vietnam veterans. In H. M. Pettinati (Ed.), *Hypnosis and memory* (pp. 265–274). New York: Guilford Press.

Kosslyn, S. M. (1981). The medium and the message in mental imagery: A theory. *Psychological Review, 88,* 46–66.

Kosslyn, S. M. (1987). Seeing and imagining in the cerebral hemispheres: A computational approach. *Psychological Review, 94,* 148–175.

Kotses, H., Rawson, J. C., Wigal, J. K., & Creer, T. L. (1987). Respiratory airway changes in response to suggestion in normal individuals. *Psychosomatic Medicine, 49,* 536–541.

Kramer, M., Lindy, J., van der Kolk, B., Hartmann, E., Kinney, L., & Scharf, M. (1986). *Post-traumatic stress syndrome: Current research.* Paper presented at the Annual Meeting of the American Psychiatric Association.

Kramer, M., Kinney, L., & Schoen, L. S. (1989, May). *Vigilance during sleep in*

PTSD. Paper presented at the Annual Meeting of the American Psychiatric Association, San Francisco.

Kripke, D. F. (1972). An ultradian biological rhythm associated with perceptual deprivation and REM sleep. *Psychosomatic Medicine, 3,* 221–234.

Kripke, D. F., & Sonnenschein, D. (1978). A biologic rhythm in waking fantasy. In K. S. Pope & J. L. Singer (Eds.), *The stream of consciousness: Scientific investigations into the flow of human experience* (pp. 321–332). New York: Plenum Press.

Kripke, D. F. (1982). Ultradian rhythms in behavior and physiology. In F. Brown & R. Graeber (Eds.), *Rhythmic aspects of behavior* (pp. 313–344). Hillsdale, NJ: Erlbaum.

Kroger, R. O. (1988). The social nature of hypnosis: An ethogenic analysis of hypnotic pain reduction. *New Ideas in Psychology, 6,* 47–66.

Kroger, W. S. (1977). *Clinical and experimental hypnosis* (2nd ed.). Philadelphia: J. B. Lippincott.

Krystal, J. H., Southwick, S. M., & Charney, D. S. (1990, May). *Yohimbine effects in PTSD patients*. Paper presented at the Annual Meeting of the American Psychiatric Association, New York.

Kumar, D., & Wingate, D. L. (1985, November 2). The irritable bowel syndrome: A paroxysmal motor disorder. *Lancet,* pp. 973–977.

Kumar, V. K., & Pekala, R. J. (1988). Hypnotizability, absorption, and individual differences in phenomenological experience. *International Journal of Clinical and Experimental Hypnosis, 36,* 80–88.

Kunst-Wilson, W. R., & Zajonc, R. B. (1980). Affective discrimination of stimuli that cannot be recognized. *Science, 207,* 557–558.

Kunzendorf, R. G., Lacourse, P., & Lynch, B. (1986–1987). Hypnotic hyperamnesia for subliminally encoded stimuli: State-dependent memory for "unmonitored sensations." *Imagination, Cognition and Personality, 6,* 365–378.

Kurtén, B. (1984). *Not from the apes: A history of man's origins and evolution*. New York: Columbia University Press.

Kuttner, L. (1988). Favorite stories: A hypnotic pain-reduction technique for children in acute pain. *American Journal of Clinical Hypnosis, 30,* 289–295.

LaBaw, W. L. (1975). Auto-hypnosis in haemophilia. *Haematologia, 9,* 103–110.

LaBerge, S. (1985). *Lucid dreaming: The power of being awake and aware in your dreams*. Los Angeles: Jeremy P. Tarcher.

LaBriola, F., Karlin, R., & Goldstein, L. (1987). EEG laterality changes from prehypnotic to hypnotic periods: Preliminary results. *Advances in Biological Psychiatry, 16,* 1–5.

Lacey, B. C., & Lacey, J. I. (1980). Cognitive modulation of time-dependent primary bradycardia. *Psychophysiology, 17,* 209–221.

Lachnit, H. (1989). Indirect suggestion as a research tool. In V. A. Gheorghiu, P. Netter, H. J. Eysenck, & R. Rosenthal (Eds.), *Suggestion and suggestibility: Theory and research* (pp. 347–350). New York: Springer-Verlag.

LaFrance, M. (1982). Posture mirroring and rapport. In M. Davis (Ed.), *Interaction rhythms: Periodicity in communicative behavior* (pp. 279–297). New York: Human Sciences Press.

Laitman, J. T., Heimbuch, R. C., & Crelin, E. S. (1979). The basicranium of fossil hominids as an indicator of their upper respiratory systems. *American Journal of Physical Anthropology, 51,* 15–34.

Lakoff, G., & Johnson, M. (1980). *Metaphors we live by.* Chicago: University of Chicago Press.

Lakoff, G. (1987). *Women, fire, and dangerous things: What categories reveal about the mind.* Chicago: University of Chicago Press.

Lakoff, G., & Turner, M. (1989). *More than cool reason: A field guide to poetic metaphor.* Chicago: University of Chicago Press.

Lambek, M. (1981). *Human spirits: A cultural account of trance in Mayotte.* Cambridge: Cambridge University Press.

Lancet (1984, December 1). Editorial: An irritable mind or an irritable bowel? *Lancet,* pp. 1249–1250.

Landau, T. (1989). *About faces.* New York: Anchor Books.

Lane, R. D., & Schwartz, G. E. (1987). Levels of emotional awareness: A cognitive-developmental theory and its application to psychopathology. *American Journal of Psychiatry, 144,* 133–143.

Lang, P. J., Kozak, M. J., Miller, G. A., Levin, D. N., & McLean, A., Jr. (1980). Emotional imagery: Conceptual structure and pattern of somato-visceral response. *Psychophysiology, 17,* 179–192.

Lange, H. (1982). EEG spectral analysis in vital depression: Ultradian cycles. *Biological Psychiatry, 17,* 3–21.

Langer, S. (1970). *Mind: An essay on human feeling* (Vol. 1). Baltimore: Johns Hopkins University Press.

Lankton, S. R., & Lankton, C. H. (1983). *The answer within: A clinical framework of Ericksonian hypnotherapy.* New York: Brunner/Mazel.

Lanzetta, J. T., Cartwright-Smith, J., & Kleck, R. E. (1976). Effects of nonverbal dissimulation on emotional experience and autonomic arousal. *Journal of Personality and Social Psychology, 33,* 354–370.

Latimer, P. R. (1983). *Functional gastrointestinal disorders: A behavioral medicine approach.* New York: Springer-Verlag.

Laurence, J.-R., & Perry, C. (1983). Hypnotically created memory among highly hypnotizable subjects. *Science, 222,* 523–524.

Laurence, J.-R., & Nadon, R. (1986a). Reports of hypnotic depth: Are they more than mere words? *International Journal of Clinical and Experimental Hypnosis, 34,* 215–233.

Laurence, J.-R., Nadon, R., Nogrady, H., & Perry, C. (1986b). Duality, dissociation, and memory creation in highly hypnotizable subjects. *International Journal of Clinical and Experimental Hypnosis, 34,* 295–310.

Lavie, P., & Kripke, D. F. (1981). Ultradian circa 1½ hour rhythms: A multioscillatory system. *Life Sciences, 29,* 2445–2450.

Lavie, P. (1985). Ultradian rhythms: Gates of sleep and wakefulness. *Experimental Brain Research, Suppl. 12,* 148–164.

LeDoux, J. E. (1982). Neuroevolutionary mechanisms of cerebral asymmetry in man. *Brain, Behavior and Evolution, 20,* 197–213.

Legewie, H., Simonova, O., & Creutzfeldt, O. D. (1969). EEG changes during performance of various tasks under open- and closed-eye conditions. *Electroencephalography and Clinical Neurophysiology, 27,* 470–479.

Lerer, B., Ebstein, R. P., Shestatsky, M., Shemesh, Z., & Greenberg, D. (1987). Cyclic AMP signal transduction in posttraumatic stress disorder. *American Journal of Psychiatry, 144,* 1324–1326.

Lerer, B., Bleich, A., & Ebstein, R. P. (1990, May). *Cyclic AMP signal transduction in PTSD.* Paper presented at the Annual Meeting of the American Psychiatric Association, New York.

Levenson, R. W., & Ditto, W. B. (1981). Individual differences in ability to control heart rate: Personality, strategy, physiological, and other variables. *Psychophysiology, 18,* 91–100.

Levenson, R. W., Ekman, P., & Friesen, W. V. (1990). Voluntary facial action generates emotion-specific autonomic nervous system activity. *Psychophysiology, 27,* 363–384.

Levin, B., Rappaport, M., & Natelson, B. (1979). Ultradian variations in plasma noradrenaline in humans. *Life Science, 25,* 621–627.

Levine, J. L., Kurtz, R. M., & Lauter, J. L. (1984). Hypnosis and its effects on left and right hemisphere activity. *Biological Psychiatry, 19,* 1461–1475.

Lewicki, P. (1986). *Nonconscious social information processing.* Orlando, FL: Academic Press.

Lewicki, P., & Hill, T. (1987). Unconscious processes as explanations of behavior in cognitive, personality, and social psychology. *Personality and Social Psychology Bulletin, 13,* 355–362.

Lewin, R. (1984). DNA reveals surprises in human family tree: The application of DNA-DNA hybridization to relationships among hominoids places humans with the chimps, while gorillas are separate. *Science, 226,* 1179–1182.

Lewis, I. M. (1989). *Ecstatic religion: A study of shamanism and spirit possession* (2nd ed.). London: Routledge.

Lewis, J. L. (1970). Semantic processing of unattended messages using dichotic listening. *Journal of Experimental Psychology, 85,* 225–228.

Lewis, J. W., Cannon, J. T., & Liebeskind, J. C. (1980). Opioid and nonopioid mechanisms of stress analgesia. *Science, 208,* 623–625.

Lewis, M., Mishkin, M., Bragin, E., Brown, R., Pert, C., & Peert, A. (1981). Opiate receptor gradients in monkey cerebral cortex: Correspondence with sensory processing hierarchies. *Science, 211,* 1166.

Libet, B. (1985). Unconscious cerebral initiative and the role of conscious will in voluntary action. *Behavioral and Brain Sciences, 8,* 529–566.

Lieberman, P. (1984). *The biology and evolution of language.* Cambridge, MA: Harvard University Press.

Liederman, J., Merola, J., & Martinez, S. (1985). Interhemispheric collaboration in response to simultaneous bilateral input. *Neuropsychologia, 23*, 673–683.

Light, K. C., Koepke, J. P., Obrist, P. A., & Willis, P. W. IV. (1983). Psychological stress induces sodium and fluid retention in men at high risk for hypertension. *Science, 220*, 429–431.

Light, P. (1979). *The development of social sensitivity*. Cambridge: Cambridge University Press.

Linden, W. (1987). A microanalysis of autonomic activity during human speech. *Psychosomatic Medicine, 49*, 562–578.

Lipman, L. S. (1985). *Hypnotizability and multiple personality*. Paper presented at the Annual Meeting of the American Psychiatric Association, Dallas.

Loewenstein, R. J., Hamilton, J., Alagna, S., Reid, N., & deVries, M. (1987). Experiential sampling in the study of multiple personality disorder. *American Journal of Psychiatry, 144*, 19–24.

Logan, R. K. (1986). *The alphabet effect: The impact of the phonetic alphabet on the development of Western civilization*. New York: William Morrow.

Lomax, A. (1982). The cross-cultural variation of rhythmic style. In M. Davis (Ed.), *Interaction rhythms: Periodicity in communicative behavior* (pp. 149–174). New York: Human Sciences Press.

Longuet-Higgins, H. C. (1979). The perception of music. *Proceedings of the Royal Society London, B205*, 307–322.

Lord, A. B. (1960). *The singer of tales*. Cambridge, MA: Harvard University Press.

Lown, B. (1982, May). *Psychophysiologic and biobehavioral factors and sudden death*. Paper presented at the Annual Meeting of the American Psychiatric Association, Toronto, Ontario.

Lum, L. C. (1983). Physiological considerations in the treatment of hyperventilation syndromes. *Journal of Drug Research, 8*, 1867–1872.

Luria, A. R. (1973). *The working brain: An introduction to neuropsychology*. Harmondsworth: Penguin Books.

Luria, A. R. (1976). *Cognitive development: Its cultural and social foundations* (M. Cole, Ed., and M. Lopez-Morillas & L. Solotaroff, Trans.). Cambridge, MA: Harvard University Press.

Lusebrink, V. B. (1987). Visual imagery: Its psychophysiological components and levels of information processing. *Imagination, Cognition and Personality, 6*, 205–218.

Lyles, J. N., Burish, T. G., Krozely, M. G., & Oldham, R. K. (1982). Efficacy of relaxation training and guided imagery in reducing the aversiveness of cancer chemotherapy. *Journal of Consulting and Clinical Psychology, 50*, 509–524.

Lynch, J. J., Long, J. M., Thomas, S. A., Malinow, K. L., & Katcher, A. H. (1981). The effects of talking on the blood pressure of hypertensive and normotensive individuals. *Psychosomatic Medicine, 43*, 25–33.

Lynn, J. G., & Lynn, D. R. (1938). Face-hand laterality in relation to personality. *Journal of Abnormal and Social Psychology, 33*, 291–322.

Lynn, J. G., & Lynn, D. R. (1943). Smile and hand dominance in relation to basic modes of adaptation. *Journal of Abnormal and Social Psychology, 38*, 250–276.

Lynn, S. J., Neufeld, V., & Matyi, C. L. (1987a). Inductions versus suggestions: Effects of direct and indirect wording on hypnotic responding and experience. *Journal of Abnormal Psychology, 96*, 76–79.

Lynn, S. J., Snodgrass, M., Rhue, J. W., Nash, M. R., & Frauman, D. C. (1987b). Attributions, involuntariness, and hypnotic rapport. *American Journal of Clinical Hypnosis, 30*, 36–43.

Lynn, S. J., Rhue, J. W., & Weekes, J. R. (1990). Hypnotic involuntariness: A social cognitive analysis. *Psychological Review, 97*, 169–184.

MacLean, P. D. (1949). Psychosomatic disease and the "visceral brain": Recent developments bearing on the Papez theory of emotion. In L. A. Gottschalk, P. H. Knapp, M. F. Reiser, J. D. Sapira, & A. P. Shapiro (Eds.), *Psychosomatic classics: Selected papers from "Psychosomatic Medicine," 1939–1958*. Basel: S. Karger AG, 1972.

MacLeod-Morgan, C. (1979). Hypnotic susceptibility, EEG theta and alpha waves, and hemispheric specificity. In G. D. Burrows, D. R. Collison, & L. Dennerstein (Eds.), *Hypnosis 1979* (pp. 181–188). Amsterdam: Elsevier-North Holland.

MacLeod-Morgan, C., & Lack, L. (1982). Hemispheric specificity: A physiological concomitant of hypnotizability. *Psychophysiology, 19*, 687–690.

MacLeod-Morgan, C. (1985). Hemispheric specificity and hypnotizability: An overview of ongoing EEG research in South Australia. In D. Waxman, P. Mizra, M. Gibson, & M. Baker (Eds.), *Modern trends in hypnosis* (pp. 169–179). New York: Plenum Press.

Maher-Loughnan, G. P., MacDonald, N., Mason, A. A., & Fry, L. (1962). Controlled trial of hypnosis in the symptomatic treatment of asthma. *British Medical Journal, 2*, 371–376.

Maher-Loughnan, G. P. (1970). Hypnosis and autohypnosis for the treatment of asthma. *International Journal of Clinical and Experimental Hypnosis, 18*, 1–14.

Maher-Loughnan, G. P. (1984). Timing of clinical response to hypnotherapy. *Proceedings of the British Society of Medical and Dental Hypnosis, 5*, 15–16.

Maier, S. F. (1986). Stressor controllability and stress-induced analgesia. In D. D. Kelly (Ed.), *Stress-induced analgesia: Annals of the New York Academy of Sciences* (Vol. 467, pp. 55–72). New York: New York Academy of Sciences.

Malmstrom, E., Ekman, P., & Friesen, M. V. (1972). *Autonomic changes with facial displays of surprise and disgust*. Paper presented at the meeting of the Western Psychological Association, Portland, OR.

Malott, J. M., Bourg, A. L., & Crawford, H. J. (1989). The effects of hypnosis upon cognitive responses to persuasive communication. *International Journal of Clinical and Experimental Hypnosis, 37,* 31–40.

Mandell, A. J. (1980). Toward a psychobiology of transcendence: God in the brain. In J. M. Davidson & R. J. Davidson (Eds.), *The psychobiology of consciousness* (pp. 379–464). New York: Plenum Press.

Mandler, G. (1982). The structure of value: Accounting for taste. In M. S. Clark & S. T. Fiske (Eds.), *Affect and cognition: The 17th Carnegie Symposium on Cognition.* Hillsdale, NJ: Erlbaum.

Manseau, C., & Broughton, R. J. (1984). Bilaterally synchronous ultradian EEG rhythms in awake adult humans. *Psychophysiology, 21,* 265–273.

Marcel, A. J. (1980). Conscious and preconscious recognition of polysemous words: Locating the selective effects of prior verbal context. In R. S. Nickerson (Ed.), *Attention and Performance* (Vol. 8). Hillsdale, NJ: Erlbaum.

Marcel, A. J. (1983). Conscious and unconscious perception: Experiments on visual masking and word recognition. *Cognitive Psychology, 15,* 197–237.

Margules, D. L. (1979). Beta-endorphin and endoloxone: Hormones of the autonomic nervous system for the conservation or expenditure of bodily resources and energy in anticipation of famine or feast. *Neuroscience and Biobehavioral Reviews, 3,* 155–162.

Margulies, D. M. (1985). Selective attention and the brain: A hypothesis concerning the hippocampal-ventral striatal axis, the mediation of selective attention, and the pathogenesis of attentional disorders. *Medical Hypotheses, 18,* 221–264.

Marino, J., Gwynn, M. I., & Spanos, N. P. (1989). Cognitive mediators in the reduction of pain: The role of expectancy, strategy use, and self-presentation. *Journal of Abnormal Psychology, 98,* 256–262.

Marks, L. E. (1987a). On cross-modal similarity: Auditory-visual interactions in speeded discrimination. *Journal of Experimental Psychology: Human Perception and Performance, 13,* 384–394.

Marks, L. E. (1987b). On cross-modal similarity: Perceiving temporal patterns by hearing, touch, and vision. *Perception and Psychophysics, 42,* 250–256.

Marks, L. E., & Bornstein, M. C. (1987c). Sensory similarities: Classes, characteristics, and cognitive consequences. In R. E. Haskell (Ed.), *Cognition and symbolic structures: The psychology of metaphoric transformation* (pp. 49–65). Norwood, NJ: Ablex.

Marr, D. (1984). *Vision: A computational investigation into the human representation and processing of visual information.* New York: W. I. T. Freeman.

Mason, J. W., Giller, E. L., Kosten, T. R., Ostroff, R. B., & Podd, L. (1986). Urinary free-cortisol levels in posttraumatic stress disorder patients. *Journal of Nervous and Mental Disease, 174,* 145–149.

Mathew, R. J., Weinman, M. L., & Largen, J. W. (1982). Sympathetic-adrenomedullary activation in migraine. *Headache, 22,* 13–19.

Mathew, R. J., Weinman, M. L., & Barr, D. L. (1984). Personality and regional cerebral blood flow. *British Journal of Psychiatry, 144,* 529–532.

Mathiot, M., & Carlock, E. (1982). On operationalizing the notion of rhythm in social behavior. In M. Davis (Ed.), *Interaction rhythms: Periodicity in communicative behavior* (pp. 175–194). New York: Human Sciences Press.

Matthews, W. J., Bennett, H., Bean, W., & Gallagher, M. (1985). Indirect versus direct hypnotic suggestions—an initial investigation. *International Journal of Clinical and Experimental Hypnosis, 33,* 219–223.

Maxwell, M. (1984). *Human evolution: A philosophical anthropology.* New York: Columbia University Press.

Mayer, D. J., Price, D. D., Barber, J., & Rafii, A. (1976). Acupuncture analgesia: Evidence for activation of a pain inhibitory system as a mechanism of action. In J. J. Bonica & D. Albe-Fessard (Eds.), *Advances in pain research and therapy* (Vol. 1). New York: Raven Press.

Mayr, E. (1982). *The growth of biological thought: Diversity, evolution, and inheritance.* Cambridge, MA: Belknap Press of Harvard University Press.

McCabe, A. (1980). *A rhetoric of metaphor.* Unpublished doctoral dissertation, University of Virginia, Charlottesville.

McCabe, A. (1983). Conceptual similarity and the quality of metaphor in isolated sentences versus extended contexts. *Journal of Psycholinguistic Research, 12,* 67–94.

McCabe, A. (1988). Effect of different contexts on memory for metaphor. *Metaphor and Symbolic Activity, 3,* 105–132.

McCarley, R. W. (1982). REM sleep and depression: Common neurobiological control mechanisms. *American Journal of Psychiatry, 139,* 565–570.

McCarley, R. W., & Massaquoi, S. (1985). The REM sleep ultradian rhythm: A limit cycle mathematical model. *Experimental Brain Research, Suppl. 12,* 288–308.

McCaul, K. D., & Malott, J. M. (1984). Distraction and coping with pain. *Psychological Bulletin, 95,* 516–533.

McCown, W., Johnson, J., & Austin, S. (1986). Inability of delinquents to recognize facial affects. *Journal of Social Behavior and Personality, 1,* 489–496.

McCue, P. A. (1988). Milton H. Erickson: A critical perspective. In M. Heap (Ed.), *Hypnosis: Current clinical, experimental and forensic practices* (pp. 257–267). London: Croom Helm.

McFall, M. E., Murburg, M. M., Veith, R. C., & Roszell, D. R. (1990, May). *Psychophysiologic investigations of PTSD.* Paper presented at the Annual Meeting of the American Psychiatric Association, New York.

McGlashan, T., Evans, F., & Orne, M. (1969). The nature of hypnotic analgesia and placebo response to experimental pain. *Psychosomatic Medicine, 311,* 227–246.

McLuhan, M. (1969). *The Gutenberg galaxy: The making of typographic man.* New York: New American Library.

McMullen, L. M. (1989). Use of figurative language in successful and unsuccessful cases of psychotherapy: Three comparisons. *Metaphor and Symbolic Activity, 4,* 203–225.

McNeill, D. (1985). So you think gestures are nonverbal? *Psychological Review, 92,* 350–371.

Means, J. R., Wilson, G. L., & Dlugokinski, L. J. (1986–1987). Self-initiated imaginal and cognitive components: Evaluation of differential effectiveness in altering unpleasant moods. *Imagination, Cognition and Personality, 6,* 219–230.

Mehrabian, A., & Ferris, S. R. (1967). Inference of attitudes from nonverbal communication in two channels. *Journal of Consulting Psychology, 31,* 248–252.

Melzack, R., & Wall, P. (1982). *The challenge of pain.* Harmondsworth: Penguin Books.

Menzel, E. W., Jr., & Halperin, S. (1975). Purposive behavior as a basis for objective communication between chimpanzees. *Science, 189,* 652–654.

Mesulam, M.-M., & Geschwind, N. (1978). On the possible role of neocortex and its limbic connections in the process of attention in schizophrenia: Clinical cases of inattention in man and experimental anatomy in monkey. *Journal of Psychiatric Research, 14,* 249–259.

Mesulam, M.-M. (1981). Dissociative states with abnormal temporal lobe EEG: Multiple personality and the illusion of possession. *Archives of Neurology, 38,* 176–181.

Mesulam, M.-M. (1983). The functional anatomy and hemispheric specialization for directed attention: The role of the parietal lobe and its connectivity. *Trends in NeuroSciences, 6,* 384–387.

Mesulam, M.-M. (1985). (Ed.), *Principles of behavioral neurology.* Philadelphia: F. A. Davis.

Mészáros, I., Bányai, E. I., & Greguss, A. C. (1985). Evoked potential correlates of verbal versus imagery coding in hypnosis. In D. Waxman, P. Mizra, M. Gibson, & M. Baker (Eds.), *Modern trends in hypnosis* (pp. 161–168). New York: Plenum.

Mészáros, I., Crawford, H. J., Szabó, C., Nagy-Kovács, A., & Révész, Z. (1989). Hypnotic susceptibility and cerebral hemisphere preponderance: Verbal-imaginal discrimination task. In V. A. Gheorghiu, P. Netter, H. J. Eysenck, & R. Rosenthal (Eds.), *Suggestion and suggestibility: Theory and research* (pp. 191–203). New York: Springer-Verlag.

Miller, L. S., & Cross, H. J. (1985). Hypnotic susceptibility, hypnosis, and EMG biofeedback in the reduction of frontalis muscle tension. *International Journal of Clinical and Experimental Hypnosis, 33,* 258–272.

Miller, M. E., & Bowers, K. S. (1986). Hypnotic analgesia and stress inoculation in the reduction of pain. *Journal of Abnormal Psychology, 95,* 6–14.

Miller, S. D. (1989). Optical differences in cases of multiple personality disorder. *Journal of Nervous and Mental Disease, 177,* 480–486.

Minsky, M. (1986). *The society of mind.* New York: Simon & Schuster.

Mitchell, G. P., & Lundy, R. M. (1986). The effects of suggestions and imagery inductions on responses to suggestions. *International Journal of Clinical and Experimental Hypnosis, 34,* 98–109.

Molfese, D. L., Buhrke, R. A., & Wang, S. L. (1985). The right hemisphere and temporal processing of consonant transition durations: Electrophysiological correlates. *Brain and Language, 26,* 49–62.

Moore-Ede, M. C., Sulzman, F. M., & Fuller, C. A. (1982). *The clocks that time us: Physiology of the circadian timing system.* Cambridge, MA: Harvard University Press.

Morais, J., Castro, S. L., Scliar-Cabral, L., Kolinsky, R., & Content, A. (1987). The effects of literacy on the recognition of dichotic words. *Quarterly Journal of Experimental Psychology, 39A,* 451–465.

Morrison, J. B. (1988). Chronic asthma and improvement with relaxation induced by hypnotherapy. *Journal of the Royal Society of Medicine, 81,* 701–704.

Moscovitch, M. (1979). Information processing and the cerebral hemispheres. In M. S. Gazzaniga (Ed.), *Handbook of behavioral neurobiology: Vol. 2. Neuropsychology* (pp. 379–446). New York: Plenum Press.

Moscovitch, M., & Olds, J. (1982). Asymmetries in spontaneous facial expressions and their possible relation to hemispheric specialization. *Neuropsychologia, 20,* 71–81.

Mott, T., & Roberts, J. (1979). Obesity and hypnosis: A review of the literature. *American Journal of Clinical Hypnosis, 22,* 3–7.

Mueser, K. T., & Butler, R. W. (1987). Auditory hallucinations in combat-related chronic posttraumatic stress disorder. *American Journal of Psychiatry, 144,* 299–302.

Mundy-Castle, A. C. (1951). Theta and beta in the electroencephalogram of normal adults. *Electroencephalography and Clinical Neurophysiology, 3,* 477–486.

Murburg, M. M., McFall, M. E., Veith, R. C., & Ko, G. N. (1990, May). *Plasma catecholamine response to stressors in PTSD.* Paper presented at the Annual Meeting of the American Psychiatric Association, New York.

Murray, E. A., & Mishkin, M. (1985). Amygdalectomy impairs crossmodal association in monkeys. *Science, 228,* 604–606.

Nadon, R., Laurence, J.-R., & Perry, C. (1987). Multiple predictors of hypnotic susceptibility. *Journal of Personality and Social Psychology, 53,* 948–960.

Nash, M., Lynn, S., & Givens, D. (1984). Adult hypnotic susceptibility, childhood punishment, and child abuse. *International Journal of Clinical and Experimental Hypnosis, 32,* 6–11.

Nash, M. R., & Lynn, S. J. (1986). Child abuse and hypnotic ability. *Imagery, Cognition, and Personality, 5,* 211–218.

Nash, M. R., Lynn, S. J., Stanley, S., & Carlson, V. (1987). Subjectively complete hypnotic deafness and auditory priming. *International Journal of Clinical and Experimental Hypnosis, 35,* 32–40.

Neff, D. F., Blanchard, E. B., & Andrasik, F. (1983). The relationship between capacity for absorption and chronic headache patient's response to relaxation and biofeedback treatment. *Biofeedback and Self-regulation, 8,* 177–183.

Neisser, U. (1976). *Cognition and reality: Principles and implications of cognitive psychology.* San Francisco: W. H. Freeman.

Neubauer, A., Schulter, G., & Pfurtscheller, G. (1988). Lateral eye movements as an indication of hemispheric preference: An EEG validation study. *International Journal of Psychophysiology, 6,* 177–184.

Nielsen, S. L., & Sarason, I. G. (1981). Emotion, personality, and selective attention. *Journal of Personality and Social Psychology, 41,* 945–960.

Nisbett, R. E., & Wilson, T. D. (1977). Telling more than we know: Verbal reports on mental processes. *Psychological Review, 84,* 231–259.

Nisbett, R. E., & Ross, L. D. (1980). *Human inference: Strategies and shortcomings.* Englewood Cliffs, NJ: Prentice-Hall.

Nolan, R. P., & Spanos, N. P. (1987). Hypnotic analgesia and stress inoculation: A critical reexamination of Miller and Bowers. *Psychological Reports, 61,* 95–102.

Nowicki, S., Jr., & Hartigan, M. (1988). Accuracy of facial affect recognition as a function of locus of control orientation and anticipated interpersonal interaction. *Journal of Social Psychology, 128*(3), 363–372.

Oakley, M. T., & Eason, R. G. (1990). Subcortical gating in the human visual system during spatial selective attention. *International Journal of Psychophysiology, 9,* 105–120.

Oden, G. C. (1977). Integration of fuzzy logical information. *Journal of Experimental Psychology: Human Perception and Performance, 3,* 565–575.

O'Hanlon, W. H. (1987). *Taproots: Underlying principles of Milton Erickson's therapy and hypnosis.* New York: W. W. Norton.

Okawa, M., Matousek, M., & Petersen, I. (1984). Spontaneous vigilance fluctuations in the daytime. *Psychophysiology, 21,* 207–211.

O'Keefe, J., & Black, A. H. (1978). Single unit and lesion experiments on the sensory input to the hippocampal cognitive map. *Functions of the Septo-Hippocampal System. Ciba Foundation Symposium, 58,* 179–191.

Oliva, J. (1982). The structure and semiotic function of paralanguage. In M. Davis (Ed.), *Interaction rhythms: Periodicity in communicative behavior* (pp. 195–203). New York: Human Sciences Press.

Olness, K., & Conroy, M. (1985). A pilot study of voluntary control of transcutaneous PO_2 by children. *International Journal of Clinical and Experimental Hypnosis, 33,* 1–5.

Olness, K., MacDonald, J. T., & Uden, D. L. (1987). Comparison of self-hypnosis and propranolol in the treatment of juvenile classic migraine. *Pediatrics, 79,* 593–597.

Olson, D. R., & Torrance, N. (1987). Language, literacy, and mental states. *Discourse Processes, 10,* 157–167.

Omer, H., Elizur, Y., Barnea, T., Friedlander, D., & Palti, Z. (1986a). Psychological variables and premature labour: A possible solution for some methodological problems. *Journal of Psychosomatic Research, 30,* 559–565.

Omer, H., Friedlander, D., & Palti, Z. (1986b). Hypnotic relaxation in the treatment of premature labor. *Psychosomatic Medicine, 48,* 351–361.

Omer, H. (1987a). A hypnotic relaxation technique for the treatment of premature labor. *American Journal of Clinical Hypnosis, 29,* 206–213.

Omer, H., & Sirkovitz, A. (1987b). Failure of hypnotic relaxation in the treatment of postterm pregnancies. *Psychosomatic Medicine, 49,* 606–609.

Ong, W. J. (1977). *Interfaces of the word: Studies in the evolution of consciousness and culture.* Ithaca, NY: Cornell University Press.

Ong, W. J. (1982). *Orality and literacy: The technologizing of the word.* London: Methuen.

Ong, W. J. (1986). Writing is a technology that restructures thought. In G. Baumann (Ed.), *The written word: Literacy in transition* (pp. 23–50). Oxford: Clarendon Press.

Orne, M. T., & McConkey, K. M. (1981). Toward convergent inquiry into self-hypnosis. *International Journal of Clinical and Experimental Hypnosis, 29,* 313–323.

Ornitz, E. M., Forsythe, A. B., Lee, J. C. M., & Hartman, D. (1973). Basic rest-activity cycle rhythms in the human auditory evoked response. *Electroencephalography and Clinical Neurophysiology, 34,* 593–603.

Ornstein, R., Herron, J., Johnstone, J., & Swencionis, C. (1979). Differential right hemisphere involvement in two reading tasks. *Psychophysiology, 16,* 398–401.

Orr, W. C., Hoffman, H. J., & Hegge, F. W. (1974). Ultradian rhythms in extended performance. *Aerospace Medicine, 45,* 995–1000.

O'Sullivan, M. (1982). Measuring the ability to recognize facial expressions of emotion. In P. Ekman (Ed.), *Emotion in the human face* (2nd ed., pp. 281–317). Cambridge: Cambridge University Press.

Overton, D. (1978). Major theories of state-dependent learning. In B. Ho, D. Richards, & D. Chute (Eds.), *Drug discrimination and state-dependent learning* (pp. 283–318). New York: Academic Press.

Oxman, A. D., & Guyatt, G. H. (1988). Guidelines for reading literature reviews. *Canadian Medical Association Journal, 138,* 697–703.

Panksepp, J., Herman, B. H., Vilberg, T., Bishop, P., & Dees-Kinazi, F. G. (1980). Endogenous opioids and social behavior. *Neuroscience and Biobehavioral Reviews, 4,* 473–487.

Panksepp, J., Siviy, S. M., & Normansell, L. A. (1985). Brain opioids and social emotions. In M. Reite & T. Field (Eds.), *The psychobiology of attachment and separation* (pp. 3–49). New York: Academic Press.

Parasuraman, R., & Beatty, J. (1980). Brain events underlying detection and recognition of weak sensory signals. *Science, 210,* 80–83.

Parry, M. (1971). *The making of Homeric verse: The collected papers of Milman Parry* (A. Parry, Ed.). Oxford: Clarendon Press.

Patel, C., & Marmot, M. G. (1988). Efficacy versus effectiveness of relaxation therapy in hypertension. *Stress Medicine, 4,* 283–289.

Pekala, R. J., Wenger, C. F., & Levine, R. L. (1985). Individual differences in phenomenological experience: States of consciousness as a function of absorption. *Journal of Personality and Social Psychology, 48,* 125–132.

Pekala, R. J., & Kumar, V. K. (1986a). The differential organization of the structures of consciousness during hypnosis and a baseline condition. *Journal of Mind and Behavior, 7,* 515–539.

Pekala, R. J., Steinberg, J., & Kumar, V. K. (1986b). Measurement of phenomenological experience: Phenomenology of consciousness inventory. *Perceptual and Motor Skills, 63,* 983–989.

Perrett, D. I., Smith, P. A. J., Potter, D. D., Mistlin, A. J., Head, A. S., Milner, A. D., & Jeeves, M. A. (1984). Neurones responsive to faces in the temporal cortex: Studies of functional organization, sensitivity to identity and relation to perception. *Human Neurobiology, 3,* 197–208.

Perrett, D. I., Smith, P. A. J., Potter, D. D., Mistlin, A. J., Head, A. S., Milner, A. D., & Jeeves, M. A. (1985). Visual cells in the temporal cortex sensitive to face view and gaze direction. *Proceedings of the Royal Society of London, B223,* 293–317.

Perry, B. D., Southwick, S., & Giller, E. J. (1989). Adrenergic receptors in PTSD. In E. L. Giller (Ed.), *Biological assessment and treatment in PTSD.* Washington, DC: APA Press.

Perry, B. D. (1990, May). *Adrenergic receptors in child and adolescent PTSD.* Paper presented at the Annual Meeting of the American Psychiatric Association, New York.

Pert, C. B., Ruff, M. R., Weber, R. J., & Herkenham, M. (1985). Neuropeptides and their receptors: A psychosomatic network. *Journal of Immunology, 135*(2, Suppl.), 820s–826s.

Pert, C. (1987). Neuropeptides: The emotions and bodymind. *Noetic Sciences Review, 2,* 13–18.

Petsche, H., Lindner, K., Rappelsberger, P., & Gruber, G. (1988). The EEG: An adequate method to concretize brain processes elicited by music. *Music Perception, 6,* 133–160.

Pettinati, H. M. (1988). Hypnosis and memory: Integrative summary and future directions. In H. M. Pettinati (Ed.), *Hypnosis and memory* (pp. 277–291). New York: Guilford Press.

Picton, T. W., & Hillyard, S. A. (1974). Human auditory evoked potentials. II. Effects of attention. *Electroencephalography and Clinical Neurophysiology, 36,* 191–199.

Pilbeam, D. R. (1978). Rearranging our family tree. *Human Nature, 1,* 38–45.

Pitman, R. K., Orr, S. P., Forgue, D. F., de Jong, J. B., & Claiborn, J. M. (1987). Psychophysiology of PTSD imagery in Vietnam combat veterans. *Archives of General Psychiatry, 44,* 970–975.

Pitman, R. K., van der Kolk, B. A., Orr, S. P., & Greenberg, M. S. (1990). Naloxone-reversible analgesic response to combat-related stimuli in post-traumatic stress disorder: A pilot study. *Archives of General Psychiatry, 47,* 541–544.

Plotkin, W. B. (1979). The alpha experience revisited: Biofeedback in the transformation of psychological state. *Psychological Bulletin, 86,* 1132–1148.

Plotkin, W. B. (1980). The role of attributions of responsibility in the facilitation of unusual experiential states during alpha training: An analysis of the biofeedback placebo effect. *Journal of Abnormal Psychology, 89,* 67–78.

Plutchik, R., & Kellerman, H. (Eds.). (1980). *Emotion: Theory, research, and experience: Vol. 1. Theories of Emotion.* New York: Academic Press.

Pompeiano. O. (1979). Cholinergic activation of reticular and vestibular mechanisms controlling posture and eye movements. In J. A. Hobson & M. A. B. Brazier (Eds.), *The reticular formation revisited* (pp. 473–572). New York: Raven.

Pöppel, E. (1988). *Mindworks: Time and conscious experience* (T. Artin, Trans.). Boston: Harcourt Brace Jovanovich.

Popper, K. R., & Eccles, J. C. (1977). *The self and its brain: An argument for interactionism.* New York: Springer-Verlag.

Porush, D. (1987). What Homer can teach technical writers: The mnemonic value of poetic devices. *Journal of Technical Writing and Communication, 17,* 129–143.

Pound, E. (1979). Treatise on metre. In H. Gross (Ed.), *The structure of verse: Modern essays on prosody* (rev. ed., pp. 234–240). New York: Ecco Press.

Preston, C. F. (1982, August). *An interactional analysis of hypnotic responsivity.* Paper presented at the International Society of Hypnosis, 9th International Congress of Hypnosis and Psychosomatic Medicine, Glasgow, Scotland.

Price, D. D., Barrell, J. J., & Gracely, R. H. (1980). A psychophysical analysis of experiential factors that selectively influence the affective dimension of pain. *Pain, 8,* 137–149.

Price, D. D., & Barber, J. (1987). An analysis of factors that contribute to the efficacy of hypnotic analgesia. *Journal of Abnormal Psychology, 96,* 46–51.

Price, K. P., & Clarke, L. K. (1979). Classical conditioning of digital pulse volume in migraineurs and normal controls. *Headache, 19,* 328–332.

Prince, R. (1982a). Shamans and endorphins: Introduction. *Ethos, 10,* 299–302.

Prince, R. (1982b). Shamans and endorphins: Hypotheses for a synthesis. *Ethos, 10,* 409–423.

Provine, R. R., Hamernik, H. B., Curchack, B. C. (1987). Yawning: Relation to sleeping and stretching in humans. *Ethology, 76,* 152–160.

Provine, R. R. (1989). Contagious yawning and infant imitation. *Bulletin of the Psychonomic Society, 27,* 125–126.

Putnam, F. W., Loewenstein, R. J., Silberman, E. J., & Post, R. M. (1984). Multiple personality disorder in a hospital setting. *Journal of Clinical Psychiatry, 45,* 172–175.

Putnam, F. W., Guroff, J. J., Silberman, E. K., Barban, L., & Post, R. M. (1986). The clinical phenomenology of multiple personality disorder: Review of 100 recent cases. *Journal of Clinical Psychiatry, 47,* 285–293.

Putnam, H. (1975). The meaning of "meaning." In K. Gunderson (Ed.), *Language, mind, and knowledge.* Minneapolis: University of Minnesota Press. Reprinted in H. Putnam (1975), *Mind, language, and reality: Philosophical Papers* (Vol. 2, pp. 215–271). Cambridge: Cambridge University Press.

Putnam, H. (1981). *Reason, truth and history.* Cambridge: Cambridge University Press.

Rachlin, H. (1985). Pain and behavior. *Behavioral and brain sciences, 8,* 43–83.

Radtke, H. L., Thompson, V. A., & Egger, L. A. (1987). Use of retrieval cues in breaching hypnotic amnesia. *Journal of Abnormal Psychology, 96,* 335–340.

Raft, D., Smith, R. H., & Warren, N. (1986). Selection of imagery in the relief of chronic and acute clinical pain. *Journal of Psychosomatic Research, 30,* 481–488.

Rainey, J. M., Jr., Aleem, A., Ortiz, A., Yeragani, V., Pohl, R., & Berchou, R. (1987). A laboratory procedure for the induction of flashbacks. *American Journal of Psychiatry, 144,* 1317–1319.

Rapkin, D. A., Straubing, M., Singh, A., & Holroyd, J. C. (1988, November). *Guided imagery and hypnosis: Effect on acute recovery from head and neck cancer surgery.* Paper presented at the Annual Meeting of the Society for Clinical and Experimental Hypnosis, Asheville, NC.

Rasmussen, D. D. (1986). Physiological interactions of the basic rest-activity cycle of the brain: Pulsatile luteinizing hormone secretion as a model. *Psychoneuroendocrinology, 11,* 389–405.

Rasmussen, J., & Goodstein, L. P. (1985). *Decision support in supervisory control.* Roskilde, Denmark: RISO National Laboratory.

Ray, W. J., & Cole, H. W. (1985). EEG alpha activity reflects attentional demands, and beta activity reflects emotional and cognitive processes. *Science, 228,* 750–752.

Reber, A. S. (1976). Implicit learning of synthetic languages: The role of instructional set. *Journal of Experimental Psychology: Human Learning and Memory, 2,* 88–94.

Reber, A. S., Allen, R., & Regan, S. (1985). Syntactic learning and judgments: Still unconscious and still abstract. *Journal of Experimental Psychology: General, 114,* 17–24.

Redfield, R. (1947). The folk society. *American Journal of Sociology, 52,* 293–308.

Redican, W. K. (1982). An evolutionary perspective on human facial displays. In P. Ekman (Ed.), *Emotion in the human face* (2nd ed., pp. 212–280). Cambridge: Cambridge University Press.

Register, P. A., & Kihlstrom, J. F. (1987). Hypnotic effects on hypermnesia. *International Journal of Clinical and Experimental Hypnosis, 35,* 155–170.

Resnick, H. S., Kilpatrick, D. G., Lipovsky, J. A., Amick, A., Best, C. L., Saunders, B. E., & Sturgis, E. (1990, May). *Sensory modalities of flashbacks: Post-trauma*. Paper presented at the Annual Meeting of the American Psychiatric Association, New York.

Reynolds, P. C. (1981). *On the evolution of human behavior: The argument from animals to man*. Berkeley: University of California Press.

Rhue, J. W., & Lynn, S. J. (1989). Fantasy proneness, hypnotizability, and absorption—a re-examination. *International Journal of Clinical and Experimental Hypnosis, 37*, 100–106.

Richards, I. A. (1979). Rhythm and metre. In H. Gross (Ed.), *The structure of verse: Modern essays on prosody* (rev. ed., pp. 68–76). New York: Ecco Press.

Rickes, W. H., Cohen, M. J., & McArthur, D. L. (1977). *A psychophysiologic study of autonomic nervous system response patterns in migraine headache patients and their headache-free friends*. Paper presented at the 19th Annual Meeting of the American Association for the Study of Headache, San Francisco.

Rinn, W. E. (1984). The neuropsychology of facial expression: A review of the neurological and psychological mechanisms for producing facial expressions. *Psychological Bulletin, 95*, 52–77.

Ritchie, J. (1973). Pain from distension of the pelvic colon by inflating a balloon in the irritable colon syndrome. *Gut, 14*, 125–132.

Rivera, M. (1989). Linking the psychological and the social: Feminism, poststructuralism, and multiple personality. *Dissociation, 2*, 24–31.

Rizzo, P. A., Amabile, G., Fiumara, R., Caporali, M., Pierelli, F., Spadaro, M., Zanasi, M., & Morocutti, C. (1980). Brain slow potentials and hypnosis. *Biological Psychiatry, 15*, 499–506.

Robles, R., Smith, R., Carver, C. S., & Wellens, A. R. (1987). Influence of subliminal visual images on the experience of anxiety. *Personality and Social Psychology Bulletin, 13*, 399–410.

Romano, S., & Gizdulich, P. (1980). Suggestion of ultradian rhythm in peripheral blood flow. *Chronobiologia, 7*, 259–261.

Rosenberg, S. D., & Tucker, G. J. (1979). Verbal behavior and schizophrenia: The semantic dimension. *Archives of General Psychiatry, 36*, 1331–1337.

Rosenthal, T. L., Wruble, L. D., Rosenthal, R. H., & Edwards, N. B. (1987). Complaint patterns of patients with irritable bowel syndrome, Crohn's disease and acute gastroenterological illness. *Behaviour Research and Therapy, 25*, 99–112.

Ross, C. A., Heber, S., Norton, G. R., & Anderson, G. (1989a). Differences between multiple personality disorder and other diagnostic groups on structured interview. *Journal of Nervous and Mental Disease, 177*, 487–491.

Ross, C. A., Heber, S., Norton, G. R., & Anderson, G. (1989b). Somatic symptoms in multiple personality disorder. *Psychosomatics, 30*, 154–160.

Ross, C. A., & Norton, G. R. (1989c). Effects of hypnosis on the features of multiple personality disorder. *American Journal of Clinical Hypnosis, 32*, 99–106.

Ross, E. D. (1985). Modulation of affect and nonverbal communication by the right hemisphere. In M.-M. Mesulam (Ed.), *Principles of behavioral neurology* (pp. 239–257). Philadelphia: F. A. Davis.

Ross, E. D., Edmondson, J. A., & Seibert, G. B. (1986). The effect of affect on various acoustic measures of prosody in tone and non-tone languages: A comparison based on computer analysis of voice. *Journal of Phonetics, 14,* 283–302.

Ross, J., & Persinger, M. A. (1987). Positive correlations between temporal lobe signs and hypnosis induction profiles: A replication. *Perceptual Motor Skills, 64,* 828–830.

Ross, R. J., Ball, W. A., Sullivan, K. A., & Caroff, S. N. (1989). Sleep disturbance as the hallmark of posttraumatic stress disorder. *American Journal of Psychiatry, 146,* 697–707.

Ross, R. J., Ball, W. A., Dinges, D. F., Kribbs, N. B., Morrison, A. R., & Silver, S. M. (1990, May). *REM sleep disturbance as the hallmark of PTSD.* Paper presented at the Annual Meeting of the American Psychiatric Association, New York.

Rossi, E. L. (1982). Hypnosis and ultradian cycles: A new state(s) theory of hypnosis? *American Journal of Clinical Hypnosis, 25,* 21–32.

Rossi, E. L. (1986a). *The psychobiology of mind-body healing: New concepts of therapeutic hypnosis.* New York: W. W. Norton.

Rossi, E. L. (1986b). Altered states of consciousness in everyday life: The ultradian rhythms. In B. Wolman & M. Ullman (Eds.), *Handbook of altered states of consciousness.* New York: Van Nostrand.

Rossi, E. L. (1987). From mind to molecule: A state-dependent memory, learning, and behavior theory of mind-body healing. *Advances, 4,* 46–60.

Rossi, E. L., & Cheek, D. B. (1988). *Mind-body therapy: Methods of ideodynamic healing in hypnosis.* New York: W. W. Norton.

Rossi, E. L., & Smith, M. (1990). The eternal quest: Hidden rhythms of stress and healing in everyday life. *Psychological Perspectives, 21*(2), 6–23.

Rothenberg, A. (1988). *The creative process of psychotherapy.* New York: W. W. Norton.

Rouget, G. (1985). *Music and trance: A theory of the relations between music and possession.* (B. Biebuyck, Trans.). Chicago: University of Chicago Press.

Roy-Byrne, P., Schmidt, P., Cannon, R. O., Diem, H., & Rubinow, D. R. (1989). Microvascular angina and panic disorder. *International Journal of Psychiatry in Medicine, 19,* 315–325.

Runeson, S., & Frykholm, G. (1983). Kinematic specification of dynamics as an informational basis for person-and-action perception: Expectation, gender, recognition, and deceptive intention. *Journal of Experimental Psychology: General, 112,* 585–615.

Russell, J. A., & Fehr, B. (1987). Relativity in the perception of emotion in facial expressions. *Journal of Experimental Psychology: General, 116,* 223–237.

Russell, M., Dark, K. A., Cummins, R. W., Ellman, G., Callaway, E., & Peeke, H. V. S. (1984). Learned histamine release. *Science, 225,* 733–734.

Saban, R. (1980). Le système des veines méningées moyennes chez deux Néandertaliens: l'Homme de La Chapelle-aux-Saints et l'Homme de La Quina, d'après le moulage endocrânien. *Comptes Rendu de l'Académie des Sciences, Paris, 1er Semestre* (T 290, no. 20), série D 1297–1300.

Saban, R. (1983). L'asymetrie du reseau des veines méningées moyennes chez les hommes fossiles et sa signification possible. In E. de Grolier (Ed.), *Proceedings of the Transdisciplinary Symposium on Glossogenetics, Paris, 1981*. Paris: Harwood Academic Press.

Sabourin, M. (1982). Hypnosis and brain function: EEG correlates of state-trait differences. *Research Communications in Psychology, Psychiatry and Behavior, 7,* 149–168.

Sabourin, M. E., Cutcomb, S. D., Crawford, H. J., & Pribram, K. (1991). EEG correlates of hypnotic susceptibility and hypnotic trance; spectra analysis and coherence. *International Journal of Psychophysiology.*

Sackeim, H. A., Gur, R. C., & Saucy, M. C. (1978). Emotions are expressed more intensely on the left side of the face. *Science, 202,* 434–436.

Sackeim, H. A. (1982). Lateral asymmetry in bodily response to hypnotic suggestions. *Biological Psychiatry, 17,* 437–447.

Sackett, D. L. (1980). The competing objectives of randomized trials. *New England Journal of Medicine, 303,* 1059–1060.

Sakai, K. (1980). Some anatomical and physiological properties of pontomesencephalic tegmental neurons with special reference to the PGO waves and postural atonia during paradoxical sleep in the cat. In J. A. Hobson & M. A. Brazier (Eds.), *The reticular formation revisited: Specifying function for a nonspecific system* (pp. 427–447). New York: Raven Press.

Saletu, B. (1987). Brain function during hypnosis, acupuncture and transcendental meditation: Quantitative EEG studies. *Advances in Biological Psychiatry, 16,* 18–40.

Salkovskis, P. M., Jones, D. R. O., & Clark, D. M. (1986). Respiratory control in the treatment of panic attacks: Replication and extention with concurrent measurement of behaviour and pCO_2. *British Journal of Psychiatry, 148,* 526–532.

Sammons, M. T., & Karoly, P. (1987). Psychosocial variables in irritable bowel syndrome: A review and proposal. *Clinical Psychology Review, 7,* 187–204.

Sanders, B., McRoberts, G., & Tollefson, C. (1989). Childhood stress and dissociation in a college population. *Dissociation, 2,* 17–23.

Sandman, C. A., O'Halloran, J. P., & Isenhart, R. (1984). Is there an evoked vascular response? *Science, 224,* 1355–1357.

Sarbin, T. R., & Slagle, R. W. (1979). Hypnosis and psychophysiological outcomes. In E. Fromm & R. E. Shor (Eds.), *Hypnosis: Developments in research and perspectives* (2nd ed., pp. 273–303). Chicago: Aldine.

Sarter, M., & Markowitsch, H. J. (1985). The amygdala's role in human mnemonic processing. *Cortex, 21,* 7–24.

Sato, P., Sargur, M., & Schoene, R. B. (1986). Hypnosis effect on carbon dioxide chemosensitivity. *Chest, 89,* 828–831.

Schacter, D. L. (1977). EEG theta waves and psychological phenomena: A review and analysis. *Biological Psychology, 5,* 47–82.

Scheflen, A. E. (1973). *Communicational structure: Analysis of psychotherapy transactions.* Bloomington: Indiana University Press.

Scheflen, A. E. (1974). *How behavior means.* New York: Doubleday.

Scheflen, A. E. (1982). Comments on the significance of interaction rhythms. In M. Davis (Ed.), *Interaction rhythms: Periodicity in communicative behavior* (pp. 13–22). New York: Human Sciences Press.

Schenk, L., & Bear, D. (1981). Multiple personality and related dissociative phenomena in patients with temporal lobe epilepsy. *American Journal of Psychiatry, 138,* 1311–1316.

Scherer, K. R. (1979). Nonlinguistic vocal indicators of emotion and psychopathology. In C. E. Izard (Ed.), *Emotions in personality and psychopathology* (pp. 495–529). New York: Plenum Press.

Scherer, K. R. (1981). Speech and emotional states. In J. K. Darby, Jr. (Ed.), *Speech evaluation in psychiatry* (pp. 189–220). New York: Grune & Stratton.

Schiff, B. B., & Lamon, M. (1989). Inducing emotion by unilateral contraction of facial muscles: A new look at hemispheric specialization and the experience of emotion. *Neuropsychologia, 27,* 923–935.

Schiffenbauer, A. (1974). Effect of observer's emotional state on judgments of the emotional state of others. *Journal of Personality and Social Psychology, 30,* 31–35.

Schlutter, L. C., Golden, C. J., & Blume, H. G. (1980). A comparison of treatments for prefrontal muscle contraction headache. *British Journal of Medical Psychology, 53,* 47–52.

Schmajuk, N. A. (1984). Psychological theories of hippocampal function. *Physiological Psychology, 12,* 166–183.

Schmitt, F. (1984). Molecular regulators of brain function: A new view. *Neuroscience, 13,* 991–1001.

Scholnick, E. K. (1987). The language of mind: Statements about mental states. *Discourse Processes, 10,* 181–192.

Schumacher, R., & Velden, M. (1984). Anxiety, pain experience, and pain report: A signal-detection study. *Perceptual and Motor Skills, 58,* 339–349.

Schuman, M. (1980). The psychophysiological model of meditation and altered states of consciousness: A critical review. In J. M. Davidson & R. J. Davidson (Eds.), *The psychobiology of consciousness* (pp. 333–378). New York: Plenum Press.

Schwartz, G. E., Ahern, G. L., & Brown, S. (1979). Lateralized facial muscle response to positive and negative emotional stimuli. *Psychophysiology, 16,* 561–571.

Schwartz, G. E., Weinberger, D. A., & Singer, J. A. (1981). Cardiovascular differentiation of happiness, sadness, anger, and fear following imagery and exercise. *Psychosomatic Medicine, 43,* 343–364.

Schwartz, M. (1963). The cessation of labor using hypnotic techniques. *American Journal of Clinical Hypnosis, 5,* 211–213.

Sexton, M. C., Harralson, T., Hulsey, T. L., & Nash, M. R. (1988, November). Hypnotizability and sexual abuse: A comparison of abused and non-abused adult women. Paper presented at the Annual Meeting of the Society for Clinical and Experimental Hypnosis, Asheville, NC.

Shagass, C., Orintz, E. M., Sutton, S., & Tueting, P. (1978). Event-related potentials and psychopathology. In E. Callaway (Ed.), *Event-related brain potentials in man.* New York: Academic Press.

Shaw, G. A. (1987). Creativity and hypermnesia for words and pictures. *Journal of General Psychology, 114,* 167–178.

Shear, M. K. (1986). Pathophysiology of panic: A review of pharmacologic provocative tests and naturalistic monitoring data. *Journal of Clinical Psychiatry, 47*(6, Suppl.), 18–26.

Sheehan, P. W., & McConkey, K. M. (1982). *Hypnosis and experience: The exploration of phenomena and process.* Hillsdale, NJ: Erlbaum.

Shepard, R. N. (1984). Ecological constraints on internal representation: Resonant kinematics of perceiving, imagining, thinking, and dreaming. *Psychological Review, 91,* 417–447.

Shields, I. W., & Knox, V. J. (1986). Level of processing as a determinant of hypnotic hypermnesia. *Journal of Abnormal Psychology, 95,* 358–364.

Siegel, R. K. (1984). Hostage hallucinations: Visual imagery induced by isolation and life-threatening stress. *Journal of Nervous and Mental Disease, 172,* 264–272.

Sigman, A. (1988). Hypnotic and biofeedback procedures for self-regulation of autonomic nervous system functions. In M. Heap (Ed.), *Hypnosis: Current clinical, experimental and forensic practices* (pp. 126–138). London: Croom Helm.

Silberman, E. K., Putnam, F. W., Weingartner, H., Braun, B. G., & Post, R. M. (1985). Dissociative states in multiple personality disorder: A quantitative study. *Psychiatry Research, 15,* 253–260.

Sitaram, N., Wyatt, R. J., Dawson, S., & Gillin, J. C. (1976). REM sleep induction by physostigmine infusion during sleep. *Science, 191,* 1281–1283.

Sletvold, H., Jensen, G. M., & Gotestam, K. G. (1986). Blood pressure responses to hypnotic and nonhypnotic suggestions in normotensive subjects. *Pavlovian Journal of Biological Science, 21,* 32–35.

Smith, D. E. (1980). Hypnotic susceptibility and eye movement during rest. *American Journal of Clinical Hypnosis, 22,* 147–155.

Smith, E. E., & Medin, D. L. (1981). *Categories and concepts.* Cambridge, MA: Harvard University Press.

Snape, W. J., Jr., Carlson, G. M., & Cohen, S. (1976). Colonic myoelectric activity in the irritable bowel syndrome. *Gastroenterology, 70,* 326–330.

Snodgrass, M., & Lynn, S. J. (1989). Music absorption and hypnotizability. *International Journal of Clinical and Experimental Hypnosis, 37*, 41–54.

Snyder, E. D., & Shor, R. E. (1983). Trance inductive poetry: A brief communication. *International Journal of Clinical and Experimental Hypnosis, 31*, 1–7.

Solomon, Z., Garb, R., Bleich, A., & Grupper, D. (1987). Reactivation of combat-related posttraumatic stress disorder. *American Journal of Psychiatry, 144*, 51–55.

Southwick, S. M., Yehudi, R., Perry, B. D., Krystal, J. H., & Charney, D. S. (1990, May). *Sympathoadrenal dysfunction in PTSD.* Paper presented at the Annual Meeting of the American Psychiatric Association, New York.

Spanos, N. P., & Barber, T. X. (1968). "Hypnotic" experiences as inferred from subjective reports: Auditory and visual hallucinations. *Journal of Experimental Research in Personality, 3*, 136–150.

Spanos, N. P., Rivers, S. M., & Gottlieb, J. (1978). Hypnotic responsivity, meditation and laterality of eye movements. *Journal of Abnormal Psychology, 87*, 566–569.

Spanos, N. P., & Bertrand, L. D. (1985a). EMG biofeedback, attained relaxation and hypnotic susceptibility: Is there a relationship? *American Journal of Clinical Hypnosis, 27*, 219–225.

Spanos, N. P., Weekes, J. R., & Bertrand, L. D. (1985b). Multiple personality: A social psychological perspective. *Journal of Abnormal Psychology, 94*, 362–376.

Spanos, N. P. (1986a). Hypnotic behavior: A social-psychological interpretation of amnesia, analgesia, and "trance logic." *Behavioral and Brain Sciences, 9*, 449–502.

Spanos, N. P., Robertson, L. A., Menary, E. P., & Brett, P. J. (1986b). Component analysis of cognitive skill training for the enhancement of hypnotic susceptibility. *Journal of Abnormal Psychology, 95*, 350–357.

Spanos, N. P., Voornevald, P. W., & Gwynn, M. I. (1986c). The mediating effects of expectation on hypnotic and nonhypnotic pain reduction. *Imagination, Cognition and Personality, 6*, 231–246.

Spanos, N. P., Weekes, J. R., Menary, E., & Bertrand, L. D. (1986d). Hypnotic interview and age regression procedures in the elicitation of multiple personality symptoms: A simulation study. *Psychiatry, 49*, 298–311.

Spanos, N. P., Brett, P. J., Menary, E. P., & Cross, W. P. (1987a). A measure of attitudes toward hypnosis: Relationships with absorption and hypnotic susceptibility. *American Journal of Clinical Hypnosis, 30*, 139–150.

Spanos, N. P., de Groh, M., & de Groot, H. (1987b). Skill training for enhancing hypnotic susceptibility and word list amnesia. *British Journal of Experimental and Clinical Hypnosis, 4*, 15–23.

Spanos, N. P., Stenstrom, R. J., & Johnston, J. C. (1988). Hypnosis, placebo, and suggestion in the treatment of warts. *Psychosomatic Medicine, 50*, 245–260.

Spellacy, F., & Wilkinson, R. (1987). Dichotic listening and hypnotizability: Variability in ear preference. *Perceptual Motor Skills, 64*, 1279–1284.

Sperry, R. (1982). Some effects of disconnecting the cerebral hemispheres. *Science, 217*, 1223–1226.

Spiegel, D., & Fink, R. (1979). Hysterical psychosis and hypnotizability. *American Journal of Psychiatry, 136*, 777–781.

Spiegel, D., & Albert, L. H. (1983a). Naloxone fails to reverse hypnotic alleviation of chronic pain. *Psychopharmacology, 81*, 140–143.

Spiegel, D., & Bloom, J. R. (1983b). Group therapy and hypnosis reduce metastatic breast carcinoma pain. *Psychosomatic Medicine, 45*, 333–339.

Spiegel, D., Cutcomb, S., Ren, C., & Pribram, K. (1985a). Hypnotic hallucination alters evoked potentials. *Journal of Abnormal Psychology, 94*, 249–255.

Spiegel, D., & Spiegel, H. (1985b). Hypnosis. In H. I. Kaplan & B. J. Sadock (Eds.), *Comprehensive textbook of psychiatry/IV* (4th ed., pp. 1389–1403). Baltimore: Williams & Wilkins.

Spiegel, D. (1986). Dissociating damage. *American Journal of Clinical Hypnosis, 29*, 123–131.

Spiegel, D., & Barabasz, A. F. (1988a). Effects of hypnotic instructions on P_{300} event-related-potential amplitudes: Research and clinical implications. *American Journal of Clinical Hypnosis, 31*, 11–17.

Spiegel, D., Bierre, P., & Rootenberg, J. (1988b, November). *Hypnotic alteration of somatosensory perception: Accompanying changes in evoked potentials.* Paper presented at the Annual Meeting of the Society for Clinical and Experimental Hypnosis, Asheville, NC.

Spiegel, D., Hunt, T., & Dondershine, H. E. (1988c). Dissociation and hypnotizability in posttraumatic stress disorder. *American Journal of Psychiatry, 145*, 301–305.

Spiegel, D., Bloom, J. R., Kraemer, H. C., & Gottheil, E. (1989a, October 14). Effect of psychosocial treatment on survival of patients with metastatic breast cancer. *Lancet*, pp. 888–891.

Spiegel, D., Frischholz, E. J., Spiegel, H., Lipman, L. S., & Bark, N. M. (1989b, May). *Dissociation, hypnotizability and trauma.* Paper presented at the Annual Meeting of the American Psychiatric Association, San Francisco.

Spiegel, H., & Spiegel, D. (1978). *Trance and treatment: Clinical uses of hypnosis.* New York: Basic Books.

Spinhoven, P. (1987). Hypnosis and behaviour therapy: A review. *International Journal of Clinical and Experimental Hypnosis, 35*, 8–31.

Spinhoven, P. (1988a). Similarities and dissimilarities in hypnotic and nonhypnotic procedures for headache control: A review. *American Journal of Clinical Hypnosis, 30*, 183–194.

Spinhoven, P., Baak, D., Van Dyck, R., & Vermeulen, P. (1988b). The effectiveness of an authoritative versus permissive style of hypnotic communication. *International Journal of Clinical and Experimental Hypnosis, 36*, 182–191.

Stacher, G., Berner, P., Naske, R., Schuster, P., Bauer, P., Starker, H., & Schulze,

B. (1975). Effect of hypnotic suggestion of relaxation on basal and betazole-stimulated gastric acid secretion. *Gastroenterology, 68,* 656–661.

Stam, H. J., McGrath, P. A., Brooke, R. I., & Cosier, F. (1986). Hypnotizability and the treatment of chronic facial pain. *International Journal of Clinical and Experimental Hypnosis, 34,* 182–191.

Stam, H. J., & Spanos, N. P. (1987). Hypnotic analgesia, placebo analgesia, and ischemic pain: The effects of contextual variables. *Journal of Abnormal Psychology, 96,* 313–320.

Stambaugh, E. E., & House, A. E. (1977). Multimodality treatment of migraine headache: A case study utilizing biofeedback, relaxation, autogenic and hypnotic treatments. *American Journal of Clinical Hypnosis, 19,* 235–240.

Stambrook, M., & Martin, D. G. (1983). Brain laterality and the subliminal perception of facial expression. *International Journal of Neuroscience, 18,* 45–58.

Stebbins, G. L. (1982). *Darwin to DNA, molecules to humanity.* San Francisco: W. H. Freeman.

Steele, J. (1989). Hominid evolution and primate social cognition. *Journal of Human Evolution, 18,* 421–432.

Steimer-Krause, E., Krause, R., & Wagner, G. (1990). Interaction regulations used by schizophrenic and psychosomatic patients: Studies on facial behavior in dyadic interactions. *Psychiatry, 53,* 209–228.

Steiner, J. E. (1973). The gustofacial response: Observation on normal and anencephalic newborn infants. In J. F. Bosma (Ed.), *Fourth Symposium on Oral Sensation and Perception* (pp. 254–278). Bethesda, MD: DHEW Pub. No. (NIH) 73-546.

Steriade, M., & Hobson, J. A. (1976). Neuronal activity during the sleep-waking cycle. *Progress in Neurobiology, 6,* 155–376.

Sterman, M. B. (1985). The basic rest-activity cycle revisited: Some new perspectives. *Experimental Brain Research, Suppl. 12,* 186–200.

Stern, D. (1977). *The first relationship.* Cambridge, MA: Harvard University Press.

Stern, D. (1982). Some interactive functions of rhythm changes between mother and infant. In M. Davis (Ed.), *Interaction rhythms: Periodicity in communicative behavior* (pp. 101–117). New York: Human Sciences Press.

Stern, D. (1985). *The interpersonal world of the infant.* New York: Basic Books.

Stern, D. B. (1977). Handedness and the lateral distribution of conversion reactions. *Journal of Nervous and Mental Disease, 164,* 122–128.

Stern, J. A., Brown, M., Ulett, G. A., & Sletten, I. (1977). A comparison of hypnosis, acupuncture, morphine, Valium, aspirin, and placebo in the management of experimentally induced pain. In W. E. Edmonston (Ed.), *Conceptual and investigative approaches to hypnosis and hypnotic phenomena. Annals of the New York Academy of Sciences, 296,* 175–193.

Sternbach, R. A. (1982). On strategies for identifying neurochemical correlates of hypnotic analgesia. *International Journal of Clinical and Experimental Hypnosis, 30,* 251–256.

Stetson, R. H. (1951). *Motor phonetics.* Amsterdam: North Holland Publishing.

Stewart, M. W., & Marks, D. F. (1990). Actual and expected hypnotizability in hypnotic analgesia. *British Journal of Experimental and Clinical Hypnosis, 7,* 47–56.

Stone, J. A., & Lundy, R. M. (1985). Behavioral compliance with direct and indirect body movement suggestions. *Journal of Abnormal Psychology, 94,* 256–263.

Strahan, C., & Zytowski, D. G. (1976). Impact of visual, vocal and lexical cues on judgments of counselor qualities. *Journal of Counseling Psychology, 23,* 387–393.

Strate, L. (1986, fall). Time-binding in oral cultures. *Et cetera,* pp. 234–246.

Strauss, E., & Moscovitch, M. (1981). Perception of facial expressions. *Brain and Language, 13,* 308–332.

Street, R. L., Jr., & Buller, D. B. (1987). Nonverbal response patterns in physician-patient interactions: A functional analysis. *Journal of Nonverbal Behavior, 11,* 234–253.

Street, R. L., Jr., & Buller, D. B. (1988). Patients' characteristics affecting physician-patient nonverbal communication. *Human Communication Research, 15,* 60–90.

Stumpf, C. (1965). Drug action on the electrical activity of the hippocampus. *International Reviews of Neurobiology, 8,* 77–138.

Stutman, R. K., & Bliss, E. L. (1985). Posttraumatic stress disorder, hypnotizability, and imagery. *American Journal of Psychiatry, 142,* 741–743.

Suberi, M., & McKeever, W. F. (1977). Differential right hemispheric memory storage of emotional and non-emotional faces. *Neuropsychologia, 15,* 757–768.

Suhor, C. (1986, summer). Jazz improvisation and language performance: Parallel competencies. *Et cetera,* pp. 133–140.

Swanson, D. W. (1984). Chronic pain as a third pathologic emotion. *American Journal of Psychiatry, 141,* 210–214.

Sweeney, C. A., Lynn, S. J., & Bellezza, F. S. (1986). Hypnosis, hypnotizability, and imagery-mediated learning. *International Journal of Clinical and Experimental Hypnosis, 34,* 29–40.

Sweetser, E. (1990). *From etymology to pragmatics.* Cambridge: Cambridge University Press.

Swirsky-Sacchetti, T., & Margolis, C. G. (1986). The effects of a comprehensive self-hypnosis training program on the use of Factor VIII in severe hemophilia. *International Journal of Clinical and Experimental Hypnosis, 34,* 71–83.

Sypher, B., & Zorn, T. (1987, May). *Individual differences and construct system content in descriptions of liked and disliked coworkers.* Paper presented at the

Annual Meeting of the International Communication Association, Organizational Communication Division, Montreal.

Taneli, B., & Krahne, W. (1987). EEG changes of transcendental meditation practitioners. *Advances in Biological Psychiatry, 16,* 41–71.

Tannen, D. (1984). *Conversational style: Analyzing talk among friends.* Norwood, NJ: Ablex.

Tannen, D., & Wallat, C. (1987). Interactive frames and knowledge schemas in interaction: Examples from a medical examination/interview. *Social Psychology Quarterly, 50,* 205–216.

Tanner, N. M. (1981). *On becoming human.* Cambridge: Cambridge University Press.

Tart, C. T. (1983). *States of consciousness.* El Cerrito, CA: Psychological Processes. (Original work published 1975)

Taylor, E. (1983). *William James on exceptional mental states: The 1896 Lowell Lectures.* New York: Charles Scribner's Sons.

Taylor, I., Darby, C., Hammond, P., & Basu, P. (1978). Is there a myoelectrical abnormality in the irritable colon syndrome? *Gut, 19,* 391–395.

Teasdale, J. D. (1983). Affect and accessibility. *Philosophical Transactions of the Royal Society of London, B302,* 403–412.

Tebēcis, A. K. (1975a). A controlled study of the EEG during transcendental meditation: Comparison with hypnosis. *Folio Psychiatrica et Neurologica Japonica, 29,* 305–313.

Tebēcis, A. K., Provins, K. A., Farnbach, R. W., & Pentony, P. (1975b). Hypnosis and the EEG: A quantitative investigation. *Journal of Nervous and Mental Disease, 161,* 1–17.

Tellegen, A., & Atkinson, G. (1974). Openness to absorbing and self-altering experiences ("absorption"), a trait related to hypnotic susceptibility. *Journal of Abnormal Psychology, 83,* 268–277.

Thayer, R. E. (1987). Problem perception, optimism, and related states as a function of time of day (diurnal rhythm) and moderate exercise: Two arousal systems in interaction. *Motivation and Emotion, 11,* 19–36.

Thigpen, C. H., & Cleckley, H. M. (1984). On the incidence of multiple personality disorder. *International Journal of Clinical and Experimental Hypnosis, 32,* 63–66.

Thorne, D. E., & Hall, H. V. (1974). Hypnotic amnesia revisited. *International Journal of Clinical and Experimental Hypnosis, 22,* 167–178.

Thorne, D. E., & Fisher, A. G. (1978). Hypnotically suggested asthma. *International Journal of Clinical and Experimental Hypnosis, 26,* 92–103.

Townsend, D. (1988). The problem of paraphrase. *Metaphor and Symbolic Activity, 3,* 37–54.

Tranel, D., & Damasio, A. R. (1985). Knowledge without awareness: An autonomic index of facial recognition by prosopagnosics. *Science, 228,* 1453–1454.

Travell, J. G. (1976). Myofascial trigger points: Clinical review. *Advances in Pain Research, 1,* 919–926.

Treisman, A. M., Squire, R., & Green, J. (1974). Semantic processing in dichotic listening? A replication. *Memory and Cognition, 2,* 641–646.

Trief, P. M., Elliott, D. J., Stein, N., & Frederickson, B. E. (1987). Functional *vs.* organic pain: A meaningful distinction? *Journal of Clinical Psychology, 43,* 219–226.

Tsuji, Y., & Kobayashi, T. (1988). Short and long ultradian EEG components in daytime arousal. *Electroencephalography and Clinical Neurophysiology, 70,* 110–117.

Tucker, D. M., Beckwith, B. E., Dopson, W. G., & Bullard-Bates, P. C. (1985). Asymmetrical facial expressions indeed: A reply to Dane and Thompson. *Cortex, 21,* 305–307.

Tucker, G. J., Price, T. R. P., Johnson, V. B., & McAllister, T. (1986). Phenomenology of temporal lobe dysfunction: A link to atypical psychosis—A series of cases. *Journal of Nervous and Mental Disease, 174,* 348–356.

Tunsater, A. (1984). Emotions and asthma, II. *European Journal of Respiratory Diseases Supplement, 136*(65), 131–137.

Turk, D. C., & Rennert, D. (1981). Pain and the terminally ill cancer patient: A cognitive social learning perspective. In H. J. Sobel (Ed.), *Behavior therapy in terminal care* (pp. 95–103). Cambridge, MA: Ballinger.

Turner, M. (1987). *Death is the mother of beauty: Mind, metaphor, criticism.* Chicago: University of Chicago Press.

Underwood, G., & Whitfield, A. (1985). Right-hemisphere interactions in picture-word processing. *Brain and Cognition, 4,* 273–286.

Van de Creek, L., & Watkins, J. T. (1972). Responses to incongruent verbal and nonverbal emotional cues. *Journal of Communication, 22,* 311–316.

van der Kolk, B. A., Greenberg, M. S., Boyd, H., & Krystal, J. (1985). Inescapable shock, neurotransmitters and addiction to trauma: Towards a psychology of post-traumatic stress. *Biological Psychiatry, 20,* 314–325.

van der Kolk, B. A., Pitman, R. K., Orr, S. P., & Greenberg, M. S. (1989, May). *Endogenous opioids and post-traumatic stress.* Paper presented at the Annual Meeting of the American Psychiatric Association, San Francisco.

Vanderwolf, C. H., & Robinson, T. E. (1981). Reticulo-cortical activity and behavior: A critique of the arousal theory and a new synthesis. *Behavioral and Brain Sciences, 4,* 459–514.

Van Dyck, R. (1980). Foreword. In J. K. Zeig (Ed.), *A teaching seminar with Milton H. Erickson.* New York: Brunner/Mazel.

van Gelder, R. S., & van Gelder, L. (1990). Facial expression and speech: Neuroanatomical considerations. *International Journal of Psychology, 25,* 141–155.

Van Gorp, W. G., Meyer, R. G., & Dunbar, K. D. (1985). The efficacy of direct versus indirect hypnotic induction techniques on reduction of experimental pain. *International Journal of Clinical and Experimental Hypnosis, 33,* 319–328.

Van Hoesen, G. W. (1982). The parahippocampal gyrus: New observations regarding its cortical connections in the monkey. *Trends in NeuroSciences, 5*(10), 345–350.

Vaughn, R., Pall, M. L., & Haynes, S. N. (1977). Frontalis EMG response to stress in subjects with frequent muscle-contraction headaches. *Headaches, 16,* 313–317.

Vogel, W., & Broverman, D. M. (1964). Relationship between EEG and test intelligence: A critical review. *Psychological Bulletin, 62,* 132–144.

Vogel, W., Broverman, D. M., & Klaiber, E. L. (1968). EEG and mental abilities. *Electroencephalography and Clinical Neurophysiology, 24,* 166–175.

Volavka, J., Matoušek, M., & Roubíček, J. (1967). Mental arithmetic and eye opening: An EEG frequency analysis and GSR study. *Electroencephalography and Clinical Neurophysiology, 22,* 174–176.

von Wright, J. M., Anderson, K., & Stenman, U. (1975). Generalization of conditioned GSRs in dichotic listening. In P. M. A. Rabitt & S. Dornic (Eds.), *Attention and performance.* New York: Academic Press.

Wadden, T. A., & Anderton, C. H. (1982). The clinical use of hypnosis. *Psychological Bulletin, 91,* 215–243.

Wallace, B. (1988). Hypnotic susceptibility, visual distraction, and reports of Necker cube apparent reversals. *Journal of General Psychology, 115*(4), 389–396.

Wallace, B. (1990). Imagery vividness, hypnotic susceptibility, and the perception of fragmental stimuli. *Journal of Personality and Social Psychology, 58,* 354–359.

Walter, D. O., Rhodes, J. M., & Adey, W. R. (1967). Discriminating among states of consciousness by EEG measurements: A study of four subjects. *Electroencephalography and Clinical Neurophysiology, 22,* 22–29.

Wapner, W., Hamby, S., & Gardner, H. (1981). The role of the right hemisphere in the apprehension of complex linguistic materials. *Brain and Language, 14,* 15–33.

Warren, L. R., & Haueter, E. S. (1981). Alpha asymmetry as a function of cognitive mode: The role of lateral eye movements. *International Journal of Neuroscience, 13,* 137–141.

Watzlawick, P., Weakland, J., & Fisch, R. (1974). *Change: Principles of problem formation and problem resolution.* New York: W. W. Norton.

Waxer, P. (1981). Channel contribution in anxiety displays. *Journal of Research in Personality, 15,* 44–56.

Waxer, P. (1984). Nonverbal aspects of psychotherapy: Discrete functions in the intercultural context. In A. Wolfgang (Ed.), *Nonverbal behavior: Perspectives, applications, intercultural insights* (pp. 229–252). Toronto: C. J. Hogrefe.

Weatherhead, A. D. (1980). Psychogenic headache. *Headache, 20,* 47–54.

Webb, W. B., & Dube, M. G. (1981). Temporal characteristics of sleep. In J. Aschoff (Ed.), *Handbook of behavioral neurobiology: Vol. 4. Biological Rhythms* (pp. 499–522). New York: Plenum Press.

Wegner, D. M., Schneider, D. J., Carter, S. R., III, & White, T. L. (1987). Paradoxical effects of thought suppression. *Journal of Personality and Social Psychology, 53,* 5–13.

Weiner, B. (1985). "Spontaneous" causal thinking. *Psychological Bulletin, 97,* 74–84.

Weisenberg, M., Aviram, O., Wolf, Y., & Raphaeli, N. (1984). Relevant and irrelevant anxiety in the reaction to pain. *Pain, 20,* 371–383.

Weitzenhoffer, A. M. (1989). *The practice of hypnotism* (Vols. 1–2). New York: John Wiley.

Welgan, P., Meshkinpour, H., & Hoehler, F. (1985). The effect of stress on colon motor and electrical activity in irritable bowel syndrome. *Psychosomatic Medicine, 47,* 139–149.

Werntz, D. A., Bickford, R. G., Bloom, F. E., & Shannahoff-Khalsa, D. S. (1981, February). *Selective cortical activation by altering autonomic function.* Paper presented at Western EEG Society, Reno.

Werntz, D. A., Bickford, R. G., Bloom, F. E., & Shannahoff-Khalsa, D. S. (1983). Alternating cerebral hemispheric activity and the lateralization of autonomic nervous function. *Human Neurobiology, 2,* 39–43.

Whitehead, W. E., Engel, B. T., & Schuster, M. M. (1980). Irritable bowel syndrome: Physiological and psychological differences between diarrhea-predominant and constipation-predominant patients. *Digestive Diseases and Sciences, 25,* 404–413.

Whitehead, W. E., Winget, C., Fedoravicius, A. S., Wooley, S., & Blackwell, B. (1982). Learned illness behavior in patients with irritable bowel syndrome and peptic ulcer. *Digestive Diseases and Sciences, 27,* 202–207.

Whitehead, W. E., & Schuster, M. M. (1985). *Gastrointestinal disorders: Behavioral and physiological basis for treatment* (pp. 125–154). New York: Academic Press.

Whorwell, P. J., Prior, A., & Faragher, E. B. (1984, December 1). Controlled trial of hypnotherapy in the treatment of severe refractory irritable-bowel syndrome. *Lancet,* pp. 1232–1234.

Whorwell, P. J., Prior, A., & Colgan, S. M. (1987). Hypnotherapy in severe irritable bowel syndrome: Further experience. *Gut, 28,* 423–425.

Wickelgren, W. A. (1979). Chunking and consolidation: A theoretical synthesis of semantic networks, configuring in conditioning, S-R versus cognitive learning, normal forgetting, the amnesic syndrome and the hippocampal arousal system. *Psychological Review, 86,* 44–60.

Wickens, C., Kramer, A., Vanasse, L., & Donchin, E. (1983). Performance of concurrent tasks: A psychophysiological analysis of the reciprocity of information-processing resources. *Science, 221,* 1080–1082.

Wilkinson, J. B. (1988a). Hyperventilation control techniques in combination with self-hypnosis for anxiety management. In M. Heap (Ed.), *Hypnosis: Current clinical, experimental and forensic practices* (pp. 115–125). London: Croom Helm.

Wilkinson, J. B. (1988b). Hypnosis in the treatment of asthma. In M. Heap (Ed.), *Hypnosis: Current clinical, experimental and forensic practices* (pp. 146–158). London: Croom Helm.

Williams, R. B., Jr., Lane, J. D., Kuhn, C. M., Melosh, W., White, A. D., & Schanberg, S. M. (1982). Type A behavior and elevated physiological and neuroendocrine responses to cognitive tasks. *Science, 218*, 483–485.

Wilmer, H. A. (1982). Post-traumatic stress disorder. *Psychiatric Annals, 12*, 995–1003.

Wilson, J. P. (1989). *Trauma, transformation, and healing: An integrative approach to theory, research, and post-traumatic therapy.* New York: Brunner/Mazel.

Wilson, L., & Kihlstrom, J. F. (1986). Subjective and categorical organization of recall during posthypnotic amnesia. *Journal of Abnormal Psychology, 95*, 264–273.

Winfree, A. T. (1980). *Biomathematics: Vol. 8. The geometry of biological time.* New York: Springer-Verlag.

Winfree, A. T. (1987). *The timing of biological clocks.* New York: Scientific American Books.

Winkelman, M. (1986). Trance states: A theoretical model and cross-cultural analysis. *Ethos, 14*, 174–203.

Winson, J., & Abzug, C. (1977). Gating of neuronal transmission in the hippocampus: Efficacy of transmission varies with behavioral state. *Science, 196*, 1223–1225.

Winson, J. (1985). *Brain and psyche: The biology of the unconscious.* Garden City, NY: Anchor Press/Doubleday.

Winson, J. (1990). The meaning of dreams. *Scientific American, 263*(5), 86–96.

Wolfgang, A. (Ed.). (1984). *Nonverbal behavior: Perspectives, applications, intercultural insights.* Lewiston, NY: C. J. Hogrefe.

Woods, D. D. (1984). Some results on operator performance in emergency events. In D. Whitfield (Ed.), *Ergonomics problems in process operations* (pp. 21–32). Elmsworth, NY: Pergamon Press.

Woods, D. L., Hillyard, S. A., Courchesne, E., & Galambos, R. (1980). Electrophysiological signs of split-second decision-making. *Science, 207*, 655–657.

Woods, S. W., Charney, D. S., Goodman, W. K., & Heninger, G. R. (1988). Carbon dioxide-induced anxiety: Behavioral, physiologic, and biochemical effects of carbon dioxide in patients with panic disorders and healthy subjects. *Archives of General Psychiatry, 45*, 43–52.

Woolson, D. A. (1986). An experimental comparison of direct and Ericksonian hypnotic induction procedures and the relationship to secondary suggestibility. *American Journal of Clinical Hypnosis, 29*, 23–28.

Yamaguchi, Y., Niwa, K., & Negi, T. (1973). Feedback of mid-frontal theta activity during mental work and its voluntary control. *Electroencephalography and Clinical Neurophysiology, 35*, 704–705.

Yaniv, I., & Meyer, D. E. (1987). Activation and metacognition of inaccessible stored information: Potential bases for incubation effects in problem solving. *Journal of Experimental Psychology: Learning, Memory, and Cognition, 13,* 187–205.

Young, A. W., Hay, D. C., & McWeeny, K. H. (1985a). Right cerebral hemisphere superiority for constructing facial representations. *Neuropsychologia, 23,* 195–202.

Young, A. W., Hay, D. C., McWeeny, K. H., & Ellis, A. W. (1985b). Familiarity decisions for faces presented to the left and right cerebral hemispheres. *Brain and Cognition, 4,* 439–450.

Young, H. F., Bentall, R. P., Slade, P. D., & Dewey, M. E. (1987). The role of brief instructions and suggestibility in the elicitation of auditory and visual hallucinations in normal and psychiatric subjects. *Journal of Nervous and Mental Disease, 175,* 41–48.

Young, J. (1978). *Programs of the brain.* New York: Oxford University Press.

Young, S. J., Alpers, D. H., Norland, C. C., & Woodruff, R. A. (1976). Psychiatric illness and the irritable bowel syndrome: Practical implications for the primary physician. *Gastroenterology, 70,* 162–166.

Yuille, J. C., & Kim, C. K. (1987). A field study of the forensic use of hypnosis. *Canadian Journal of Behavioral Science, 19,* 418–429.

Yunis, J. J., & Prakash, O. (1982). The origin of man: A chromosomal pictorial legacy. *Science, 215,* 1525–1530.

Zajonc, R. (1984). On the primacy of affect. *American Psychologist, 37,* 117–123.

Zajonc, R. B. (1985). Emotion and facial efference: A theory reclaimed. *Science, 228,* 15–21.

Zajonc, R. B., Adelmann, P. K., Murphy, S. T., & Niedenthal, P. M. (1987). Convergence in the physical appearance of spouses. *Motivation and Emotion, 11,* 335–346.

Zamansky, H. S., & Bartis, S. P. (1984). Hypnosis as dissociation: Methodological considerations and preliminary findings. *American Journal of Clinical Hypnosis, 26,* 246–251.

Zamansky, H. S., & Bartis, S. P. (1985). The dissociation of an experience: The hidden observer observed. *Journal of Abnormal Psychology, 94,* 243–248.

Zamansky, H. S., & Clark, L. E. (1986). Cognitive competition and hypnotic behavior: Whither absorption? *International Journal of Clinical and Experimental Hypnosis, 34,* 205–214.

Zeig, J. K. (1980). *Teaching seminar with Milton H. Erickson, M.D.* New York: Brunner/Mazel.

Zeig, J. K., & Lankton, S. R. (1988). *Developing Ericksonian therapy: State of the art.* New York: Brunner/Mazel.

Zeltzer, L., LeBaron, S., & Zeltzer, P. M. (1984). The effectiveness of behavioral intervention for reduction of nausea and vomiting in children and adolescents receiving chemotherapy. *Journal of Clinical Oncology, 2,* 683–690.

Ziller, R. C. (1988). Orientations: The cognitive link in person situation interaction. *Journal of Social Behavior and Personality, 3,* 1–9.

Zimmermann, P., Gortelmeyer, R., & Wiemann, H. (1983). Diurnal periodicity of lateral asymmetries of the visual evoked potential in healthy volunteers. *Neuropsychobiology, 9,* 178–181.

Zlotogorski, Z., Hahnemann, L. E., & Wiggs, E. A. (1987). Personality characteristics of hypnotizability. *American Journal of Clinical Hypnosis, 30,* 51–56.

Zubin, D., & Köpcke, K.-M. (1986). Gender and folk taxonomy: The indexical relation between grammatical and lexical categorization. In C. Craig (Ed.), *Categorization and noun classification* (pp. 139–180). Philadelphia: Benjamins North America.

INDEX